Psoriasis

CHARLES CAMISA MD
Head, Section of Clinical Dermatology
Vice Chairman, Department of Dermatology
The Cleveland Clinic Foundation
Cleveland, Ohio; Associate Professor
Department of Internal Medicine
Ohio State University College of Medicine
Columbus, Ohio

WITH CONTRIBUTIONS FROM

THOMAS N. HELM MD
Departments of Dermatology and Pathology
The Cleveland Clinic Foundation

ARUN L. PATHY MD
Department of Dermatology
The Cleveland Clinic Foundation

MICHAEL E. SAYERS DO
Department of Rheumatic and Immunologic Disease
The Cleveland Clinic Foundation

WILLIAM S. WILKE MD
Head, Section on Subspecialty Clinics
Department of Rheumatic and Immunologic Disease
The Cleveland Clinic Foundation

BOSTON

BLACKWELL SCIENTIFIC PUBLICATIONS

OXFORD LONDON EDINBURGH

MELBOURNE PARIS BERLIN VIENNA

Editorial Offices:
238 Main Street, Cambridge
Massachusetts 02142, USA
Osney Mead, Oxford OX2 0EL,
England
25 John Street, London WC1N 2BL
England
23 Ainslie Place, Edinburgh EH3 6AJ
Scotland
54 University Street, Carlton, Victoria
3053, Australia

Other Editorial Offices:
Librairie Arnette SA
2, rue Casimir-Delavigne
75006 Paris
France

Blackwell Wissenschafts-Verlag GmbH
Düsseldorfer Str. 38
D-10707 Berlin
Germany

Blackwell MZV
Feldgasse 13
A-1238 Wien
Austria

First published 1994

Set by Setrite Typesetters Ltd, Hong Kong
Printed and bound by Dah Hua Printing Press
Co. Ltd, Hong Kong

94 95 96 97 5 4 3 2 1

DISTRIBUTORS

USA
Blackwell Scientific Publications, Inc.
238 Main Street
Cambridge, Massachusetts 02142
(*Orders*: Tel: 617 876–7000
800 759–6102)

Canada
Times Mirror Professional Publishing, Ltd
130 Flaska Drive
Markham, Ontario L6G 1B8
(*Orders*: Tel: 800 268–4178
416 470–6739)

Australia
Blackwell Scientific Publications Pty Ltd
54 University Street
Carlton, Victoria 3053
(*Orders*: Tel: 03 347–5552)

Outside North America and Australia
Marston Book Services Ltd
PO Box 87
Oxford OX2 0DT
England
(*Orders*: Tel: 0865 791155
Fax: 0865 791927
Telex: 837515)

Library of Congress
Cataloging-in-Publication Data

Camisa, Charles.
Psoriasis/Charles Camisa. — 1st ed.
p. cm.
Includes bibliographical references and index.
ISBN 0–86542–247–8
1. Psoriasis. I. Title.
[DNLM: 1. Psoriasis. WR 205 C183p 1994]
RL321.C26 1994
616.5′26 — dc20

Contents

Preface

Psoriasis is a very common and perplexing disease. As a result, primary-care physicians, dermatologists, and rheumatologists are involved in the care of patients. This textbook is written by practitioners for practitioners and every chapter contains practical information. Dermatologists-in-training will probably want to read it through prior to completing residency. Others may use it for reference to a particular treatment their patient is currently using or when contemplating a new one. Chapter 2, Pathogenesis, often the most intimidating chapter in a monograph on psoriasis, is written with relevance to treatment always in mind. Chapter 4, Evaluation, considers the myriad published protocols employed in the evaluation of psoriasis with a critical look at the popular psoriasis area and severity index (PASI). Chapter 8, Psoriatic Arthritis, consists of a scholarly review of the subject by an internationally known authority, Dr William S. Wilke, that should appeal equally to generalists and specialists. Chapter 9 covers the pertinent topic of psoriasis and related arthropathic syndromes associated with human immunodeficiency virus infection and includes three case studies.

Chapters 13–16 and 18 contain case studies of actual patients treated by the authors at the Cleveland Clinic. These have been selected to illustrate pitfalls in treatment, adverse reactions, noncompliance, and serendipity, as well as success stories evolving from the orderly progression of choices of modalities and, occasionally, innovative combinations used with appropriate followup and practical monitoring. It is acknowledged that every case is different and is managed individually. The book provides only the ingredients and some examples; you must provide the creativity.

Over the years, I have benefited from the knowledge and experience of pioneers and geniuses in the field of dermatology by reading, attending conferences, and from personal communications. The chapters are referenced for detailed review of recent or historical articles, but not so heavily, I hope, as to be distracting to the reader. On the other hand, let me apologize in advance to the hundreds of doctors and patients who have taught me but who cannot all be included here. I would like to gratefully acknowledge the inspiration of Edmund D. Lowney, Robert Auerbach, Constantin Orfanos, and Henry H. Roenigk Jr. I thank Thomas N. Helm for taking the photomicrographs in Chapter 5, Dr Wilke for critically revising Chapter 15, Carl Allen for permission to use Figs 5.34 and 5.35b, and Jacob W.E. Dijkstra for review and helpful discussion of Chapter 12 and his kind permission to use Tables 12.1 and 12.2. I am most appreciative of the clinical photography of Ms Flora Williams and the use of the extensive Cleveland Clinic Department of Dermatology teaching files. Finally, this book would not have been possible without the expert typing of the manuscript by Ms Kathy Willis.

Notice The indications and dosages of all drugs in this book have been recommended in the medical literature and conform to the practices of the general medical community. The medications described do not necessarily have specific approval by the Food and Drug Administration for use in the diseases and dosages for which they are recommended. The package insert for each drug should be consulted for use and dosage as approved by the FDA. Because standards of usage change, it is advisable to keep abreast of revised recommendations, particularly those concerning new drugs.

Part one

Overview of Psoriasis for the Clinician

one Introduction

Psoriasis is at once a common and complex disease. The prevalence of psoriasis in the population of the USA and UK is estimated to be 1–2%. Its severity ranges from a single fingernail pit to some small blemished fraction of skin surface area to the total body skin disfigurement associated with crippling arthritis. It has been said that psoriasis does not take lives; it ruins them. This book is dedicated to those lives; thus physicians, dermatologists, and general practitioners, can review and select one or more of the many good therapies available that are suitable for the individual patient.

The cause of this vexing condition is still unknown, although it is agreed that the clinical lesions represent the end result of hyperproliferation and abnormal differentiation of the epidermis. Many hypotheses of the pathogenesis of psoriasis have been advanced. Some have been disproved or have fallen out of favor with the cognoscenti; others remain viable candidates to explain the primary pathophysiologic alterations or they are considered secondary phenomena.

Before the advent of modern science with its sophisticated instrumentation and technology for identifying and quantitating small and large molecules in skin, dermatologists relied on clinical and histopathologic morphology for correlating cause and cure to a skin disease (Table 1.1).

Some dermatologic diseases have a long list of available treatments, none of which is consistently effective. However, although many different treatments exist for psoriasis, they are individually and in combination frequently effective and nearly completely so in some subsets of psoriatic patients. Goeckerman wrote, "The comparative frequency with which this disease occurs demands that not only the specialist but the general practitioner should be familiar with effective therapeutic measures directed against it." Psoriasis accounts for the third most common reason for office visits to dermatologists (behind acne and warts). In the USA it is estimated that 150 000–260 000 new cases of psoriasis occur annually [1]. It is likely that as many as two-thirds of cases of psoriasis are encountered initially and managed by primary care physicians [2] further emphasizing

Table 1.1 Clinicopathologic correlations of psoriasis

Clinical morphology	Histopathologic morphology	Treatment
Scales	Hyperkeratosis/parakeratosis	Keratolytics, emollients
Thickness	Acanthosis ("psoriasiform hyperplasia")	Coal tar, anthralin, phototherapy
Redness	Dilated capillaries Lymphocytes in dermis	Corticosteroids Cyclosporine
Pustules	Neutrophils in epidermis	Retinoids, methotrexate

the importance of recognizing psoriasis in practice and treating it competently. A study comparing the ability of primary care physicians to diagnose the 20 most common skin diseases from color slides gave an overall score of 54% (compared to >90% for dermatologists). However, psoriasis was recognized 85% of the time compared to 100% for dermatologists. Computerized diagnostic algorithm systems do not improve on this and cannot replace the trained human eye and touch [3].

If it is appropriate to define a disease morphologically and/or by its response to specific therapy, then it would be fair to say that "psoriasis" represents a common skin reaction pattern to different stimuli, a thesis analogous to "eczema" which may be atopic, nummular, asteatotic, stasis, contact allergic, etc.

For the purposes of this book we will consider "psoriasis" as a single disease with several morphologic variants, and a full range of severity and expression based on:

1 certain genetic influences (HLA type).
2 environmental factors (such as trauma and climate).
3 associated diseases (particularly infections) and concomitant medications.
4 immunologic status of the host.

The first three factors mentioned have been studied by direct observation, simple laboratory techniques, and statistical analysis; the fourth had to await the development of *in vitro* assays of cellular function and the accurate measurement of nanomolar quantities of substances elaborated by cells in blood and skin. Historically, polymorphonuclear leukocytes and mononuclear phagocytes were examined first because they were readily retrieved and purified in large quantities from circulating blood. The roles of lymphocytes and Langerhans cells were subsequently explored by *in situ* monoclonal antibody labeling techniques. It was soon recognized that differences in the microenvironment of skin could be influenced by soluble mediators secreted by all of the cell types involved including the keratinocyte itself. A "new" skin cell with antigen-processing capability, the dermal dendrocyte, has been proposed as the pivotal cell type in the autoimmune pathogenesis of psoriasis. The ability of immunosuppressive drugs used in organ transplantation (e.g., cyclosporine and FK506) to block interleukin-2 production and the cascade of cytokines and receptors before slowing hyperproliferation and the concomitant inflammatory responses suggest that an aberration in the regulation of interleukins, growth factors, or adhesion molecules could be the primary pathologic process in psoriasis. Like many others preceding it, this theory may be partially or completely debunked in time, perhaps before the publication date of this book, or indeed it may be accepted as the cornerstone of the psoriatic phenomenon at which future therapies will be directed.

Where then does arthritis fit into this picture? Although less common than the skin disease, occurring in 1–40% of cases of psoriasis, psoriatic arthritis by its nature can be more disabling. A joint space is about as far removed anatomically and functionally from a hyperproliferative epidermis as one can get. Mucous membranes and the eye are more closely related to skin embryologically than synovium and are rarely if ever affected by psoriasis. Is psoriasis a multisystem inflammatory disease? Other than the skin and the articular involvement in a minority of cases, it is dubious that other organ systems such as the liver and kidney are affected in psoriasis. The hypothesis of aberrant immunoregulatory control combined with genetic and environmental factors may help to explain the accumulation of inflammatory cells in such disparate sites, but the pathogenesis of the skin and joint disease may in fact be different.

The total annual expenditure for psoriasis treatment in the USA exceeded $1.5 billion even before the use of cyclosporine, which is currently the most expensive systemic treatment available. When tailoring therapy to the individual patient, selections should be based on efficacy, toxicity, accessibility, and cost. Sander and colleagues [1] determined that excellent results can be achieved at high cost with the Goeckerman regimen in a psoriasis day-treatment center (although less expensive than hospitalization) and that methotrexate was the most cost-effective systemic treatment. While a cure for psoriasis is still wanting as we draw toward the end of the twentieth century, the treatments discussed in this book offer incalculable advantages to patients and clinicians when compared to those of Pusey and Goeckerman's day: "six doses of emetin, 0.75 grain each, three doses of arsphenamin, simultaneous intramuscular injections of mercury, twenty-five injections of staphylococcus and streptococcus vaccine, Fowler's solution, five injections of autoserum, a seven months' course of nonprotein diet, a few roentgen-ray exposures, removal of the tonsils, and extraction of seven teeth within a period of three years, produced no therapeutic effect [4]."

REFERENCES

1 Sander HM, Morris LF, Phillips CM, *et al.* The annual cost of psoriasis. *J Am Acad Dermatol* 1993;28:422–5.

2 Ramsay DL, Fox AB. The ability of primary care physicians to recognize the common dermatoses. *Arch Dermatol* 1981;117:620–2.

3 Brooks GJ, Ashton RE, Pethybridge RJ. DERMIS: a computer system for assisting primary-care physicians with dermatological diagnosis. *Br J Dermatol* 1992;127: 614–9.

4 Goeckerman WH. The treatment of psoriasis. *Northwest Med* 1925;24:229–31.

two Pathogenesis

INTRODUCTION

While it is true that the pathogenesis of psoriasis is unknown, more is known about the pathophysiology of psoriasis than any other skin disease.

Psoriasis is the result of hyperproliferation of the epidermis, concomitant inflammation, and vascular changes, which occur in response to the proper combination of genetic and environmental pressures. Hyperproliferation results in an epidermis with a germinative layer that is two times thicker than normal and in which all the cells enter the growth fraction. The result is a cell cycle shortened from 311 to 36 hours and an epidermal turnover time, the time it takes a basal cell to reach the stratum corneum, accelerated from 27 days to 4 days [1]. These experimentally derived time periods help to explain the rapid redevelopment of scale within 24 hours of debridement. They were first reported from *in vivo* experiments in the 1960s and reconfirmed in the 1980s. Interestingly, hyperproliferation of psoriatic keratinocytes cannot be duplicated under the conditions of cell culture techniques, which suggests that the influence of circulating or dermal components is necessary. Moreover, in xenografts of psoriasis lesions and uninvolved skin to athymic nude mice, epidermal hyperproliferation continues, but there is no maintenance or development of a "psoriasiform" lesion.

Psoriatic epidermis had 26.6% of the proliferative cells in the DNA synthesis (S) phase compared to 7.8% of normal skin. The main defect in epidermal kinetics is the overall eightfold increase in the germinative cell cycle compared to normal. The increase in the growth fraction from 60 to 100% and the doubling in size of the proliferative population of cells are less important contributory factors to the aberrant kinetics in psoriasis.

The understanding of the kinetic abnormalities identified in psoriasis has been exploited in the development of therapeutic modalities. Treatments in this category include the antimetabolites methotrexate (MTX), hydroxyurea, 6-thioguanine, 5-fluorouracil, as well as photochemotherapy with 8-methoxypsoralen plus UVA. In some cases, a mechanism of action including inhibition of DNA synthesis has been deduced long after the empiric use of the agent. The latter category includes anthralin, coal tar, and UVB phototherapy.

Abnormalities in polyamine synthesis and their rate-limiting [2] biosynthetic enzyme ornithine decarboxylase (ODC) have been detected in psoriasis and other hyperproliferative states. Significantly increased levels of spermine, spermidine, and ODC have been detected in both involved and uninvolved psoriatic compared to normal epidermal shave biopsies, indicating that the abnormality is generalized to the entire skin surface in psoriasis [3]. The stimulus for hyperproliferation of the epidermis in psoriasis is therefore continuous. While changes in polyamine metabolism are not primary to the pathogenesis of psoriasis, some treatments may act in part by inhibiting ODC activity and decreasing polyamine levels in skin including anthralin, topical corticosteroids, and etretinate.

KERATINOCYTE DIFFERENTIATION

Another pathomechanism involved in psoriasis is abnormal keratinocyte (KC) differentiation, in contrast to proliferation. Histopathologically, the granular cell layer is reduced or absent, and hyperkeratosis and parakeratosis develop. Cytokeratin expression is altered compared to normal skin and atopic dermatitis. Involucrin and membrane-bound transglutaminase appear prematurely in psoriatic epidermis. Involved psoriatic skin revealed little or no reaction of antifilagrin antibody in the stratum corneum or granular layer. Involucrin staining appeared paradoxically in the lower cell layer. The staining pattern of uninvolved psoriatic epidermis was the same as normal skin [4]. Fifty-four and 57 kDa keratin is detected in lesional psoriasis only, not in uninvolved or normal skin [5]. These filaments had reduced glycine content (60% of normal). The 50 kDa cytokeratin or K14 is localized to the basal cell layer of normal skin. The level of K14 is considerably higher in psoriatic lesional skin [6] and is distributed throughout the whole thickness of the epidermis. Normalization of the K14 staining pattern was obtained after treatment with anthralin, betamethasone diproprionate, and psoralen UVA (PUVA) [7]. In psoriatic epidermis there is apparently a downregulation of K1 and K10 and upregulation of K6 and K16. Quantitative differences in cytokeratins result from a delay in the differentiation of the basal cell layer in psoriatic epidermis [8]. Thus, the earliest sign of epidermal differentiation that has been detected to date, the appearance of K1 and K10 in the suprabasal cell compartment, is delayed in psoriasis. It is suspected but not yet shown that these alterations originate at the level of keratin gene promoters.

These findings have prompted interest in vitamin D_3 and analogs in the therapy of psoriasis because it promotes the terminal differentiation of cultured murine epidermal cells. 1,25-Dihydroxy vitamin D_3 inhibited growth and DNA synthesis in a dose-dependent fashion in cell cultures of normal, psoriatic involved and uninvolved KCs [9]. Vitamin D promotes intestinal absorption of calcium, and hypocalcemia has been associated with relapses of pustular psoriasis. Calmodulin, a calcium-binding protein, is increased in involved psoriatic epidermis and falls to normal levels after various palliative treatments [10]. There was also a significant reduction in calmodulin levels in the uninvolved epidermis of the patients who cleared following anthralin or MTX treatment [11].

Cyclic adenosine monophosphate (cAMP) has been implicated as a modulator of cellular growth and differentiation in many cell systems and was thought to be involved in the pathogenesis of psoriasis because of reduced levels measured in involved skin. Later, epidermal levels were shown to be normal or higher overall with a relative reduction of cAMP in the basal proliferative compartment. Basal cAMP levels were significantly lower in cultured psoriatic compared to control fibroblasts [11]. Stimulation by β-adrenergic agonists had much less stimulatory effect and addition of phosphodiesterase inhibitor had no effect. Vasoactive intestinal polypeptide (VIP) and peptide histidine methonine (both found in unmyelinated nerve fibers in human skin) had no effect on dermal fibroblasts from normals or lesions of psoriasis. These findings relate to the observation that lithium and propanolol, which inhibit cAMP production, can initiate or exacerbate psoriasis. The effects of these drugs do not occur in all patients, therefore other mechanisms must also be involved.

The adenylate cyclase system is far more complex than originally suspected. Cyclic AMP-dependent protein kinases are deficient in cultured fibroblasts and uncultured red blood cells (RBCs) [12]. The binding of cAMP to the regulatory subunits of protein kinase A in fibroblasts and erythrocytes is abnormal. There was a significant negative correlation between the level of binding and psoriasis area and severity index (PASI) score. In some normal first-degree relatives of psoriatic patients binding was lower than the normal mean. Retinoid treatment in four patients produced a decrease in the PASI score and an increase in the ability of the RBC regulatory subunit to bind a cAMP analog.

POLYMORPHONUCLEAR LEUCOCYTES

Ever since the identification of polymorphonuclear leukocytes (PMNLs) in histologic sections of psoriasis (Fig. 2.1) taken together with the development of localized (Fig. 2.2) or generalized pustulation (Fig. 2.3) evolving from stable plaque disease after certain stimuli, interest has piqued concerning the role of circulating PMNLs in the pathogenesis of psoriasis. The functions studied by numerous investigators have included chemokinesis (random migration), chemotaxis (directed migration), lysosomal enzyme release, morphology, adherence, generation of oxidation intermediates such as superoxide anion, hydroxyl radical, and hydrogen peroxide, phagocytosis, chemiluminescence, and antibody-dependent cytotoxicity. In some of the studies monocyte functions were also assayed. Various stimuli were used, and cells were incubated with buffer or serum from psoriatics or normal controls. The results add up to a confusing array ranging from decreased to increased response of psoriatic cells to stimuli; inhibiting to enhancing effects of psoriatic sera; and strong correlation to no correlation

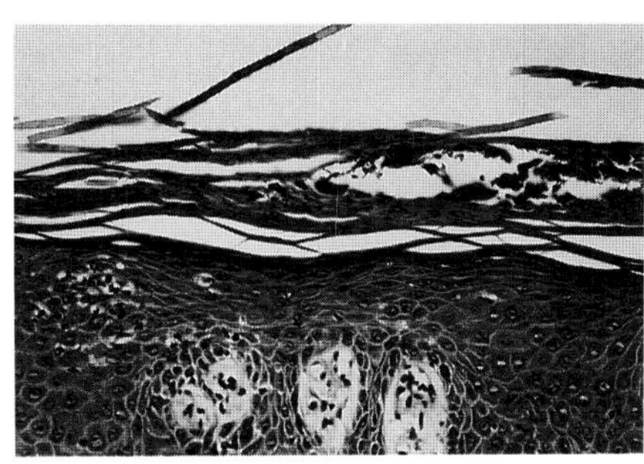

Fig 2.1 Polymorphonuclear leukocyte aggregations in the stratum corneum (Munro microabscess) and the stratum spinosum (spongiform pustule of Kogoj).

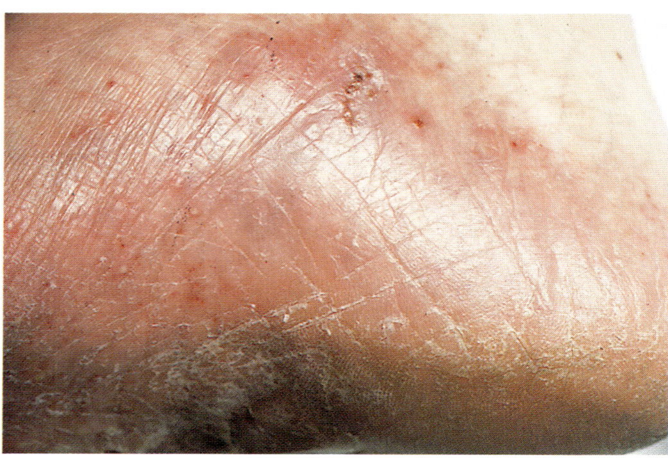

Fig 2.2 Small pustules forming at periphery of localized plaque psoriasis.

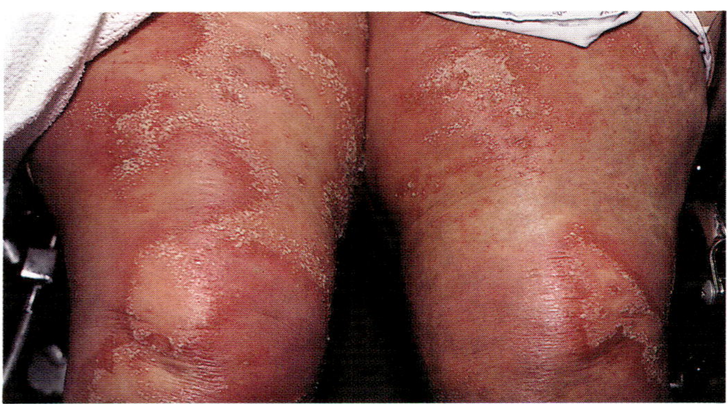

Fig 2.3 Generalized pustular psoriasis.

with disease activity or severity. Unfortunately, these results are of little practical value to the clinician except when they are evaluated in the context of simultaneous response to therapy, that is, PMNL function and the clearing of psoriasis. Such experiments may help to answer whether the abnormalities identified are intrinsic to the disease process or are merely a signatory epiphenomenon analogous to an elevated erythrocyte sedimentation rate or C-reactive protein level in systemic lupus erythematosus. In one study difference was found in PMNL chemotaxis; however, the enhancing effect of psoriatic serum on normal PMNL chemotaxis was significantly increased [13]. After PUVA, chemotaxis remained unchanged, but the activity of psoriatic serum returned to normal values. In another study, chemotaxis for psoriatic PMNLs and monocytes (MNCs) was significantly increased before treatment but remained unaltered by PUVA treatment [14]. Increased chemotaxis of PMNLs and MNCs occurs as well as an enhancing effect of psoriatic plasma before treatment [15]. The chemotaxis activity of the cells normalized after 4–6 weeks of anthralin or PUVA. The plasma properties normalized after only 2 weeks of either treatment. Langner and coworkers [16] selected seven patients out of 15 with abnormally high chemotaxis who normalized after obtaining a good clinical response with anthralin treatment. Of the remaining eight patients, four had no change and four had abnormally low values that increased during clinical improvement. This study demonstrates the randomness of chemotaxis values because if all the results were compared in aggregate (as they should be), there would be no difference in the means before and after treatment.

Long-term MTX treatment normalizes enhanced PMNL and MNC chemotaxis before clinical resolution of psoriasis is noted. Conversely, lithium increases migrational activity of PMNLs possibly by lowering cAMP levels and has been reported to induce psoriasis or exacerbate preexisting disease. cAMP and cyclic guanosine monophosphate (cGMP) levels have been found to be normal in psoriatic PMNLs and MNCs. Moreover, responses of MNCs to stimulatory agents did not differ from normal and did not correlate to the severity of disease [17].

Some reasonable conclusions that can be drawn from experimental evidence found in this large body of work are listed below.

1 PMNLs from psoriatics may be more sensitive to the usual chemoattractants employed in experimental assays.

2 Potent chemoattractants are passively trapped or produced *de novo* in the psoriatic epidermis. Candidates include immune complexes detected in the stratum corneum by direct immunofluorescence, serine proteinases, cytokines produced by MNCs such as tumor necrosis factor, granulocyte-macrophage-colony stimulating factor, a 12 kDa chemotactic factor found in psoriatic scales, C5 cleavage products, leukotriene B_4 (LTB_4), and more recently, neutrophil activating peptide-1 or interleukin-8 (IL-8).

3 Psoriatic serum may contain high levels of chemoattractants, the result of diffusion from the skin or generated in the circulation by activated PMNLs and MNCs.

4 Treatment of psoriasis may be successful in part by reducing the epidermal synthesis of chemoattractants or inactivating them and therefore preventing the accumulation of PMNLs in the skin.

5 Pustular psoriasis, a model of exaggerated PMNL accumulation in skin, is most appropriate for closer scrutiny because more homogeneous groups of patients in terms of activity (severe) and extent (generalized, localized, or palmoplantar) can be compared.

While hemodialysis and hemofiltration have not successfully treated psoriasis, continuous peritoneal dialysis (CPD) dramatically improved four of five severe psoriatics in a sham-controlled study [18]. The authors suggested the mechanism was the removal of a "psoriatic factor" from the blood by dialysis. Complete remission of psoriasis occurred in five of 16 patients treated with CPD who lost more than 100×10^9 PMNLs during treatment [19]. The investigators noted that the higher the number of PMNLs eliminated through the peritoneal cavity, the better the clinical effect of treatment. Neutral proteinases in peripheral blood PMNLs in patients with active psoriasis were significantly greater than in stationary psoriasis or normal controls. The quantity of neutral proteinases in the peritoneal PMNLs was two to five times lower in comparison to circulating PMNLs and decreased with the duration of peritoneal dialysis. A patient with widespread treatment-resistant psoriasis was treated with seven leukapheresis procedures during a 4-week period which yielded an average of 3.13×10^{10} white blood cells (WBC) (69% PMNLs). "Complete relief from the itching and burning ... and considerable resolution of his lesions" was obtained lasting at least 3 months [20]. Lest we get too comfortable with the concept of a role for PMNLs in the development of psoriasis, consider the case of psoriasis evolving during the leukocyte nadir induced by chemotherapy [21].

NEUROPEPTIDES

Based on clinical experience and questionnaire surveys of psoriatic populations, psychologic stress or "worry" is believed to exacerbate the skin disease of some patients. This effect may be considered an "endogenous Koebner phenomenon" if inflammation and/or proliferation is evoked by the release of peptides from cutaneous nerve fibers [22]. Indirect evidence for this derives from anecdotal case reports involving surgical procedures to underlying joints and organs, which sever nerves and result in local clearing of psoriasis without affecting the contralateral side [23]. When sensation returns to the area, that is, when the nerve endings regenerate, the psoriasis recurs. While it has been proposed that extirpation of abnormal microvasculature or dermal growth factors are the mechanisms by which carbon dioxide laser vaporization or keratome excisions "cured" psoriasis, it is also plausible that severing nerve endings contributed to the result.

The symmetry of psoriasis has also been postulated to favor a neurogenic origin of the disease although symmetry is clearly not constant. "Worry" was cited by 30% of patients to precipitate psoriasis, but this subjective feeling is difficult to define, and impossible to quantify. It should be mentioned that the 30% figure cited closely approximates to the proportion of improvement in psoriatic populations generally attributed to the "placebo-effect".

Biochemical and histochemical data have been sought. VIP and substance P (SP) were detected in suction blisters induced over psoriatic plaques [24]. Two studies demonstrated that the immunocytochemical localization of neuropeptides was similar for lesional, nonlesional, and control skin. There was a low but similar frequency of nerve fibers: SP was found in dermal papillae parallel to the dermoepidermal junction and VIP was found in the deeper dermis around eccrine glands and parallel to the skin surface [25].

There was no difference in the plasma levels of these neurotransmitters by radioimmunoassay (RIA) between psoriatics and normal controls and no correlation with area of body surface involvement suggesting that if they play any role in the pathogenesis of psoriasis, it is probably at the local level.

Using double-labeling immunohistochemical stains, Naukkarinen and colleagues [26] found both mast cells and mast cell–nerve contacts were markedly more frequent in the basement membrane zone and papillary dermis of psoriatic lesional skin compared to healthy control skin and lichen planus. Increased contact between mast cells and sensory nerves strongly suggests a role for neurogenic inflammation in psoriasis because both VIP and SP can degranulate mast cells. VIP probably has nonspecific vasodilatory and proinflammatory effects because it is also elevated in biopsies of atopic dermatitis, allergic contact dermatitis, and irritant contact dermatitis compared to the corresponding anatomic sites in normal control subjects.

Both SP and VIP were significantly elevated in skin biopsies of psoriasis lesions compared to nonlesional and control skin (expressed as picomoles per gram weight tissue) [27]. By contrast, other investigators found that VIP was significantly elevated and SP was significantly decreased in lesional skin compared to nonlesional and normal skin [28]. The techniques used and the absolute values obtained are similar; the reason for the divergent results is unexplained.

VIP stimulated KC proliferation in culture in a dose-dependent fashion; SP did not stimulate growth and blocked VIP-induced proliferation [29]. When added to cultures of adult KC, however, either VIP or SP enhanced the modest mitogenicity of LTB_4. The biologic relevance of SP effects in skin is further suggested by the demonstration of specific binding of ^{125}I-labeled SP in the epidermis and dermal papillae of normal skin. An imbalance in the quantity of VIP and SP *in vivo* taken together with disparate effects on KC proliferation *in vitro* suggest that neurotransmitters are probably involved in the pathogenesis of psoriasis by exerting modulatory influences on growth and inflammatory mediators.

Various hypotheses have been advanced suggesting that psoriasis is under the neuroendocrine control of human growth hormone (HGH), prolactin, epidermal growth factor (EGF), insulin growth factor-1 (IGF-1) (somatomedin-C), and insulin. Serum growth hormone levels are not elevated in psoriasis, nor are those of IGF-1 through which HGH effects are mediated. Any association between psoriasis and acromegaly or pituitary hyperplasia is coincidental. Somatostatin (SOM) and analogs have improved psoriasis and psoriatic arthritis but not via HGH or IGF-1 [30]. Plasma EGF levels were reduced by SOM in one series. SOM inhibits the release of many pituitary and gastrointestinal hormones including insulin, producing mild carbohydrate intolerance. Carbohydrate metabolism is otherwise normal in psoriatics as are basal SOM levels in plasma. Bromocriptine, which has been reported to be active in psoriasis, may act by inhibiting prolactin release. Interestingly, prolactin actually competes with cyclosporine for the same receptor [31].

EGF receptors are normally found in the basal and lower spinous cell layers of the epidermis. In psoriasis they persist from the basal layer to the stratum corneum resulting in a net increase in receptors. These receptors are biologically active *in vivo*. Regression of the psoriatic phenotype in lesional skin transplanted to nude mice could be induced by topical application of a high concentration of EGF (50 μg/ml) to the grafts [32]. This could be attributed to suppression of autocrine sources of transforming growth factor-α (TGF-α) produced within lesions.

IGF-1 receptors are confined to the basal cell layer where proliferative cells normally reside. IGF-1 or high-dose insulin transmodulates the expression of EGF receptors by cultured KCs via the IGF-1 receptor, increasing EGF binding an average 1.8 times [33]. The EGF receptors may then bind to TGF-α produced by KCs. This finding may be relevant to hyperproliferation of psoriatic epithelium.

A randomized double-blind, placebo-controlled trial of subcutaneous injections of a SOM analog, octreotide acetate, was performed in 150 patients [34]. Octreotide was superior to placebo as monotherapy for mild to moderate psoriasis. There was no change in body surface area of involvement, however, and 90% experienced gastrointestinal side effects (diarrhea, steatorrhea, abdominal cramping, nausea, etc.). Even more alarming was that 10% of patients developed a new onset of gallstones after 12 weeks of therapy; this was determined by ultrasound. Some of the patients with gallstones suffered further complications such as biliary colic, cholecystitis, and pancreatitis necessitating discontinuation of octreotide and, in some cases, medical or surgical intervention. Therefore, we do not recommend that octreotide injections be used in the treatment of psoriasis.

Capsaicin depletes nerve endings of SP and other peptides and prevents their reuptake. Topical capsaicin cream (Zostrix) 0.25% was tested in bilateral paired comparisons and resulted in 68% overall clinical improvement compared to 44% on the vehicle side [35]. Scaling and erythema were diminished. Burning, stinging, itching, and redness were experienced by nearly half the subjects upon initial application of the capsaicin cream. These reactions, graded as moderate to severe, diminished with time but may have introduced "open-label bias" into the study thereby disrupting the double-blind design. Capsaicin cream has not been accepted as a treatment for psoriasis.

Peptide T, a VIP agonist, is mitogenic toward KCs in culture at higher concentrations and might be expected to adversely affect psoriasis. However, intravenous infusions of peptide T, 1 mg b.i.d., have improved psoriasis in some patients with or without HIV infection [36,37]. When approximately 40 ng of peptide T was infused directly into lesions of psoriasis, significant clinical and histologic improvement occurred after 2 weeks compared to saline controls [38]. While these reports are encouraging, double-blind placebo-controlled trials must be carried out before the clinical use of peptide T can be recommended.

In summary, no effective treatment for psoriasis has yet emerged from the neurotransmitter hypothesis. SOM and bromocriptine have an unacceptable side-effect profile and probably should not be used outside of carefully controlled trials. Topical capsaicin produces intolerable local reactions and seems to be only weakly active against psoriasis. Peptide T deserves further study. Development of VIP antagonists would be the next logical step in these investigations.

ARACHIDONIC ACID METABOLITES

Arachidonic acid (AA) is found esterified to certain phospholipids that constitute the lipid bilayer of the cell membrane. The membrane-bound enzyme phospholipase A_2 (PLA_2) cleaves the esterified AA from the phospholipid, and now free AA can be metabolized to either the prostaglandins and thromboxanes or the leukotrienes and eicosanoids via the cyclooxygenase pathway or via a series of lipoxygenase enzymes, respectively (see Fig. 8.13, p. 129). Several lines of evidence have suggested that these enzymes and their resulting inflammatory mediator products may cause development of the psoriatic lesion.

First, PLA_2 activity in keratome slices is significantly elevated in both involved and uninvolved psoriatic specimens compared to normal controls [39]. Involved and uninvolved psoriatic epidermis also shows increased transformation of AA via 5-lipoxygenase and 12-lipoxygenase. LTB_4, a 5-lipoxygenase product, increases both random and directed migration of human neutrophils *in vitro* at physiologic concentrations ($10^{-9}-10^{-7}$ mol/l), and is as potent as C5a. Neutrophils have specific receptors for LTB_4. Application of 35 ng LTB_4 to normal or uninvolved psoriatic skin produced heavy collections of neutrophils in the epidermis (Munro microabscesses) within 24 hours [40]. A proliferative response of KCs was also observed 72–96 hours after LTB_4 application. There was no difference observed in the effects between psoriatics and healthy controls. Because the hyperproliferation occurred 32–56 hours after application, the authors concluded that it was a consequence of the physical disruption of the stratum corneum accompanying rupture of microabscesses and desquamation, analogous to the Koebner phenomenon induced by cellophane tape-stripping the skin. 12-Lipoxygenase activity is enhanced and its product, 12-hydroxyheptadecatrienoic acid (12-HETE), is markedly elevated (81-fold) in psoriatic skin [41]. Epidermal cells possess specific high affinity binding sites for 12-HETE. AA and 12-HETE stimulated increased levels of guanylate cyclase (two- to threefold) in involved and uninvolved skin of psoriasis but not in normal skin, suggesting that elevated cGMP is a consequence of the altered cyclic nucleotide metabolism in psoriasis [42].

The keratome sampling techniques utilized make it impossible to specifically localize LTB_4 to the KC or dermal/epidermal leukocytes. Moreover, while application of 12-HETE and LTB_4 to symptomless skin of psoriatics produces erythema and attracts neutrophils, they do not reproduce the psoriatic lesion. The relative sparcity of microabscesses in chronic plaques of psoriasis compared to the dramatic appearance of numerous microabscesses richly populated with PMNLs suggests that this is an interesting experimental artifact. That PLA_2 is elevated in uninvolved as well as involved skin implies that we are missing an important piece of the puzzle or that inhibitors of the enzyme must be active *in vivo*.

Some clinical evidence has been used to help support the theory that products of the lipoxygenase pathway exacerbate psoriasis. In a single perhaps too often cited study, indomethacin exacerbated psoriasis [43]. Indomethacin is a nonsteroidal antiinflammatory drug (NSAID) and is a potent inhibitor of cyclooxygenase. In topical form, indomethacin prevented the slight improvement of psoriatic plaques secondary to its emollient vehicle [44]. Although it did not aggravate the lesion, the authors concluded that indomethacin caused more AA to be shunted to the lipoxygenase enzyme pathways. A more recent study showed that oral indomethacin treatment during an Ingram regimen had no effect compared to placebo [45], a finding more in keeping with the experience of the Cleveland Clinic rheumatology and dermatology services. We do not believe the assertion that indomethacin, or any NSAID for that matter, including aspirin and ibuprofen, which our patients regularly take, alters the response of psoriasis to treatment. A recent report demonstrated that enhanced *in vitro* aggregation of platelets from psoriatic patients was related to increased cyclooxygenase activity [46].

Meclofenamate is similar to indomethacin in that it is a potent inhibitor of cyclooxygenase and a modest inhibitor of 5-lipoxygenase activity. After an initial anecdotal report that meclofenamate cleared psoriasis, a 4-week double-blind, placebo-controlled trial was performed which showed that there was no difference in the response of psoriasis between the group taking meclofenamate and the group taking placebo [47]. The authors concluded that it is therefore an appropriate choice for psoriatic arthritis. Benoxaprofen, on the other hand, a NSAID which is a potent inhibitor of 5-lipoxygenase, was very effective in about 75% of patients with severe psoriasis [48]. While benoxaprofen is no longer available for further study, another putative oral inhibitor of leukotriene biosynthesis (MK886) had no clinical effect on psoriasis and did not change lesional LTB_4 levels [49]. However, a slight decrease in epidermal PMNL accumulation was observed. We do not hesitate to recommend the use of any NSAID for psoriatic arthropathy or other concomitant diseases if the drugs are indicated.

Based on the finding of increased levels of free AA, 12-HETE, PGE_2, $PGF_{2\alpha}$, and LTB_4, LTC_4, LTD_4, an attempt has been made to modify the metabolism of AA by supplementing the diet of psoriatic patients with fish oil containing large amounts of eicosapentaenoic acid (EPA), a fatty acid relative of AA. It was hoped that other fatty acids incorporated into the cell membrane might lead to the formation of less "psoriagenic" metabolites or that they might compete directly with AA as substrates. Five of 13 patients who completed an early trial had moderate improvement in the severity of lesions [50]. These results might have been attributed to the open, unblinded nature of the study. Fish oil supplementation used as adjuvant treatment will be covered in subsequent chapters.

COMPLEMENT

Autoantibodies to stratum corneum are present in all sera and there are no differences in titer between normal controls and psoriatic patients. Albumin and IgG are present in extracts of psoriatic scales and normal callus. IgA, IgM and C3 were also found in psoriatic scales including patients with erythroderma and arthritis. Anti-IgG factors were found in psoriatic scales, but not in normal callus [51]. Apparently, passive diffusion occurs of serum proteins into the epidermis. In two patients with a severe flare of erythroderma, the titers of stratum corneum antibodies dropped and rose again during resolution of the crisis. Absorption of sera with extracts of either psoriatic scales or normal callus suggests that the former contain unique antigenic determinants on the basis of amino acid composition and localization on cell envelopes [52].

Circulating immune complexes (CICs) were measured by the Raji cell and C1q binding assays in psoriatics and controls. All were negative with the Raji method, but 31% of psoriatics were positive by C1q binding compared to 7% of controls and 55% of SLE patients [53] indicating that the classical complement pathway may be activated in psoriasis. Hall and colleagues [54] detected IgA-containing CICs at some time during the course of the disease in 14 of 21 (67%) psoriatics compared to only one of 25 (4%) patients with other disorders of keratinization using the Raji IgA RIA. In contrast to the previous study cited above [53], only one of 19 (5%) had evidence of IgG- or IgM-containing CICs using the C1q binding assay. There was no correlation between clinical improvement and the presence or level of IgA-containing CICs after treatment with etretinate, indicating that CICs probably do not play a primary role in the pathogenesis of psoriasis. The detection of elevated levels of complement fragments C4d and Bb in psoriatic scale extracts suggests that both the classical and alternative pathways are activated, respectively, in lesional skin [55]. It is possible that these reactions are secondary to the colonization of psoriatic skin by staphylococci, streptococci, and pityrosporum yeasts.

Direct immunofluorescence studies of psoriatic skin reveal strongly positive focal deposits of IgG, IgA, IgM, complement components and fibrin in the stratum corneum. This finding is considered evidence for the only antigen-specific immunologic reactions that occur *in vivo* in 100% of patients with active psoriasis. Beutner and coworkers [56] hypothesized that a massive Arthus-type reaction occurs in the stratum corneum which activates complement, attracts and stimulates PMNLs to produce AA metabolites which in turn induce epidermal hyperproliferation.

IMMUNOLOGY/CYTOKINE NETWORK

The development of cyclosporine A as an effective immunosuppressive agent (that is neither cytotoxic nor myelosuppressive) and its efficacy in treating the most recalcitrant cases of psoriasis has placed T-cell activation center-stage and focused attention on psoriasis as an autoimmune disease. One of the difficulties inherent with proving this hypothesis has been that routine histopathology of psoriasis does not resemble a cell-mediated immune reaction and cannot differentiate individual cell-types nor identify their specific products. These obstacles have lately been overcome by advances in technology, which include monoclonal antibodies, sensitive immunoassays of biologic activity, messenger RNA (mRNA) transcripts coding for cytokines by Northern blot hybridization, polymerase chain reaction, and *in situ* hybridization.

Cyclosporine suppresses inflammation and immune-based reactions in a generic fashion by diminishing transcription of cytokines such as IL-2, IL-4, and interferon-γ (IFN-γ). Interleukin receptor mRNA transcription is not directly affected by cyclosporine, nor does it specifically target any unique autoreactive T-cell clones. Cyclosporine is thus clinically useful in many inflammatory skin diseases, e.g., chronic graft-vs-host reaction, lichen planus, atopic dermatitis, etc. It may also have a direct inhibitory effect on epidermal proliferation based on KC cultures [57].

Cytokines are potent multifunctional glycoproteins capable of influencing their target cell by binding to specific cell surface receptors at picomolar concentrations. The term "cytokine" now encompasses lymphokines, monokines, interleukins, interferons, and growth factors. More than 20 cytokines have been identified. KCs, T lymphocytes, and macrophages (antigen-presenting cells) communicate by a complex, bidirectional, functional cascade that is distinct for psoriasis. Some investigators [58,59] believe that psoriasis is an autoimmune disease caused by a genetic defect in one or more of these chief cell types. The isolation of the genetic lesion and the antigen-specific T cells remain elusive at present. Their discovery will bring more specific and safer therapy. That the defect lies with the immunocyte is supported by a report of two patients with long-standing psoriasis and leukemia who achieved and maintained complete remission of both diseases 4 years after allogeneic bone marrow transplantation [60]. The immediate etiologic stimuli in the genetically susceptible host are diverse and apparently unrelated: exogenous — epidermal injury such as scratching and tape-stripping, i.e., the Koebner phenomenon; endogenous — chemically unrelated drugs, e.g., lithium, β-adrenergic blockers, antimalarials, corticosteroids; neuropeptides, streptococcal-related immune complexes, and HIV infection. The common final pathway must therefore involve the KC and its response to cytokines.

Evidence of autoimmunity in psoriasis derives from experiments of lymphocyte transformation when T cells are mixed with autologous non-T cells such as keratinocytes, B cells, macrophages, and dendritic cells. Lymphocyte transformation was significantly increased when mixed with autologous KCs from psoriatics compared to normal subjects and (surprisingly) patients with lichen planus, which is generally considered to represent a cell-mediated immune reaction to the basal cell layer. Psoriatic, but not normal or lichen planus KC, stimulated the release of a leukocyte migration-inhibition factor [60]. An apparently contradictory result was found in autologous mixed lymphocyte reactions (MLRs) in psoriasis with non-T mononuclear cells which were significantly lower than normal subjects or patients with atopic dermatitis [62]. Lymphocyte transformation increased significantly after successful treatment of psoriasis. The reduced MLR in these experiments may be explained in part by inhibitory factors in the relatively high concentration (20%) of autologous psoriatic serum used or by an intrinsic suppressor cell dysfunction in psoriasis.

The dermal dendrocyte (macrophage) may be the pivotal cell involved because of its strategic anatomic location between epidermal KCs and dermal microvascular endothelial cells (ECs) and their intercommunication via tumor necrosis factor-α (TNF-α) [58]. The genesis of an immune reaction such as psoriasis may be initiated by nonspecific proinflammatory stimuli but the specific immune-mediated reaction includes activation of subsets of T cells by contact with an adhesion molecule bearing intercellular adhesion molecule-1 (ICAM-1) positive stimulatory cell. This cell expresses a specific antigenic determinant (self or nonself). The T cell can bind to the macrophage via the CD3 molecular complex and to cytokine-activated KCs by the accessory surface molecules CD2 and CD18 (Table 2.1). There is evidence to support a critical role for TNF-α in psoriasis: TGF-α which acts via EGF receptors and affects angiogenesis, is elevated in psoriatic epidermis compared to nonlesional skin. Elevated IL-6 is expressed in psoriatic but not normal epidermis. IL-6 receptor has been demonstrated only in the transitional zone [63]. Neutrophil-activating peptide-1 (NAP-1)/IL-8 was increased 50 times in psoriatic scales compared to normal callus [64]. NAP-1/IL-8 has potent chemotactic activity for PMNLs and T cells and promotes epidermal cell proliferation [65]. Dermal blood vessels express the TNF-α-inducible adhesion molecules ICAM-1, endothelial leukocyte adhesion molecule-1 (ELAM-1), and vascular cell adhesion molecule-1 (VCAM-1) which facilitate binding of leukocytes and extravasation into the lesion including skin homing CD4 memory T cells.

Serum concentrations of TNF-α tended to be higher than controls although not significantly [66]. IFN-γ levels were elevated and rapidly returned to normal with etretinate or cyclosporine treatment before any clinical improvement was documented [67]. TNF-α tended to decrease during etretinate and increase during cyclosporine therapy. Psoriatic lesions developed at the site of intradermal IFN-γ and IFN-α injections. Systemic administration of interferons may improve or aggravate psoriasis. Psoriasis and psoriatic arthritis have been induced by either systemic IFN-α [68,69] or IFN-γ [70] therapy.

Systemic administration of TNF may be effective in clearing psoriasis. Recombinant human TNF has been used to treat severe psoriasis. Of five patients treated, three had complete clearing, one partial resolution, and one no change [71,72]. Significant toxicity (fever, chills, hypertension, hypotension, elevated serum transaminases) may occur at higher doses.

ICAM-1 can be induced by IFN-γ and psoriatic KCs are not as inhibited by IFN-γ as are normal KCs. Soluble ICAM-1 is significantly increased in

Table 2.1 Model for the immunopathogenesis of psoriasis. Adapted from Nickoloff [58]

I	Response to nonspecific injury: induction of acute-phase inflammatory reactants
II	Recruitment of leukocytes: cytokine induction of adhesion molecules, chemotaxins
III	Regenerative wound-healing response:induction of growth factors
IV	Revelation of psoriasis mutation: interaction between cytokine-activated keratinocytes and T cells with return to the circulation of autoreactive T cells
V	Repetition of II–IV with propagation of lesions both locally and at remote sites via skin-seeking (epidermotropic) autoreactive T cells

the serum of psoriatic patients compared with normal controls: ICAM-1 levels were directly proportional to the PASI score [73]. The hypothesis is that overactivation of the growth stimulatory pathway (TGF-α) or inactivation of the growth inhibitory pathway (IFN-γ receptors) occurs. Active EGF receptors (also the receptor for TGF-α) persist from the basal layer to the stratum corneum in psoriasis (normally only basal and lower spinous layers).

The relative contributions of epidermal proliferation and immunologic activation to the maintenance of active psoriatic lesions have been studied by examining the specific effects of cyclosporine treatment on these cells *in vivo* [74]. Cyclosporine treatment (2–7.5 mg/kg per day) reduced the number of IL-2 receptor (IL-2R) positive T cells in plaques, decreased HLA-DR expression in KCs, and decreased IFN-γ-induced protein-10 (chemoattractant and mitogenic cytokine). Increased expression of P-10 may result from IFN-γ produced by activated lymphocytes. On the other hand, markers of KC growth activation, TGF-α and IL-6, did not change after 1–3 months of cyclosporine treatment. Most patients (five of eight) continued to express the hyperproliferative keratin marker K16 after cyclosporine treatment. Petzelbauer and colleagues [75] reported slightly different results after 2 weeks of cyclosporine treatment at 5 mg/kg per day. HLA-DR expression by KC was not altered, but ICAM-1 expression by endothelial cells lining the elongated and tortuous vessels within tips of dermal papillae was markedly reduced in five of seven patients who improved clinically but persisted in two who failed to respond. Because IFN-γ induces both HLA-DR and ICAM-1 expression by KCs, the authors doubted that cyclosporine affected ICAM-1 expression via IFN-γ. There was an increase in the density of intraepidermal Langerhans cells and a decrease in IL-2R positive cells. The density of CD3, CD4, and CD8 cells did not change.

Soluble IL-2R levels in serum are elevated in patients with psoriasis and atopic dermatitis [76]. The data indicated the effect of nonspecific T-cell activation in both diseases. There was a strong positive correlation between IL-2R level and PASI. As patients improved with various treatments, UVB + tar [77], PUVA, or cyclosporine [78], the IL-2R level was reduced significantly. Similar results were obtained in patients with psoriatic arthritis responding to cyclosporine but not in the nonresponders [79].

Three patients have had definite but transient improvement of severe psoriasis when treated by CD4 monoclonal antibody infusion [80]. After 2 weeks, there was no change in endothelial cell ICAM-1 expression, but HLA-DR positive KCs and intraepidermal CD4 cells were decreased. Epidermal Langerhans cells increased.

The predominant *in vivo* effect of cyclosporine was to decrease immune activation; KC growth activation was less sensitive. The inability of cyclosporine treatment to decrease TGF-α and IL-6 levels in plaques as well as the persistence of hyperproliferative keratin helps to explain the recurrence of disease to pretreatment activity after cesssation of cyclosporine. Moreover, cyclosporine did not inhibit NAP-1/IL-8 synthesis or secretion by

MNCs [81]. These studies suggest that immune activation is important in the pathogenesis of psoriasis and that agents which interfere with T-cell activation and/or inhibit cytokine secretion will play a major role in the future therapy of psoriasis. In Chapter 16, the details of current recommendations for systemic cyclosporine treatment of severe psoriasis will be covered including a discussion of the structurally unrelated but similar acting immunosuppressive compound FK506 (Tacrolimus).

REFERENCES

1 Weinstein GD. Epidermal cell kinetics. In Fitzpatrick TB, Eisen AZ, Wolff K, *et al.* eds. *Dermatology in General Medicine*, 3rd edn. New York: McGraw-Hill, 1987:154–65.

2 Kaur I, Kaur S, Valshnavi C, *et al.* Epidermal calmodulin levels in psoriasis before and after therapy. *Indian J Med Res* 1991;94:130–3.

3 Lowe NJ, Breeding J, Russell D. Cutaneous polyamines in psoriasis. *Br J Dermatol* 1982;107:21–6.

4 Watanabe S, Wagatsuma K, Ichikawa E, Takahashi H. Abnormal distribution of epidermal protein antigens in psoriatic epidermis. *J Dermatol* 1991;18:143–51.

5 Thaler M, Fukuyama K, Epstein WL, Fisher KA. Comparative studies of keratins isolated from psoriasis and atopic dermatitis. *J Invest Dermatol* 1980;75:156–8.

6 Thewes M, Stadler R, Korge B, Mischke D. Normal psoriatic epidermis expression of hyperproliferation-associated keratins. *Arch Dermatol Res* 1991;283:465–71.

7 Fedi AM, Lotti T, Meo AL, *et al.* Immunohistochemical study on the pattern of 50 kd cytokeratin in psoriasis. *Int J Dermatol* 1992;31:30–2.

8 Bernerd F, Magnaldo T, Darmon M. Delayed onset of epidermal differentiation in psoriasis. *J Invest Dermatol* 1992;98:902–10.

9 Hashimoto K, Matsumoto K, Higashiyama M, *et al.* Growth-inhibitory effects of 1,25-dihydroxy vitamin D_3 on normal and psoriatic keratinocytes. *Br J Dermatol* 1990;123:93–8.

10 Tucker WFG, MacNeil S, Dawson RA, *et al.* Calmodulin levels in psoriasis: the effect of treatment. *Acta Derm Venereol* 1986;66:241–4.

11 Eedy DJ, Canavan JP, Shaw C, Trimble ER. Beta-adrenergic stimulation of cyclic AMP is defective in cultured dermal fibroblasts of psoriatic subjects. *Br J Dermatol* 1990;122:477–83.

12 Raynaud F, Gerbaud P, Enjolras O, *et al.* A cAMP binding abnormality in psoriasis. *Lancet* 1989;i:1153–6.

13 Guillot B, Guilhou JJ, Vendrel JP, Meynadier J. Neutrophil chemotaxis in psoriasis before and after PUVA therapy. *Arch Dermatol Res* 1983;275:19–22.

14 Silny W, Pehamberger H, Zielinsky C, Gshnait F. Effect of PUVA treatment on the locomotion of polymorphonuclear leukocytes and mononuclear cells in psoriasis. *J Invest Dermatol* 1980;75:187–8.

15 Ternowitz T. The enhanced monocyte and neutrophil chemotaxis in psoriasis is normalized after treatment with psoralens plus ultraviolet A and anthralin. *J Am Acad Dermatol* 1987;16:1169–75.

16 Langner A, Chorzelski TP, Fraczykowska M, *et al.* Effect of anthralin on stratum corneum antigenicity and polymorphonuclear leukocyte chemotaxis. *Br J Dermatol* 1981;105(Suppl. 20):62–3.

17 Herlin T, Kragballe K. Enhanced monocyte and neutrophil cytotoxicity and normal cyclic nucleotide levels in severe psoriasis. *Br J Dermatol* 1981;105:405–14.

18 Whittier FC, Evans DH, Anderson PC, Nolph KD. Peritoneal dialysis for psoriasis: a controlled study. *Ann Intern Med* 1983;99:165–8.

19 Glinski W, Zarebska Z, Jablonska S, *et al.* The activity of polymorphonuclear

leukocyte neutral proteinases and their inhibitors in patients with psoriasis treated with a continuous peritoneal dialysis. *J Invest Dermatol* 1980;75:481–7.

20 Jupe DML, Nightingale RF. Leukapheresis for the treatment of psoriasis (Letter). *Arch Dermatol* 1983;119:629–30.

21 Paslin D. Psoriasis without neutrophils. *Int J Dermatol* 1990;29:37–40.

22 Farber FM, Rein G, Lanigan SW. Stress and psoriasis: psychoneuroimmunologic mechanisms. *Int J Dermatol* 1991;30:8–12.

23 Raychaudhuri SP, Farber EM. Are sensory nerves essential for the development of psoriatic lessons? *J Am Acad Dermatol* 1993;28:488–9.

24 Wallengren J, Ekman R, Sundler F. Occurrence and distribution of neuropeptides in human skin. An immunocytochemical and immunochemical study on normal skin and blister fluid from inflamed skin. *Acta Derm Venereol* 1987;67:185–92.

25 Johansson O, Han SW, Enhamre A. Altered cutaneous innervation in psoriatic skin as revealed by PGP 9.5 immunohistochemistry. *Arch Dermatol Res* 1991;283: 519–23.

26 Naukkarinen A, Harvima IT, Aalto ML, *et al*. Quantitative analysis of contact sites between mast cells and sensory nerves in cutaneous psoriasis and lichen planus based on a histochemical double staining technique. *Arch Dermatol Res* 1991;283: 433–7.

27 Eedy DJ, Johnston CF, Shaw C, Buchanan KD. Neuropeptides in psoriasis: an immunocytochemical and radioimmunoassay. *J Invest Dermatol* 1991;96:434–8.

28 Pincelli C, Fantini F, Romualdi P, *et al*. Substance P is diminished and vasoactive intestinal peptide is augmented in psoriatic lesions and these peptides exert disparate effects on the proliferation of cultured human keratinocytes. *J Invest Dermatol* 1992;98:421–7.

29 Rabier M, Wilkinson DI, Farber EM. Peptide T behaves as a vasoactive intestinal agonist towards cultured keratinocytes. *J Invest Dermatol* 1991;96:628(Abstract).

30 Camisa C. Somatostatin therapy. In Roenigk HH Jr, Maibach HI, eds. *Psoriasis*, 2nd edn. New York: Marcel Dekker, Inc., 1991:829–46.

31 Paus R. Does prolactin play a role in skin biology and pathology? *Med Hypotheses* 1991;36:33–42.

32 Nanney LB, Yates RA, King LE Jr. Modulation of epidermal growth factor receptors in psoriatic lesions during treatment with topical EGF. *J Invest Dermatol* 1992;98: 296–301.

33 Krane JF, Murphy DP, Carter M, Krueger JG. Synergistic effects of epidermal growth factor (EGF) and insulin-like growth factor/somatomedin C (IFG-1) on keratinocyte proliferation may be mediated by IGF-1 transmodulation of the EGF receptor. *J Invest Dermatol* 1991;96:419–24.

34 Camisa C, Bagatell F, Bainbridge C, *et al*. Somatostatin analogue (octreotide acetate) vs placebo in the treatment of psoriasis. *J Invest Dermatol* 1990;94:511 (Abstract).

35 Bernstein JE, Parish LC, Rapaport M, *et al*. Effects of topically applied capsaicin on moderate and severe psoriasis vulgaris. *J Am Acad Dermatol* 1986;15:504–7.

36 Marcusson JA, Talme T, Wetterberg L, Johansson O. Peptide T, a new treatment for psoriasis? A study of nine patients. *Acta Derm Venereol* 1991;71:479–83.

37 Delfino M, Fabbrocini, Brunetti B, *et al*. Peptide T in the treatment of severe psoriasis. *Acta Derm Venereol* 1992;72:68–9.

38 Farber EM, Cohen EN, Trozak DJ, Wilkinson DI. Peptide T improves psoriasis when infused into lesions in nanogram amounts. *J Am Acad Dermatol* 1991;25: 658–64.

39 Verhagen A, Berger SM, Van Erp PEJ, *et al*. Confirmation of raised phospholysase A_2 activity in the uninvolved skin of psoriasis. *Br J Dermatol* 1984;110:731–2.

40 Bauer FW, Van de Kerkhof PCM, Maasen-de Grood RM. Epidermal hyperproliferation following the induction of microabscesses by leukotriene B_4. *Br J Dermatol* 1986;114:409–12.

41 Voorhees JJ. Leukotrienes and other lipoxygenase products in the pathogenesis and therapy of psoriasis and other dermatoses. *Arch Dermatol* 1983;119:541–7.
42 Cantieri JS, Graff G, Goldberg ND. Cyclic GMP metabolism in psoriasis: activation of soluble epidermal guanylate cyclase by arachidonic acid and 12-hydroxy-5,8,10, 14-eicosatetraenoic acid. *J Invest Dermatol* 1980;74:234–7.
43 Katayama H, Kawada A. Exacerbations of psoriasis induced by indomethacin. *J Dermatol* 1981;8:323–7.
44 Fallon JD, Ellis CN, Voorhees JJ. Topical indomethacin prevents the therapeutic effects of emollients in psoriasis. *Clin Res* 1983;31:811(Abstract).
45 Sheehan-Dare RA, Goodfield MJD, Rowell NR. The effect of oral indomethacin on psoriasis treated with the Ingram regime. *Br J Dermatol* 1991;125:253–5.
46 Vila L, Cullare C, Sola J, *et al.* Cyclooxygenase activity is increased in platelets from psoriatic patients. *J Invest Dermatol* 1991;97:922–6.
47 Ellis CN, Goldfarb MT, Roenigk HH Jr, *et al.* Effects of oral meclofenamate therapy in psoriasis. *J Am Acad Dermatol* 1986;14:49–52.
48 Kragballe K, Herlin T. Benoxaprofen improves psoriasis. A double-blind study. *Arch Dermatol* 1983;119:548–52.
49 deJong EM, van Vlijmen IM, Scholte JC, *et al.* Clinical and biochemical effects of an oral leukotriene biosynthesis inhibitor (MK886) in psoriasis. *Skin Pharmacol* 1991;4:278–85.
50 Ziboh VA, Cohen KA, Ellis CN, *et al.* Effects of dietary supplementation of fish oil on neutrophil and epidermal fatty acids. *Arch Dermatol* 1986;122:1277–82.
51 Krogh HK, Tonder O. Antibodies in psoriatic scales. *Scand J Immunol* 1973;2: 45–51.
52 Qutaishat SS, Kumar V, Beutner EH, Jablonska S. A distinct stratum corneum antigen in psoriasis and its reactions with stratum corneum antibodies. *Acta Pathol Microbiol Immunol Scand* 1992;100:341–6.
53 Karsh J, Espinoza LR, Dorval G, *et al.* Immune complexes in psoriasis with and without arthritis. *J Rheumatol* 1978;5:314–9.
54 Hall RP, Peck GL, Lawley TJ. Circulating IgA immune complexes in patients with psoriasis. *J Invest Dermatol* 1983;80:465–8.
55 Takematsu H, Tagami H. Activation of the alternative pathway of complement in psoriatic lesional skin. *Dermatologica* 1990;181:289–92.
56 Beutner EH, Jablonska S, Hebborn P, Kumar V. Autoimmunity in psoriasis. In Beutner EH, Chorzelski TP, Kumar V, eds. *Immunopathology of the Skin*, 3rd edn. New York: Wiley & Sons, 1987:703–26.
57 Khandke L, Krane JF, Ashinoff R, *et al.* Cyclosporine in psoriasis treatment. *Arch Dermatol* 1991;127:1172–9.
58 Nickoloff BJ. The cytokine network in psoriasis. *Arch Dermatol* 1991;127: 871–84.
59 Baker BS, Fry L. The immunology of psoriasis. *Br J Dermatol* 1992;126:1–9.
60 Yin JA, Jowitt SN. Resolution of immune-mediated diseases following allogeneic bone marrow transplantation for leukemia. *Bone Marrow Transplant* 1992;9:31–3.
61 Steinmuller D, Zinsmeister AR, Rogers RS III. Cellular autoimmunity in psoriasis and lichen planus. *J Autoimmun* 1988;1:279–98.
62 Terui T, Rokugo M, Aiba S, *et al.* Autologous mixed lymphocyte reaction is reduced in patients with psoriasis. *Br J Dermatol* 1990;123:325–31.
63 Ohta Y, Katayama I, Funato T, *et al.* *In situ* expression of messenger RNA of interleukin-1 and interleukin-6 in psoriasis: interleukin-6 involved in formation of psoriatic lesions. *Arch Dermatol Res* 1991;283:351–6.
64 Schroder JM, Gregory H, Young J, Christophers E. Neutrophil-activating proteins in psoriasis. *J Invest Dermatol* 1992;98:241–7.
65 Tuschil A, Lam C, Haslberger A, Lindley I. Interleukin-8 stimulates calcium transients and promotes epidermal cell proliferation. *J Invest Dermatol* 1992;99: 294–8.

66 Gomi T, Shiohara T, Munakata T, *et al.* Interleukin 1 alpha, tumor necrosis factor alpha and interferon gamma in psoriasis. *Arch Dermatol* 1991;127:827–30.
67 Shiohara T, Imanishi K, Sagawa Y, Nagashima M. Differential effects of cyclosporine and etretinate on serum cytokine levels in patients with psoriasis. *J Am Acad Dermatol* 1992;27:568–74.
68 Jucgla A, Marcoval J, Curco N, Servitje O. Psoriasis with articular involvement induced by interferon alpha (Letter). *Arch Dermatol* 1991;127:910–1.
69 Funk J, Langeland T, Schrumpf E, Hanssen LE. Psoriasis induced by interferon-alpha. *Br J Dermatol* 1991;125:472–4.
70 O'Connel PG, Gerber LH, DiGiovanna JJ, Peck GL. Arthritis in patients with psoriasis treated with gamma interferon. *J Rheumatol* 1992;19:80–2.
71 Creaven PJ, Stoll HL Jr. Response to tumor necrosis factor in two cases of psoriasis. *J Am Acad Dermatol* 1991;24:735–7.
72 Takematsu H, Ozawa H, Yoshimura T, *et al.* Systemic TNF administration in psoriatic patients: a promising therapeutic modality for severe psoriasis. *Br J Dermatol* 1991;24:209–10.
73 Schopf RE, Naumann S, Rehder M, Morsches B. Soluble intercellular adhesion molecule-1 levels in patients with psoriasis. *Br J Dermatol* 1993;128:34–7.
74 Gottlieb AB, Grossman RM, Khandke L, *et al.* Studies of the effect of cyclosporine in psoriasis *in vivo*: combined effects of activated T lymphocytes and epidermal regenerative maturation. *J Invest Dermatol* 1992;98:302–9.
75 Petzelbauer P, Stingl G, Wolff K, Volc-Platzer B. Cyclosporin A suppresses ICAM-1 expression by papillary endothelium in healing psoriatic plaques. *J Invest Dermatol* 1991;96:362–9.
76 Kapp A, Neuner P, Krutmann J, *et al.* Production of interleukin-2 by mononuclear cells *in vitro* in patients with atopic dermatitis and psoriasis. Comparison with serum interleukin-2 receptor levels. *Acta Derm Venereol* 1991;71:403–6.
77 Betti R, Rosti A, Lodi A, *et al.* Effect of UVB plus tar therapy on serum levels of interleukin-2 receptors in patients with psoriasis. *Clin Exp Dermatol* 1991;16: 364–6.
78 Duncan JI, Horrocks C, Ormerod AD, *et al.* Soluble IL-2 receptor and CD25 cells in psoriasis: effects of cyclosporin A and PUVA therapy. *Clin Exp Immunol* 1991;85:293–6.
79 Salvarani C, Macchioni P, Boiardi L, *et al.* Low dose cyclosporine A in psoriatic arthritis: relation between soluble interleukin 2 receptors and response to therapy. *J Rheumatol* 1992;19:74–9.
80 Nicolas J-F, Rizova H, Demidem A, *et al.* CD4 antibody therapy and cyclosporin A differentially affect HLA-DR and ICAM-1 expression in psoriatic skin. *J Invest Dermatol* 1992;98:943–4.
81 Mrowietz U, Sticherling M, Mielke V, *et al.* Neutrophil-activating peptide 1/interleukin 8 mRNA expression and protein secretion by human monocytes: effect of cyclosporin A. *Cytokine* 1991;3:322–6.

three

Concurrent Diseases, Associations, and Drugs

CONCURRENT DISEASES AND ASSOCIATIONS

Almost any other disease or condition can coexist with psoriasis (Table 3.1). Some associations have unarguable pathogenetic relationships with psoriasis, such as psoriatic arthritis and Reiter's syndrome because of morphology and association with HLA-B27. Common genetic factors may help to explain the relationship between and among psoriasis, peripheral arthropathy, sacroiliitis, ankylosing spondylitis, and inflammatory bowel diseases. In a case-control study, the prevalence of psoriasis was significantly higher in patients with ulcerative colitis (5.7%) and Crohn's disease (11.2%) compared to the control group (1.5%) (Fig. 3.1) [1]. Diseases like palmoplantar pustulosis (PPP) and subcorneal pustular dermatosis are highly associated with ordinary psoriasis and may alternate between the original state and generalized pustular psoriasis.

The group of diseases considered "autoimmune" occurs infrequently in association with psoriasis, e.g., systemic lupus erythematosus (SLE) [2] and the vesiculobullous diseases [3], in part because they are uncommon in the general population. These associations suggest that psoriasis is an

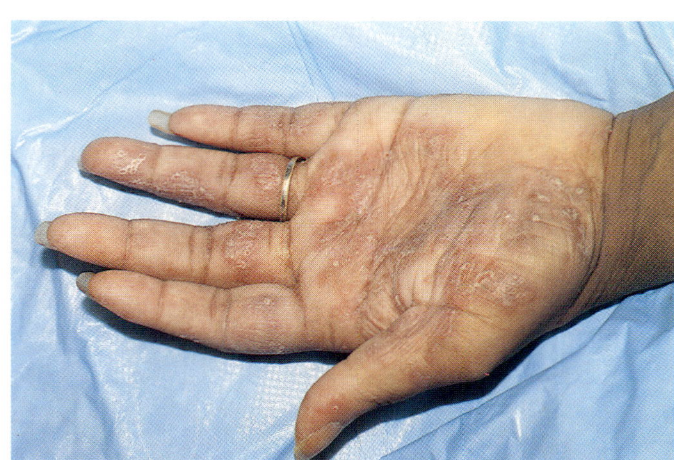

Fig 3.1 A patient with Crohn's disease who developed pustular psoriasis of the palms upon withdrawal of prednisone.

Table 3.1 Diseases coexisting with psoriasis

Probable pathogenetic relationship
Psoriatic arthritis
Reiter's syndrome
Palmoplantar pustulosis
Subcorneal pustular dermatosis
Inflammatory bowel diseases
Crohn's disease
Ulcerative colitis
Possible pathogenetic relationship
Bullous diseases
Bullous pemphigoid
Pemphigus vulgaris
Pemphigus foliaceus
Benign familial chronic pemphigus
Remote pathogenetic relationship
Lichen planus
Lichen striatus
Vitiligo
Atopic dermatitis
Other autoimmune diseases
Systemic and discoid lupus erythematosus
Hashimoto's thyroiditis
Myasthenia gravis
Sjögren's syndrome

autoimmune disease, which are known to have a tendency to cluster together [4].

Because of the past and present treatment of patients with potential and known carcinogens including arsenic, ionizing radiation, sunlight, artificial UV light, coal tar, and psoralen UVA (PUVA), the relative risks of all types of cancers have been sought in patients with psoriasis. Smoking and drinking patterns may be influenced by the disease or be causally related to the activity of psoriasis and increase the risk of serious morbidity from respiratory cancers and liver cirrhosis, respectively.

As most cases of severe or complicated psoriasis are cared for by dermatologists, concurrent cutaneous conditions are more likely to be found on long-term observation of the skin. If the findings are curious, create an unusual juxtaposition of lesions, or a puzzling diagnostic or treatment dilemma, the cases are likely to be presented and discussed at meetings and eventually published. On the other hand, common skin diseases in association with psoriasis are probably ignored and therefore underreported. For example, almost every case of psoriasis coexisting with pemphigus vulgaris is reported in the literature, while it is doubtful that any cases of concomitant acne or atopic eczema would be published as such. As a result one might erroneously conclude that the psoriasis and pemphigus occur together frequently while the combination of psoriasis and acne is rare.

Bullous pemphigoid

Most cases of psoriasis reported in association with autoimmune bullous diseases have had bullous pemphigoid (BP). In all cases, the psoriasis preceded BP. Therefore, antipsoriatic treatment, which is proinflammatory has been implicated as the cause including radiation therapy, PUVA, UVB, sun exposure, tar, anthralin, and salicylic acid [3]. The chronology of occurrence is to be expected based on the mean age of onset of psoriasis (28 years) and BP (60 years). An almost equal number of cases of coexisting psoriasis and BP have been reported without a suspected cause. Blisters have occurred on psoriatic and uninvolved skin. Psoriasis can arise as a Koebner response to a pemphigoid lesion. The treatment of BP in these circumstances is problematic because an effort should be made to avoid systemic steroids in psoriasis. In a patient with long-standing psoriatic arthritis without skin lesions who developed BP, psoriatic plaques appeared for the first time after oral steroid therapy was withdrawn [3]. If topical steroids and oral antibiotics are unsuccessful at preventing blisters, dapsone 100 mg daily [5], cyclosporine 5 mg/kg per day [6], and cyclosporine 3 mg/kg per day plus oral steroids [7] may be effective. Methotrexate (MTX), azathioprine, and cyclophosphamide may be considered as alternative steroid-sparing agents. BP has a tendency to combine with arthritis and autoimmune thyroid disease, and these associations should be sought [8].

Pemphigus

The blisters of the superficial forms of pemphigus, foliaceus and erythematosus, occur in a subcorneal location and may resemble subcorneal pustular dermatosis, pustular psoriasis or psoriasis vulgaris when the lesions appear dry, red, and scaly (Fig. 3.2). These diseases have been reported in association with psoriasis [9]. Biopsy and immunofluorescence studies can usually differentiate all forms of autoimmune pemphigus and psoriasis. If systemic steroids are used to treat pemphigus, and they are often indicated, a steroid-sparing agent may be required to prevent a rebound flare of

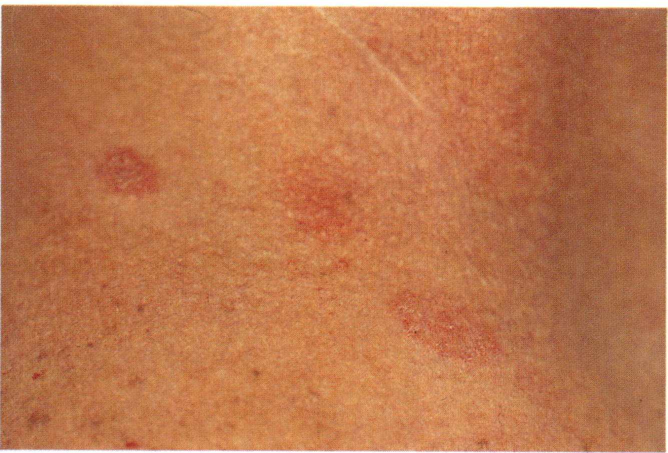

Fig 3.2 Pemphigus erythematosus. The patient has superficial scaling guttate lesions.

psoriasis [10]. A suppressor T-cell deficit or dysfunction in psoriasis has been proposed as the mechanism that allows the production of autoantibodies in coexisting bullous diseases. Plasminogen activator (PA), which is believed to be crucial in the development of acantholysis, is found to be markedly increased in the involved epidermis of psoriasis, BP and benign familial chronic pemphigus (Hailey–Hailey disease). PA activity was normal or modestly elevated in pemphigus vulgaris or foliaceus [11].

Hailey–Hailey disease

In Hailey–Hailey disease, the intertriginous exudative lesions may be confused with atypical flexural psoriasis. Phototherapy may aggravate it. A positive family history and/or histopathology showing acantholysis are necessary for the diagnosis. Immunofluorescence studies are negative. The course of benign chronic pemphigus may be altered by topical steroids and antimicrobials, broad-spectrum systemic antibiotics, or dapsone [12].

Urticaria, candidiasis, atopic dermatitis, and vitiligo

Among common skin diseases, urticaria [13] and candidiasis [14] showed an excess rate in psoriasis patients, but in the past psoriasis has been believed to be mutually exclusive of atopic dermatitis, vitiligo, and lichen planus (LP). In a large prospective study, systematic examinations in a dermatology clinic revealed that 16.7% of atopic dermatitis patients had psoriasis and 9.5% of psoriatic patients had atopic dermatitis [15]. Clearly, the two diseases frequently coexist in the same patient. Chronologically, the atopic dermatitis generally preceded the onset of psoriasis, and both diseases respond well to similar treatments. Vitiligo was also thought to be rarely associated with psoriasis until reports in 1982–83 showed it to be as prevalent in psoriasis patients as in the general population (0.55%) [16,17]. The converse was also true. Vitiligo usually appeared first. Psoriasis lesions were distributed randomly with respect to the depigmented skin (Fig. 3.3). The coexistence of vitiligo with psoriasis apparently increases

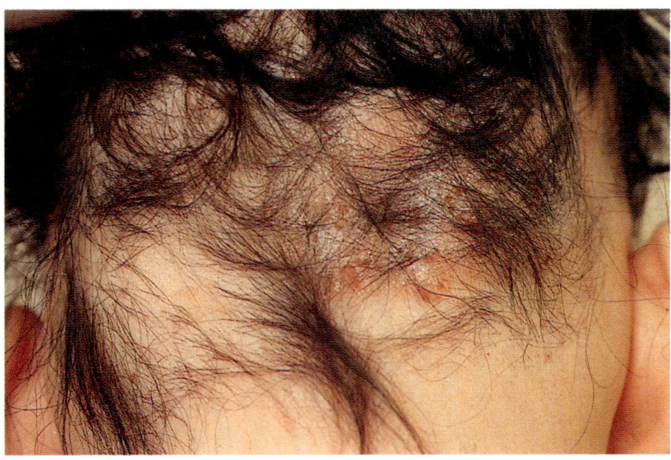

Fig 3.3 Coexisting alopecia areata and psoriasis. The patient was receiving intralesional triamcinolone injections for both diseases.

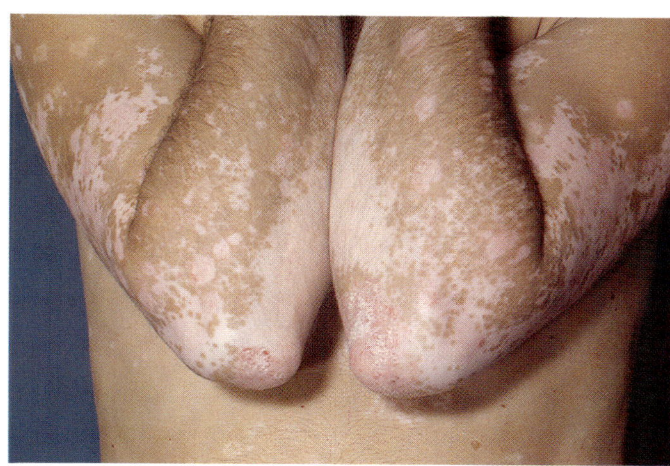

Fig 3.4 Coexisting vitiligo and psoriasis. Note that psoriasis occurs within vitiliginous areas of skin.

the incidence of additional putative autoimmune diseases: arthritis, thyroid disease, diabetes, ulcerative colitis, pernicious anemia, lupus, and alopecia areata (Fig. 3.4) [18]. Occasionally, both vitiligo and psoriasis will respond to potent topical steroids, but PUVA is an ideal treatment for both diseases if one is extensive enough to warrant the effort, expense, and risks involved.

Lichen planus

Considering the high prevalence of psoriasis and both skin and mucous membrane LP in general dermatology practices, their coexistence does seem underrepresented in the literature. A case was reported in which long-standing psoriasis improved during the development of LP, and exacerbation of psoriasis was associated with resolution of LP [19]. The authors suggested that the two diseases might be mutually exclusive because of immunologic and pathogenetic interrelationships. For example, local production of interferon-γ by lymphocytes in the inflammatory infiltrate is believed to play a role in the expression of HLA-DR on keratinocytes, which is more marked in LP than in psoriasis. Therapy of psoriasis with interferons has given mixed results, but there are examples of definite exacerbation by both local and systemic administration of interferons. The epidermal kinetics are vastly different with hyperproliferation in psoriasis and markedly reduced proliferation in LP resulting in the characteristic histologic picture of hypergranulosis and orthokeratosis [20]. One similarity, however, is that both diseases demonstrate the classic Koebner phenomenon. Naldi and colleagues [21] disputed the rarity of the coexistence of psoriasis and LP. They performed a case-control study of LP in Italy. Of 711 patients with LP, 12 (1.7%) reported a diagnosis of psoriasis. Among the controls with other skin diseases except LP, 2.7% reported a diagnosis of psoriasis. The difference between the two groups was not statistically significant. Among 19 recently reported cases of lichen striatus in children, three had psoriasis including one with an unusual eruptive variant on the contralateral side [22,23]. We have seen at least two cases of erythema annulare centrifugum coexisting with psoriasis vulgaris (Fig. 3.5).

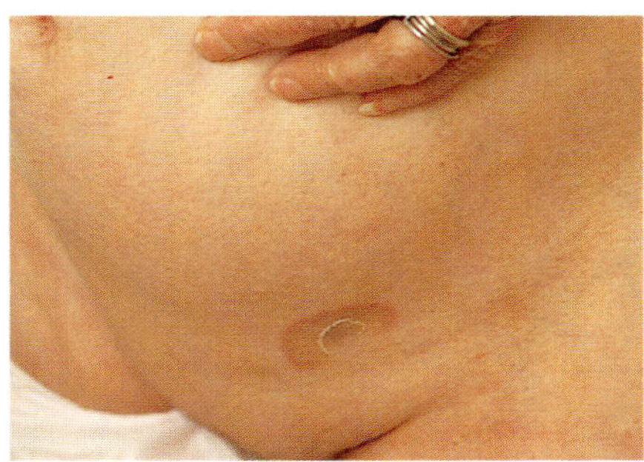

Fig 3.5 Erythema annulare centrifugum on the abdomen in association with psoriasis on the hand, navel, and thigh.

Lupus erythematosus

Based on their prevalence in the population the coexistence of all forms of lupus with psoriasis seems to be less than expected. Dubois [24] reported that 0.6% of 520 patients with SLE had concurrent psoriasis. The coexistence of psoriasis and lupus (Fig. 3.6) raises issues of diagnosis and treatment. Forty-three percent of patients with SLE are photosensitive, and 80% of patients with psoriasis improve with sunlight [25,26]. However, a subset of "photosensitive psoriasis" comprises about 5.5% of all cases [27]. These patients have a significantly higher frequency of skin type I, and 50% have preceding polymorphous light eruption developing into psoriasis. Subacute cutaneous lupus erythematosus (SCLE) lesions are either annular or psoriasiform. Biopsy, immunofluorescence, and serologic testing are necessary to distinguish SCLE from psoriasis. Some of these patients, especially those with circulating Ro (SS-A) antibodies, may be exquisitely photosensitive [28]. The action spectrum for lupus is generally considered to be UVB, but some patients may flare after UVA exposures received in tanning salons or from sunlight filtered through window glass.

The control of SLE often requires systemic steroids, especially for renal and CNS involvement. A rebound flare of psoriasis is always possible upon withdrawal of steroids. Antimetabolites used as steroid-sparing agents may prevent this as well as improve psoriasis. Phototherapy is contraindicated in patients with lupus, but PUVA is indicated for "photosensitive psoriasis" if it is severe [27]. Screening for antinuclear antibodies including Ro and La is necessary prior to treating any photosensitive patient with light [2]. The antimalarials are now the drugs of choice in the treatment of the cutaneous and joint manifestations of lupus, but chloroquine and hydroxychloroquine may precipitate drug reactions or flares of psoriasis [29]. The retinoids isotretinoin and etretinate have been used successfully to treat cutaneous lupus erythematosus in open trials. Recently, double-blind trials confirmed the efficacy of acitretin (50 mg/day) or hydroxychloroquine (400 mg/day) in 50% of cases of cutaneous lupus erythematosus [30].

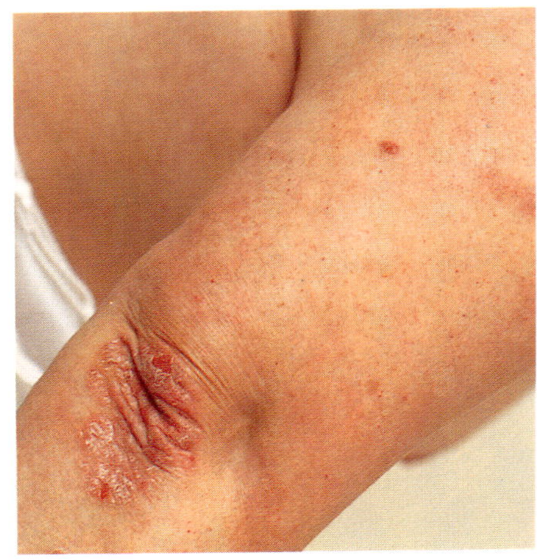

Fig 3.6 The dusky lesions on the arm represent subacute cutaneous lupus lesions. The elbow shows typical psoriasis.

Alcohol and smoking

In a Swedish population study including 372 psoriatics, ankylosing spondylitis and iritis (but not together) were overrepresented in males; there was an excess of obesity and lung cancer in females [13]. Liver cirrhosis and alcoholism showed excess rates in both sexes, but only three of the alcoholics had cirrhosis. After 10 years of prospective study of a cohort of 1380 American patients treated with PUVA, there were more deaths caused by cirrhosis than expected in the general population (11% vs 2.9%) [31]. The investigator found that having two alcoholic drinks per day increased the risk of death threefold whereas prior MTX treatment was not a risk factor.

Alcohol consumption has been investigated in recall questionnaire surveys using patients with other skin diseases as controls. A Finnish study showed a dramatic increase in the daily consumption of alcohol by 129 psoriatics (55 g vs 20 g) and the annual frequency of intoxication (58 vs 37) compared to 238 controls [32]. In a similar but larger ($n = 215$) Italian study, there was a trend for increased relative risk of psoriasis: 1.3 for one to two drinks daily and 1.6 for three or more drinks daily compared to nondrinkers [33]. One major difference between the two studies is the duration of skin manifestations, 12 years or less in the former [32] and 2 years or less in the latter [33]. If chronic psoriasis sustains drinking, then the daily consumption may increase over time. Gupta and coworkers [34] showed that alcohol abuse interferes with the response of psoriasis to aggressive inpatient therapy. More studies are needed to clarify whether alcohol consumption is a risk factor for the development of psoriasis or an epiphenomenon of the disease which increases the morbidity and mortality of this population by causing liver cirrhosis.

Case-control studies of cigarette smoking have also been performed. In a study of 216 patients with PPP 80% were smokers at the onset of disease compared to 36% of controls, an odds ratio of 7.2 [35]. Mills and coworkers [36] surveyed 108 psoriatics including 16 with PPP. There were 46.2% current smokers compared to 23.6% matched controls. The relative risk of psoriasis was greatest (5.3) for those currently smoking more than 20 cigarettes per day. This was confirmed by Naldi and coworkers [33] who reported that current smokers were at higher risk of psoriasis than "never-smokers" and that the relative risk became significant (2.1) for people smoking 15 or more cigarettes per day. However, no difference in the mean number of cigarettes smoked (12 daily) prior to onset of skin disease was found in the Finnish study [32], but again there was a much longer recall time for patients completing this questionnaire.

The dose–response relationship between the number of cigarettes smoked and the development of psoriasis have suggested a "cause and effect" relationship. The higher prevalence of current smoking among psoriatics is probably an indicator of a stressful life-style. In either case, these patients take on the additional risks of cardiovascular diseases, respiratory ailments, and certain cancers.

Stern and coworkers [31] found no increase in cardiovascular disease in their PUVA cohort. A study of 372 psoriatics from a defined population of 159 200 Swedes showed a significant association with lung cancer in women [13]. In another Swedish population of 20 328 living persons with psoriasis, there was no increase in the overall number of cancers or lung cancers [37]. However, there was a statistically significant excess of kidney cancers in women. In a more selective series of 4799 PUVA patients from Sweden [38], (which probably includes some of the same patients from the two previously cited studies) [13,37], respiratory cancer in both sexes, kidney and colonic cancer in women, and pancreatic cancer in men were significantly increased. Stern's group [31] also found increased colonic cancer in their PUVA cohort. A Danish study of 6910 patients with psoriasis revealed excesses of lung cancer in men and women, cancers of the larynx and pharynx in men, and cancers of the colon and kidney in women [39]. No increased frequency of bladder cancer, another neoplasm linked to smoking, was found. A Scottish study reported the same incidence of lung cancer and bladder cancer among 8400 psoriatics diagnosed between 1968 and 1979 as expected in the general population [40].

The concordance of the findings of excess numbers of respiratory cancers in both sexes and colon and kidney cancers in women, especially in the nonoverlapping national studies, is worrisome. It is possible that the genetic makeup of individuals with psoriasis, related behavioral patterns including diet, smoking, and alcohol intake, and the various treatments used contributed to these risks. More prospective case-control studies are needed to resolve these questions.

Skin cancer

All of the population studies linked to cancer registries and the long-term prospective PUVA followup studies have shown that the incidence of malignant melanoma in psoriatics is the same as expected in the general population. Nonmelanoma skin cancers were not significantly increased in Scotland (1.17) [40] or in Sweden (1.48) [37], but lesions on the trunk and extremities had an unusually higher prevalence. In Norway, where squamous cell carcinoma (SCC) is apparently more common than basal cell carcinoma (BCC), the relative risk was increased 2.5 and the usual anatomic distribution was altered [39]. When the PUVA cohort is selected out of the Swedish series, the relative risk of cutaneous SCC increases to sixfold [38]. Men who received a greater than 1200 J/cm^2 cumulative dose or more than 200 PUVA treatments had 27–30 times the incidence of SCC in the general population. In the American PUVA cohort, the relative risk for developing SCC or BCC after more than 200 PUVA treatments was 37–62 and 5–7, respectively [41]. The latter two studies indicate that PUVA has definite carcinogenic effects on the skin.

DRUGS THAT EXACERBATE OR INDUCE PSORIASIS

It is well known that antipsoriatic treatments have the potential to exacerbate psoriasis by irritating uninvolved skin (coal tar, anthralin), by UV-induced burns (sunburn, UVB, PUVA) or by their reduction or withdrawal (superpotent topical and systemic corticosteroids) [42].

When psoriasis flares upon withdrawal of potent systemic agents like MTX, etretinate, and cyclosporine, it probably represents resumption of the natural course of severe disease. Therefore, if it is necessary to stop treatment, it is advisable to taper the dose and convert to PUVA or another alternative treatment simultaneously. Whenever possible, systemic corticosteroids should be avoided in psoriatic patients. Their use accounts for most cases of extremely unstable psoriasis and the conversion of ordinary psoriasis into generalized pustular and erythrodermic psoriasis. Moreover, systemic corticosteroids are not particularly effective in treating the most severe forms of psoriasis.

The nonsteroidal antiinflammatory drugs (NSAIDs), cyclooxygenase inhibitors, are widely used for fever, pain, and inflammation. Specifically, they are effective in stabilizing or diminishing the activity of peripheral psoriatic arthropathy. The implication that NSAIDs exacerbate psoriasis is anecdotal and not substantiated by experience or in the literature. In fact, the only double-blind studies of these drugs in psoriasis have shown no effect (meclofenomate) or significant improvement (benoxaprofen).

There are at least three classes of drugs that have been implicated in the induction or aggravation of preexisting psoriasis on the weight of cumulative case reports since the 1960s and 1970s to the present. These are the β-adrenergic blockers, lithium carbonate, and the antimalarials. To my knowledge, no prospective study has been published in which psoriatics were treated with a specific drug and evaluated objectively at intervals for 1 or more years by dermatologists unaware of which drug the patient was taking together with a case-control population matched for baseline severity, sex, age, and duration of disease. There are, however, hypothetical reasons to explain the putative associations as well as some supporting but inconclusive biochemical and immunologic data.

β-blocking drugs

Both the cardioselective (β_2-adrenergic receptor) and noncardioselective (β_1-adrenergic-receptor) β-blockers can cause variable cutaneous eruptions described as maculopapular, lichenoid, eczematous, and psoriasiform in patients without psoriasis after an average 10–12 months of therapy. The appearance of a psoriasiform rash or aggravation of psoriasis occurs within several weeks to months in patients with established psoriasis. Many of the earlier cases were reported with practolol, a β_2-blocker which has been withdrawn from the market. When oral challenge tests have been done, the cutaneous eruption recurred within 5 days. Hu and colleagues [43] reported a generalized pustular flare of chronic plaque-type psoriasis 3 days after taking propanolol (prototype β_2-blocker) and on the occasion of two oral provocation tests. This reaction may be classified as acute generalized exanthematous pustulosis (Chapter 5), which is usually caused by antibiotics.

In a retrospective study of 26 selected patients receiving UVB or PUVA in 1986–87, there was a total of 29 exposures to β-blocking drugs and 21 (72%) self-reported exacerbations of psoriasis [44]. The authors recognized the design flaws of their study, but it is interesting because while propanolol was most often taken, both β_1- and β_2-blockers were represented, and nadolol was first reported to exacerbate psoriasis.

The β-blockers have many uses in medicine today: angina, arrhythmias, hypertension, postmyocardial infarction, migraine headache prophylaxis, open-angle glaucoma, essential tremor, and thyrotoxicosis. Therefore, they are not contraindicated in patients with concomitant psoriasis. When consulting on a patient with a new psoriasiform eruption or flaring of stable psoriasis who is also taking a β-blocker, it would be wise to ask the primary physician if it is feasible to switch from a noncardioselective (β_2) blocker to a cardioselective (β_1) blocker (Table 3.2). If the patient is

Table 3.2 Generic and brand names of β-adrenergic receptor blocking drugs in the USA. Adapted from Anonymous [45]

Generic name	Brand name
Noncardioselective (β_2)	
Propanolol	Inderal
Pindolol	Visken
Timolol	Blocadren, Timoptic
Nadolol	Corgard
Carteolol	Cartrol
Penbutolol	Levatol
Labetalol (+ selective α_1-blocking)	Normodyne, Trandate
Cardioselective (β_1)	
Acebutolol	Sectral
Atenolol	Tenormin
Metoprolol	Lopressor
Betaxolol	Kerlone

already taking a β_1-blocker, switch to another drug in that class as they may not cross-react.

A recent report suggested that alternative antihypertensive agents, the angiotensin-converting enzyme (ACE) inhibitors, may exacerbate psoriasis [46].

Lithium

Lithium carbonate is used in the treatment of manic disorders and for the prophylaxis and treatment of psychotic depression. Lithium is a cation that substitutes incompletely for other extra- and intracellular cations, notably sodium, in metabolic reactions. It also interferes with cyclic adenosine monophosphate (cAMP)-mediated processes. Cutaneous reactions are common with lithium particularly folliculitis and acneiform eruptions. The first cases of preexisting psoriasis exacerbated by lithium were reported in 1972. This finding was confirmed in 1976 with the report of three patients flaring after a few weeks and a new case of psoriasis appearing a few months after starting lithium [47]. The largest single series reported from Denmark included 12 patients who developed psoriasis *de novo* during lithium therapy [48]. The mean latency period was 10 months (range 1–24 months). Oral provocation with lithium induced the reappearance of psoriasis in two patients after 5 and 21 days when the original latency was 7 and 15 months, respectively. In three patients preexisting mild to moderate psoriasis was aggravated and became treatment resistant after 1 week, 1 month, and 6 months, respectively. Thus, it would seem that the latency period is shorter for aggravating preexisting psoriasis or provoking a recurrence of psoriasis upon oral rechallenge than for including psoriasis for the first time. Because psoriasis has been associated with psychic factors, it should be emphasized that the new onset and exacerbation of psoriasis in patients taking lithium generally occurred without relation to changes in mood or after the mental illness had actually improved. Notwithstanding, lithium carbonate is not contraindicated in patients with psoriasis. It does not aggravate all cases of preexisting psoriasis, but if it does, an attempt should be made to lower the dose before discontinuing lithium and substituting another drug. Interestingly, the popular antidepressant fluoxetine, which selectively inhibits serotonin reuptake, reportedly induced psoriasis in two patients [49]. The latency period was 6 months and 1 year, respectively; one case improved after reducing the dose of fluoxetine.

Mechanisms of β-blockers and lithium carbonate

These chemically diverse compounds may induce or aggravate psoriasis through a final common pathway but by different mechanisms. Human keratinocytes have β_2-adrenergic receptors. Pharmacologic blockade of the β-adrenergic pathway may lead to a decrease in the adenylate cyclase–cAMP cascade, decreased intracellular cAMP and free calcium, which is associated with increased rates of proliferation and insufficient epidermal differentiation, both features of psoriasis [50]. The adenyl cyclase system of psoriatic involved skin has a markedly decreased response to epinephrine and prostaglandin E_2 (PGE_2) *in vitro*. Lithium carbonate was shown to inhibit adenyl cyclase stimulation by epinephrine in pig epidermis [49]. Basal levels of cAMP were not altered after a 24-hour incubation with lithium. The authors also showed that the involved and uninvolved epidermis from a psoriatic patient taking lithium carbonate generated less cAMP than the mean values of patients not on lithium therapy [49]. The ability of lithium to inhibit the same adenyl cyclase receptors that are defective in lesional epidermis may amplify the defect and produce flares of psoriasis. Lithium carbonate also increases the total mass of polymorphonuclear leukocytes (PMNLs) in the circulation. Decreases in intracellular cAMP can enhance mobility and phagocytosis of PMNLs [52]. The increased migration of activated PMNLs into the skin and their products may attract more PMNLs and stimulate epidermal hyperproliferation.

Antimalarials

All of the antimalarial drugs currently used to treat dermatologic diseases, quinacrine, chloroquine, and hydroxychloroquine, have been associated with drug eruptions and aggravation of preexisting psoriasis [29]. The structurally related antiarrhythmic agent quinidine may also rarely exacerbate psoriasis [53]. The antimalarials are indicated for lupus erythematosus and rheumatoid arthritis but are used for many other purposes including psoriatic arthritis.

In the 1950s and 1960s evidence mounted that the antimalarials caused acute flares of psoriasis, sometimes exfoliative dermatitis, and were to be avoided in the treatment of psoriatic arthritis. There was a resurgence in the use of hydroxychloroquine for psoriatic arthritis after a report treating 50 patients showed no exacerbation of psoriasis; however, four patients (8%) experienced generalized maculopapular eruptions [54]. In this study 34 (68%) of patients achieved remission, improvement, or stabilization of psoriatic arthritis after 3–4 months of therapy.

Isolated reports of exacerbation of psoriasis [55], exfoliative erythroderma [56], and a new case of pustular psoriasis associated with hydroxychloroquine [57] continue to be reported, however. Eighteen percent of patients had "worsening of psoriasis" within 1 month of taking the antimalarial drug, most commonly chloroquine [56]. Quinacrine was responsible for the greatest frequency of acute generalized eruptions. A new case of psoriasis with pustules developed 3 weeks after treating a man with quinacrine for actinic reticuloid [58]. A markedly lower incidence of worsening psoriasis and drug eruptions was found with hydroxychloroquine. Malarial prophylaxis is not contraindicated for psoriatics traveling to endemic areas [59]. Hydroxychloroquine may be used with caution in the treatment of psoriatic arthritis because the risk of flare-ups of skin disease recalcitrant to conventional therapy is low. A Canadian group found no difference in the number of patients experiencing a flare-up of psoriasis while receiving chloroquine for psoriatic arthritis compared with a control group taking no remittive agents [60].

The mechanism of action of antimalarials in all diseases with the possible exception of prophyria cutanea tarda is unknown [29]. Antiinflammatory (stabilization of lysosomal membranes and inhibition of PMNL chemotaxis) and immunosuppressive (inhibition of lymphocyte response to mitogens) effects have been reported *in vitro* with chloroquine. Recently, it was shown that chloroquine impaired the allostimulatory properties of fresh normal epidermal antigen-presenting cells (EAPCs) to activate T cells but had no such effect on these cells from psoriatic skin [61]. In fact, the investigators noted that in some experiments the chloroquine-treated psoriatic EAPCs displayed significantly enhanced abilities to activate allogeneic T cells. While not directly applicable to clinical situations, this study emphasizes a constitutive difference between normal and psoriatic EAPCs that may be relevant to the exacerbation of psoriasis experienced by some patients while receiving chloroquine.

REFERENCES

1 Yates VM, Watkinson G, Kelman A. Further evidence for an association between psoriasis, Crohn's disease and ulcerative colitis. *Br J Dermatol* 1982;106:323–30.

2 Hays SB, Camisa C, Luzar MJ. The coexistence of systemic lupus erythematosus and psoriasis. *J Am Acad Dermatol* 1984;10:619–22.

3 Grunwald MH, David M, Feuerman EJ. Coexistence of psoriasis vulgaris and bullous diseases. *J Am Acad Dermatol* 1985;13:224–8.

4 Nogita T, Aramoto Y, Terajima S, *et al.* The coexistence of psoriasis vulgaris, Sjögren's syndrome, and Hashimoto's thyroiditis. *J Dermatol* 1992;19:302–5.

5 Hisler B, Blumenthal NC, Aronson PJ, *et al.* Bullous pemphigoid in psoriatic lesions. *J Am Acad Dermatol* 1989;20:683–4.

6 Boixeda JP, Soria C, Medina S, Ledo A. Bullous pemphigoid and psoriasis: treatment with cyclosporine (Letter). *J Am Acad Dermatol* 1991;24:152.

7 Bianchi L, Gatti S, Nini G. Bullous pemphigoid and severe erythrodermic psoriasis: combined low-dose treatment with cyclosporine and systemic steroids (Letter). *J Am Acad Dermatol* 1992;27:278.

8 Smith WD, Jones MS, Stewart TW, Fernando MU. Bullous pemphigoid occurring in psoriatic plaques in association with Hashimoto's thyroiditis. *Clin Exp Dermatol* 1991;16:389–91.

9 Lee CW, Ro YS, Kim JH. Concurrent development of pemphigus foliaceus and psoriasis. *Int J Dermatol* 1985;24:316–7.

10 Yokoo M, Oka D, Ueki H. Coexistence of psoriasis vulgaris and pemphigus foliaceus. *Dermatologica* 1989;179:222–3.

11 Jensen PJ, Baird J, Morioka S, *et al.* Epidermal plasminogen activator is abnormal in cutaneous lesions. *J Invest Dermatol* 1988;90:777–82.

12 Heaphy MR, Winkelmann RK. Coexistence of benign familial pemphigus and psoriasis vulgaris. *Arch Dermatol* 1976;112:1571–4.

13 Lindegard B. Diseases associated with psoriasis in a general population of 159 200 middle-aged, urban, native Swedes. *Dermatologica* 1986;172:298–304.

14 Henseler T. Associated diseases in psoriatic patients. *Proceedings of the Fifth International Psoriasis Symposium, San Francisco*, July 1991: p. 82.

15 Beer WE, Smith AE, Kassab JY, *et al.* Concomitance of psoriasis and atopic dermatitis. *Dermatology* 1992;184:265–70.

16 Koransky JS, Roenigk HH Jr. Vitiligo and psoriasis. *J Am Acad Dermatol* 1982;7: 183–9.

17 Powell FC, Dicken CH. Vitiligo and psoriasis (Letter). *J Am Acad Dermatol* 1983;8:137.

18 Humbert P, Dupond JL, Vuitton D, Agache P. Dermatological autoimmune diseases and the multiple autoimmune syndromes. *Acta Derm Venereol* 1989;148(Suppl.): 2–8.

19 Shiohara T, Hayakawa J, Nagashima M. Psoriasis and lichen planus: coexistence in a single patient. Are both diseases mutually exclusive? *Dermatologica* 1989;179: 178–82.

20 Camisa C. Lichen planus and related conditions. *Adv Dermatol* 1987;2:47–70.

21 Naldi L, Sena P, Cainelli T. About the association of lichen planus and psoriasis (Letter). *Dermatologica* 1990;181:79–80.

22 Taieb A, el Youbi A, Grosshans E, Maleville J. Lichen striatus: a Blaschko linear acquired inflammatory skin eruption. *J Am Acad Dermatol* 1991;25:637–42.

23 Menni S, Grimalt R, Caputo R. Unilateral eruptive psoriasis and lichen striatus. *Pediatr Dermatol* 1991;8:322–4.

24 Dubois EL. *Lupus Erythematosus*, 2nd edn. Los Angeles: University of Southern California Press, 1974.

25 Tan EM, Cohen AS, Fries JE, *et al.* The 1982 revised criteria for the classification of systemic lupus erythematosus. *Arthritis Rheum* 1982;25:1271–7.

26 Farber EM, Nall L. Epidemiology: natural history and genetics. In Roenigk HH Jr, Maibach HI, eds. *Psoriasis*, 2nd edn. New York: Marcel Dekker, Inc., 1991: 209–58.

27 Ros A-M, Wennersten G. Photosensitive psoriasis. In Roenigk HH Jr, Maibach HI, eds. *Psoriasis*, 2nd edn. New York: Marcel Dekker, Inc., 1991:149–56.

28 Kulick KB, Mogavero H Jr, Provost TT, Reichlin M. Serologic studies in patients with lupus erythematosus and psoriasis. *J Am Acad Dermatol* 1983;8:631–4.

29 Camisa C. Antimalarials. In Wolverton SE, Wilkin JK, eds. *Systemic Drugs for Skin Diseases*. Philadelphia: WB Saunders, 1991:265–84.

30 Ruzicka T, Sommorburg C, Goerz G, *et al.* Treatment of cutaneous lupus erythematosus with acitretin and hydroxychloroquine. *Br J Dermatol* 1992;127:513–8.

31 Stern RS, Lange R, and Members of the Photochemotherapy Follow-up Study. Cardiovascular disease, cancer, and cause of death in patients with psoriasis: 10 years prospective experience in a cohort of 1380 patients. *J Invest Dermatol* 1988;91:197–201.
32 Poikolainen K, Reunala T, Karvonen J, *et al.* Alcohol intake: a risk factor for psoriasis in young and middle aged men? *Br Med J* 1990;300:780–3.
33 Naldi L, Parazzini F, Brevi A, *et al.* Family history, smoking habits, alcohol consumption and risk of psoriasis. *Br J Dermatol* 1992;127:212–7.
34 Gupta MA, Schork NJ, Gupta AK, Ellis CN. Alcohol intake and treatment responsiveness of psoriasis: A prospective study. *J Am Acad Dermatol* 1993;28:730–2.
35 O'Doherty CJ, MacIntyre C. Palmoplantar pustulosis and smoking. *Br Med J* 1985;291:861–4.
36 Mills CM, Srivastava ED, Harvey IM, *et al.* Smoking habits in psoriasis: a case control study. *Br J Dermatol* 1992;127:18–21.
37 Lindelof B, Eklund G, Liden S, Stein RS. The prevalence of malignant tumors in patients with psoriasis. *J Am Acad Dermatol* 1990;22:1056–60.
38 Lindelof B, Sigurgeirsson B, Tegner E, *et al.* PUVA and cancer: a large-scale epidemiological study. *Lancet* 1991;338:91–3.
39 Olsen JH, Moller H, Frentz G. Malignant tumors in patients with psoriasis. *J Am Acad Dermatol* 1992;27:716–22.
40 Alderson MR, Clarke JA. Cancer incidence in patients with psoriasis. *Br J Cancer* 1983;47:857–9.
41 Stern RS, Lange R, and Members of the Photochemotherapy Follow-up Study. Non-melanoma skin cancer occurring in patients treated with PUVA five to ten years after first treatment. *J Invest Dermatol* 1988;91:120–4.
42 Abel EA, DiCicco LM, Orenberg EK, *et al.* Drugs in exacerbation of psoriasis. *J Am Acad Dermatol* 1986;15:1007–22.
43 Hu C-H, Miller AC, Peppercorn R, Farber EM. Generalized pustular psoriasis provoked by propariol. *Arch Dermatol* 1985;121:1326–7.
44 Gold MH, Holy AK, Roenigk HH Jr. Beta-blocking drugs and psoriasis. A review of cutaneous side effects and retrospective analysis of their effects on psoriasis. *J Am Acad Dermatol* 1988;19:837–41.
45 Anonymous. Betaxolol for hypertension. *Med Lett* 1990;32(821):61–2.
46 Gilleaudeau P, Vallat VP, Carter DM, Gottlieb AB. Angiotensin-converting enzyme inhibitor as possible exacerbating drugs in psoriasis. *J Am Acad Dermatol* 1993; 28:490–2.
47 Bakker JB, Pepplinkhuizen L. More about relationship of lithium to psoriasis. *Psychosomatics* 1976;17:143–6.
48 Skoven I, Thormann J. Lithium compound treatment and psoriasis. *Arch Dermatol* 1979;115:1185–7.
49 Hemlock C, Rosenthal JS, Winston A. Fluoxetine-induced psoriasis. *Ann Pharmacother* 1992;26:211–2.
50 Steinkraus V, Steinfath M, Mensing H. Beta-adrenergic blocking drugs and psoriasis. *J Am Acad Dermatol* 1992;27:266–7.
51 Di Giovanna JJ, Aoyagi T, Taylor JR, Halprin KM. Inhibition of epidermal adenylcyclase by lithium carbonate. *J Invest Dermatol* 1981;76:259–63.
52 Lazarus GS, Gilgor RS. Psoriasis, polymorphonuclear leukocytes, and lithium carbonate. An important clue. *Arch Dermatol* 1979;115:1183–4.
53 Harwell WB. Quinidine-induced psoriasis (Letter). *J Am Acad Dermatol* 1983;9:278.
54 Kammer GM, Soter NA, Gibson DJ, *et al.* Psoriatic arthritis: a clinical, immunologic, and HLA study of 100 patients. *Semin Arthritis Rheum* 1979;9:75–95.
55 Luzar M. Hydroxychloroquine in psoriatic arthropathy: exacerbations of psoriatic skin lesions. *J Rheumatol* 1983;9:462–4.

56 Slagel GA, James WD. Plaquenil-induced erythroderma. *J Am Acad Dermatol* 1985;12:857–62.
57 Friedman SJ. Pustular psoriasis associated with hydroxychloroquine (Letter). *J Am Acad Dermatol* 1987;16:1256–7.
58 Stone MS, Tschen JA. Psoriasis with pustules and actinic reticuloid. *J Am Acad Dermatol* 1986;14:888–92.
59 Kuflik EG. Effect of antimalarial drugs on psoriasis. *Cutis* 1980;26:153–5.
60 Gladman DD, Blake R, Brubactier B, Farewell VT. Chloroquine therapy in psoriatic arthritis. *J Rheumatol* 1992;19:724–6.
61 Demidem A, Taylor JR, Grammer SF, Streilein JW. Effects of chloroquine on antigen-presenting functions of epidermal cells from normal and psoriatic skin. *J Invest Dermatol* 1992;98:181–6.

four Evaluation

As you read through this book, you will encounter a bewildering array of evaluation scoring and assessment methods reported in the literature, which make our task of critically interpreting those studies all the more difficult.

One of these, the psoriasis area and severity index (PASI), was introduced for studies of the synthetic retinoids in 1978 [1]. It has been employed in numerous clinical trials to assess differences before and after treatment in a fairly rigorous and consistent manner that is reproducible between investigators and centers. The four main anatomic sites are assessed: the head (h), upper extremities (u), trunk (t) and lower extremities (l) roughly corresponding to 10, 20, 30 and 40% of body surface area (BSA), respectively. The PASI score is calculated from:

$$\begin{aligned} \text{PASI} = {} & 0.1\,(E_h + I_h + D_h)\,A_h + 0.2\,(E_u + I_u + D_u)\,A_u \\ & + 0.3\,(E_t + I_t + D_t)\,A_t + 0.4\,(E_l + I_l + D_l)\,A_l \end{aligned}$$

where E = erythema, I = induration, D = desquamation, and A = area. E, I, and D are assessed according to a 4-point scale where

0 = no symptoms;
1 = slight;
2 = moderate;
3 = marked;
4 = very marked.

A is assigned a numerical value based on the extent of lesions in a given anatomic site:

1 (< 10%);
2 (10–29%);
3 (30–49%);
4 (50–69%);
5 (70–89%);
6 (90–100%).

The PASI varies in steps of 0.1 units from 0.0 to 72.0. The highest score represents complete erythroderma of the severest possible degree.

Such a complex and detailed assessment is generally not necessary or practical in a busy outpatient office setting. It is most useful for the inpatient, day-care, or pharmaceutical research setting. It is more popular with European than American investigators. The PASI score is good but not infallible for the following reasons.

1 Experienced clinicians may differ in their estimates of body area involved, which could alter the resulting PASI score and make comparisons to the same study performed in other centers or in the literature invalid.

2 There is high interobserver variability in the calculation of the area involved. The same clinician must calculate the PASI score on a given patient throughout the entire study or treatment period.

3 PASI does not apply as well to the less common but more severe types of psoriasis such as erythroderma and pustular compared to plaque-type disease. For example, erythroderma with moderate erythema, slight induration and scaling could have the same score as chronic plaque-type psoriasis involving 10–30% BSA with marked erythema, induration, and desquamation [2].

4 The evaluation of the physical signs or parameters of psoriatic lesions is purely subjective on the part of the investigator.

5 The PASI score does not take into account the patient's subjective symptoms such as itching or pain and the level of disability.

Estimation of BSA involved is not as accurate as objective measures which utilize a computer image analyzing system. In one study, all four observers overestimated the area involved compared to the computerized image analysis of traced plaque outlines (planimetric method) [3]. A greater degree of error was made when assessing patients with small plaque disease (overestimated 3.8 times) compared to large plaque psoriasis (overestimated 1.7 times). Individual observers were surprisingly consistent in their overestimates with differences of only 1–2% between days 1 and 2, suggesting that the estimates have some clinical value if recorded sequentially by the same observer. Computerized image analysis of whole body photographs gave results similar to those achieved by the planimetric method, which is probably the most accurate way of assessing area when the lesions are sharply demarcated from normal skin. There was no interobserver error. Hairbearing scalp and genitalia still had to be estimated by the human eye. These techniques required hours of work as well as acquisition of the image analysis systems and are not practical for most large pharmaceutical studies let alone office-based practices. Bahmer [4] suggested the use of an old and simpler technique of "point counting" which allows area estimation with "astonishing accuracy." The crossover points in a lattice grid falling on the lesion are counted. The area (A) to be estimated is calculated by the formula:

$$A = n \times a$$

where n is the number of points falling onto the lesion and a is the known area of each box in the grid employed. The ratio of the number of points falling on to the lesion to number falling on to the total body skin area yields an estimate of the percentage of involved skin independent from magnification or scale. For evaluating individual lesions of modest size, the grids can be made on photographic high contrast film or from drawings photocopied on to overhead foils [5]. For determining the extent (%BSA) of psoriasis on the entire body or a segment of it, the grid has to be copied on to the film when the clinical photograph is taken. To determine the actual area of the lesions a calibration bar on the film is necessary.

To estimate %BSA involved, the "rule of nines" may be used: head (9%), anterior trunk (upper 9%, lower 9%), posterior trunk (upper 9%, lower 9%), legs (18% each), arms (9% each). A "modified rule of nines" allocates BSA as follows: head (3%), scalp (6%), anterior trunk (14%), posterior trunk (16%), genitalia or perineum (1%), leg (16% each), dorsum foot (2% each), sole (2% each), arm (7% each), dorsum hand (1.5% each), palm (1.5%). The area of one side of a flat closed hand has been used to measure 1% of BSA, but that is also an overestimate. The actual value calculated by a planimetric method was 0.70–0.76% of BSA [6].

To highlight the wide variation in assessment methods of psoriasis, Marks and colleagues [7] analyzed 30 articles published in 1985 and 1986: 18 gave an assessment of individual signs (only two used the PASI) and in 13 there was a global assessment or an assessment of clearing. Erythema, scaling, and induration (thickness) received a step grade ranging from 0 to 9. The number of sites at which physical signs were recorded varied from 1 to 7. The symptom of pruritus was recorded in only four of 30 studies. The definition of "clearing" differed widely. The percentage area of body involvement was estimated in nine studies. In only one article were late assessments made independent of earlier records. Seven different formulae distinct from the PASI were used resulting in a wide range of incompatible and noncomparable totals.

Marks *et al.* [7] gave "honorable mentions" to the articles which evaluated:

1 erythema, scaling, thickness, and pruritus on a scale of 0–3 at seven sites = maximum score of 84; "clearing" = less than 10% of the initial score;

2 erythema, scaling, thickness on a scale of 0–6 at four sites = maximum score of 72; independent global score on visual analog scale as a check on total score;

3 erythema, scaling, thickness on a scale of 0–3 and estimated BSA involved.

None of the 30 studies objectively measured the three common physical signs of psoriasis. Thickness could be quantified by instrumentation, but erythema and scaling fluctuate rapidly after minor stimuli. They may reflect ambient temperature, humidity, and the recent use of emollients. Thickness or induration is probably the most reliable parameter to assess because it reflects epidermal thickness, edema, and cellular infiltrate. Calipers can be used, but A-scan ultrasound and magnetic resonance imaging are more accurate for the determination of skin thickness. The conflicting and confusing results of clinical trials in psoriasis are evidence of our need for objective clinical measurements. Clinical photography can be evaluated later for erythema, scaling, and extent but not thickness by an independent panel. Similarly, skin biopsies can be reviewed by a dermatopathologist not involved in the treatment of the patients under study. The ocular micrometer can be used to measure acanthosis. The cellular infiltrate can be graded on a scale of 1, 2, 3+. The presence or absence of dermal edema and neutrophils in the dermis can be noted.

Anderson [8] wrote, "Improvement clinically should be apparent to all observers and objectively measurable. Psoriasis is best evaluated by measuring the disability primarily and the skin lesions secondarily."

Distillation of various questionnaires administered to outpatients before and at 3 months of treatment revealed that the two most useful questions were: "Does the state of your psoriasis affect your life in any way?" and "Have you had to stop your usual sports or hobbies because of your skin?" The combination of responses to these questions were the best predictors of overall disease severity scores in the judgment of the patient or doctor [9]. The severity score was derived by asking the patient to grade the following six features of their psoriasis on a scale of 0–4 (none to severe):

1 amount of body with psoriasis;
2 degree of itch;
3 pain or discomfort;
4 scaliness;
5 embarrassment;
6 stopping you doing what you want to do.

The authors found that a considerable number of patients (25–37%) considered their symptoms of itch, irritation, or scaliness to be the worst aspect of their psoriasis. The patient's assessment is not included in the PASI, therefore this should be documented in an alternative way.

In an audit of consultations for psoriasis in two teaching hospitals, most of the case notes showed a surprising lack of an estimation of extent or distribution of lesions including routine use of an anatomic diagram (Fig. 4.1), as well as any reference to patients' symptoms or disability [10]. The auditors also found it difficult to determine whose assessment of treatment was being recorded at followup visits, the patient's or the doctor's. Without baseline documentation of extent of disease, symptoms, and disability, it would not be possible to compare the outcome of different treatment strategies.

The UK sickness impact profile (SIP), a questionnaire with 136 questions, which evaluates how disease affects a patient's physical and emotional state, but registered the same score regardless of extent or severity of psoriasis. Psychosocial activities were most severely impaired whereas physical ability was least impaired. Psoriasis had a major impact on patients' ability to sleep, work, manage their homes, and participate in recreational activities. Their overall quality of life was adversely affected to about the same degree as patients with cardiovascular disease [11]. There was good correlation between SIP score and the psoriasis disability index (PDI), a more compact questionnaire consisting of 15 questions answered on a linear analog scale from 1 ("not at all") to 7 ("very much"). Ten of the

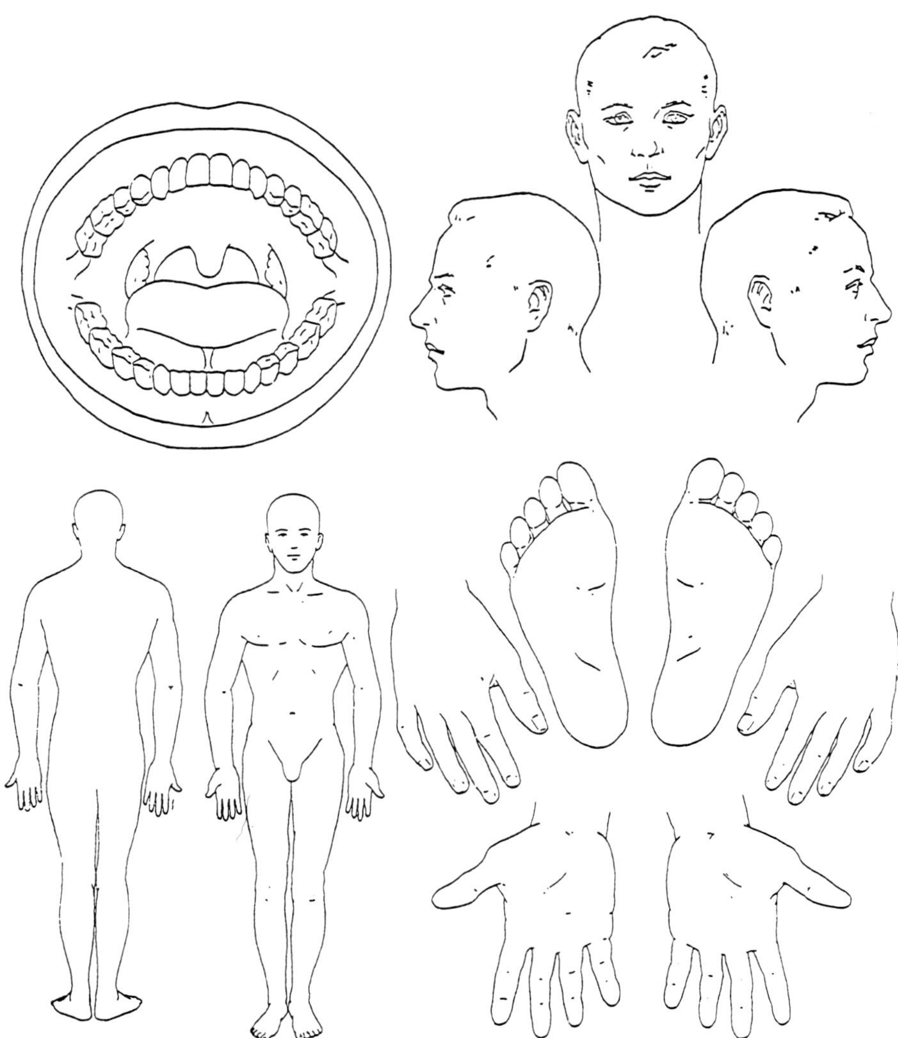

Fig 4.1 Anatomic diagram used for documenting extent of psoriasis in the Cleveland Clinic Department of Dermatology.

most efficient questions based on the most recent 4 weeks are listed in Table 4.1. Overall PDI scores, but not overall SIP scores, correlated well with PASI scores. The PDI provides a simple rapid overall measure of psoriasis disability [12]. The PASI score did not correlate with the patients' global rating of their overall health, probably because they might include symptoms and emotional effects not accounted for by the PASI. The PDI is a practical way of monitoring the effect of treatment on functional impairment together with visual documentation of psoriasis morphology and extent. Since unemployment is an important issue among psoriatic patients, return to work may be a more critical and attainable goal than clearing or cure of psoriasis.

In the USA many physicians use the "**SOAP**" method for documenting patient encounters: **s**ubjective, **o**bjective, **a**ssessment, **p**lan. "**S**" includes the patient's symptoms, perceived disability, and reference to current and previously used medications: "**O**" includes the morphologic description of rash, distribution, and estimation of percentage body area involvement: the use of self-sticking labels or rubber stamps of anatomic diagrams facilitates the graphic representation of this information (Fig. 4.1); "**A**" is the diag-

Table 4.1 Psoriasis disability index questionnaire. Adapted from Finlay and Kelly [12]

1 How much has your psoriasis interfered with you carrying out work around the house or garden?
2 How often have you worn different types or colors of clothes because of your psoriasis?
3 How much more do you have to change or wash your clothes?
4 Has your psoriasis been much of a problem at the hairdressers?
5 Has your psoriasis resulted in you having to take more baths than usual?
6 Has your career been affected by your psoriasis (promotion refused, lost a job, asked to change a job)?
7 Is your psoriasis making it difficult to do any sport?
8 Have you been unable to use, criticized while using, or stopped from using communal bathing or changing facilities?
9 Has your psoriasis resulted in you smoking or drinking alcohol more than you would normally?
10 To what extent has your psoriasis or treatment made your home messy or untidy?

nosis, qualifying variant, and the physician's impression of whether it is mild, moderate, or severe disease.

On followup visits "S" includes the patient's subjective assessment of progress, and "A" is the physician's impression of progress based on integration of the patient's symptoms and results of the physical examination compared to the previous one. "P" includes the choice of medical and/or physical therapies, documentation of any verbal or written information dispensed about the disease or its treatment (e.g., your own psoriasis sheet, the manufacturer's brochure on etretinate, the National Psoriasis Foundation's booklet on methotrexate). If you are the consultant, a copy of a brief summary report to the referring physician or agency should be maintained in the record. Medical record-keeping is held to high standards which continue to rise in a cost-conscious and litigious society. Thus, the records are important not only for the obvious clinical and research purposes, but also for administrative, medicolegal, and economic concerns.

It has been assumed that psychologic stressors such as anxiety, depression, work, family, or friend-related dysfunctions can exacerbate psoriasis. However, the evidence for this is only anecdotal or else derived from questionnaire studies. Biofeedback training, relaxation exercises, psychotherapy, psychopharmaceuticals, and hypnosis have been suggested as adjuncts to the traditional medical treatments of psoriasis [13].

Group meetings of psoriatic patients led by a dermatologic nurse or physician are fairly easy to organize in existing psoriasis treatment centers. Such groups become forums for dissemination of general information about psoriasis and its treatments and for discussion of anecdotal experience with the disease, social situations, specific treatments, and professional staff. Familiarity with the environment, clinic, staff, and other people with psoriasis presumably reduces anxiety and any sense of stigmatization. While it may be valuable for patients to learn what areas of their life are stressful, how to reduce stressful issues and cope with them more effectively (i.e., develop defense mechanisms), there is no convincing proof that psychotherapy, insight-oriented or otherwise, has any biologic effect on the cutaneous lesions of psoriasis. Price and colleagues [14] selected a group of patients to participate in 90-minute meetings with a clinical psychologist weekly for 8 weeks and complete several psychologic assessment tests at three separate time points.

Perhaps it is a measure of patient interest and acceptance of such an approach to therapy that only 31 of 82 (38%) of invited patients agreed to participate. Of these, eight of 31 (26%) did not complete all requirements of the 6-month study. The authors found that the remaining 23 patients in the study, by now self-selected, comprised a "noticeably anxious" group. Psychologic testing indicated that patients were not depressed and had a relatively high self-esteem. Patients considered their psoriasis to cause impairment in the area of social leisure activities but not work, home management, or private leisure activities.

The patients who took part in the group therapy sessions were taught relaxation techniques including self-hypnosis and were encouraged to practice these at home and whenever under stress. They showed a fall in anxiety scores after the group sessions, which persisted at the 6 months' followup visit. The control group showed no change. The authors noted a paradoxical significant negative correlation between anxiety and severity of disease suggesting that a patient's anxiety may be out of proportion to the extent of disease. Patients with extensive disease may become better adjusted to its chronicity than those with mild disease who may have unrealistic expectations of a cure. Group therapy sessions had no demonstrable clinical benefit on the clearing of psoriasis compared to the control group. In a separate study, improvement in the symptoms of scalp psoriasis was obtained with meditation in a few patients leading the authors to conclude that stress reduction techniques should be a component of the overall treatment of psoriasis [15]. Interestingly, perceived stress increased the most in psoriasis during the stressor exposure but tended to normalize faster in psoriatics compared to control groups of atopic dermatitis patients or healthy subjects [16]. Coping style and other cognitive factors were found to be more significant discriminators between the groups than psychosocial stress or the specific skin disease. Stress apparently affects skin reactivity but cognitive factors modulate these effects.

On the basis of these and other studies, I believe that routine psychologic consultation is not indicated for psoriatic patients unless requested by the individual patient or if a patient demonstrates unusual aggressiveness or suicidal tendency. Educational information can be disseminated to patients verbally or by virtue of literature and videotapes. Group discussions with patients may be led by the treating dermatologist or other professional staff on the team such as nursing personnel.

A recent survey of more than 10 000 psoriasis patients by the National Psoriasis Foundation revealed that "self-consciousness or embarrassment" ranked as one of the three most common complaints. Respondents said they were helped most by physicians who were frank about the incurability of the disease yet encouraging and hopeful in their approach to management.

While the disease does not overtly affect established social relationships, it can certainly interfere with the social development of children with psoriasis and adults who are initiating sexual relationships. Children may become withdrawn, angry, and frustrated if their self-image is poor. They may not be able to benefit from exposure to natural sunlight because of avoidance of public pools and beaches for fear of stares and questions concerning contagion. Because the genitalia are so often affected by psoriasis, an explanation that it is not a venereal disease is usually required.

The sexual relations of married couples may be adversely affected during flares when ointments must be worn to bed or when scales accumulate between the sheets and on the floors of bedroom and bathroom. Because there is a greater emphasis on female beauty in Western culture, women may be more emotionally disturbed by psoriasis. Sexual relations may be avoided altogether until remission occurs. All patients openly express fear to their doctors of developing lesions in exposed areas such as the face and hands, but they may not mention lesions in the genital area that already exist.

If the sympathetic physician is comfortable discussing emotional and sexual problems, a special longer session, possibly together with the partner, should be arranged for more open communication. If either the physician or patient is uncomfortable discussing these matters, then referral to a psychologist, sex therapist, or psychiatrist with an interest in the "psychocutaneous diseases" is indicated. Supportive group therapy would be ideal for discussing feelings of shame or guilt arising from psoriasis, isolation, and appearing sexually unattractive because these emotions are probably common to most psoriasis patients at some time during the course of their disease. In group and private sessions, advice and treatment concerning abuse of drugs, tobacco, caffeine, alcohol, and irregular eating habits which can increase stress and theoretically aggravate psoriasis can be dispensed. Aerobic exercise should be promoted to help obese patients lose weight, improve the cardiovascular system, increase high density lipoprotein-cholesterol, and improve their sense of well-being by improving self-image and raising endorphin levels.

In conclusion, calculation of the PASI score is far too cumbersome for ordinary office practice although it is excellent and should be required for publications. However, as a minimum, the clinician should include in his/her evaluation an estimate of the overall BSA involved in percentage or displayed graphically, a record of symptoms such as pruritus or pain, and a determination of the level of disability by directed verbal queries or the PDI questionnaire.

REFERENCES

1 Fredriksson T, Pettersson U. Severe psoriasis. Oral therapy with a new retinoid. *Dermatologica* 1978;157:238–44.

2 Van de Kerkhof PCM. On the limitations of the psoriasis area and severity index (PASI) (Letter). *Br J Dermatol* 1992;126:205.
3 Ramsay B, Lawrence CM. Measurement of involved surface area in patients with psoriasis. *Br J Dermatol* 1991;124:565–70.
4 Bahmer F. The size of lesions, or point counting as a step toward the solution of the PASI problem (Letter). *Arch Dermatol* 1989;125:1282–3.
5 Bahmer FA, Smolle J. Morphometry in clinical dermatology. *Acta Derm Venereol* 1992;72:52–7.
6 Long CC, Finlay AY, Averill RW. The rule of hand: 4 hand areas = 2 FTU = 1 g. *Arch Dermatol* 1992;128:1129–30.
7 Marks R, Barton SP, Shuttleworth D, Finlay AY. Assessment of disease progress in psoriasis. *Arch Dermatol* 1989;125:235–40.
8 Anderson PC. Reply to Dialysis and psoriasis (Letter). *J Am Acad Dermatol* 1983;8:427.
9 McHenry PM, Doherty VR. Psoriasis: an audit of patients' views on the disease and its treatment. *Br J Dermatol* 1992;127:13–17.
10 Shuttleworth D, Finlay AY, Rademaker M, *et al.* Psoriasis consultation audit: a two-centre study. *Br J Dermatol* 1990;123:99–105.
11 Finlay AY, Khan GK, Luscombe DK, Salek MS. Validation of sickness impact profile and psoriasis disability index in psoriasis. *Br J Dermatol* 1990;123:751–6.
12 Finlay AY, Kelly SE. Psoriasis — an index of disability. *Clin Exp Dermatol* 1987;12:8–11.
13 Kantor SD. Stress and psoriasis. *Cutis* 1990;46:331–2.
14 Price ML, Mottahedin I, Mayo PR. Can psychotherapy help patients with psoriasis? *Clin Exp Dermatol* 1991;16:114–7.
15 Gaston L, Crombez JC, Lassonde M, *et al.* Psychological stress and psoriasis: experimental and prospective correlational studies. *Acta Derm Venereol* 1991; 156(Suppl.):37–43
16 Arnetz BB, Fjellner B, Eneroth P, Kallner A. Endocrine and dermatological concomitants of mental stress. *Acta Derm Venereol* 1991;156(Suppl.):9–12.

Part two

Clinical Presentations of Psoriasis

five Variants of Psoriasis

INTRODUCTION

The prevalence of psoriasis in the USA is 1–2%, owing chiefly to the northwest European ancestry of most white Americans. The prevalence of psoriasis is much lower in native Americans, African-Americans, and Asians. Most African-Americans have ancestors in West Africa where the prevalence of psoriasis is 0.7% [1]. There are between 150 000 and 260 000 new cases of psoriasis per year in the USA [2]. There is an equal sex incidence, although some studies have shown a predominance of males with psoriasis. The mean age of onset is 28 years with the range of human life from newborn to 100 years. Females may be affected earlier in life than males.

The most common pattern of psoriasis is that of a symmetric inflammatory papulosquamous disease (Figs 5.1 and 5.2). Recognition of the classical morphology of the skin lesions by an experienced clinician is usually sufficient for confirmation of the diagnosis, but simple diagnostic maneuvers such as potassium hydroxide examination of scales for hyphal elements, serologic testing for syphilis, and skin biopsy may be necessary to

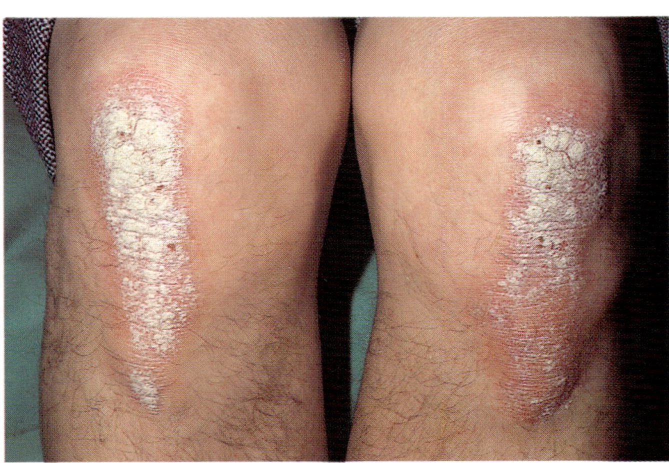

Fig 5.1 Symmetrical chronic plaques of psoriasis on the knees.

rule out other considerations. The pathogenesis of psoriasis, however, remains unexplained.

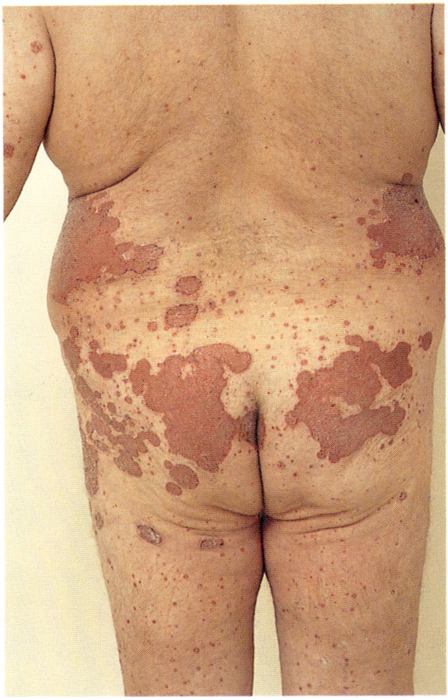

Fig 5.2 More or less symmetric plaques of psoriasis evolving from eruptive guttate psoriasis.

KOEBNER PHENOMENON

One of the hallmarks of psoriasis is the Koebner phenomenon or isomorphic response, which occurs in some patients with unstable or flaring psoriasis [3]. Physical trauma results in linear or figurate patterns of psoriasis, which conform to the localization of injury from a scratch, burn, or surgical incision (Fig. 5.3). The isomorphic response is not unique to psoriasis: it can occur in lichen planus (LP) (Fig. 5.4), vitiligo, lichen nitidus, and other skin diseases. Apparently, injury to the epidermis alone can induce the Koebner phenomenon: the technique of "tape stripping" commonly used by investigators results in the removal of the entire stratum corneum, leaving the granular layer and stratum spinosum intact. A recent study examined the phenotypes of infiltrating cells in Koebner-positive skin at 5 min and 24 hours [4]. The authors found a predominance of cytotoxic T cells in the epidermis and dermis. They hypothesized that these lymphocytes are activated by heat shock proteins and directly induce lytic changes in keratinocytes. Alternative explanations include degranulation of mast cells and release of proteases by macrophages. Normal trauma may be partly responsible for the prominent involvement of scalp, elbows, knees, hands, fingernails, sacrum, and genitalia. Because the scales of about 50% of psoriatic plaques are colonized by pathogenic staphylococci, it is recommended to clear psoriasis as much as possible prior to elective surgery, particularly orthopedic, in order to reduce the risks of postoperative infection and developing psoriasis in the healing incision.

Certain drugs have been associated with a kind of "endogenous Koebner phenomenon," notably, lithium, antimalarials, and β-blockers, which can

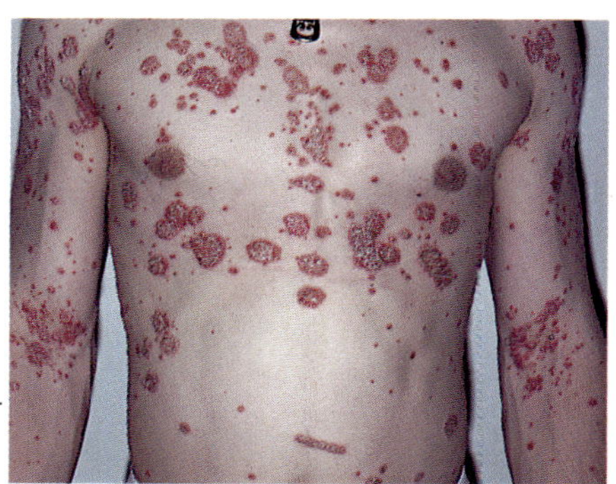

Fig 5.3 Generalized plaque psoriasis with linear lesion above umbilicus secondary to laceration (Koebner phenomenon).

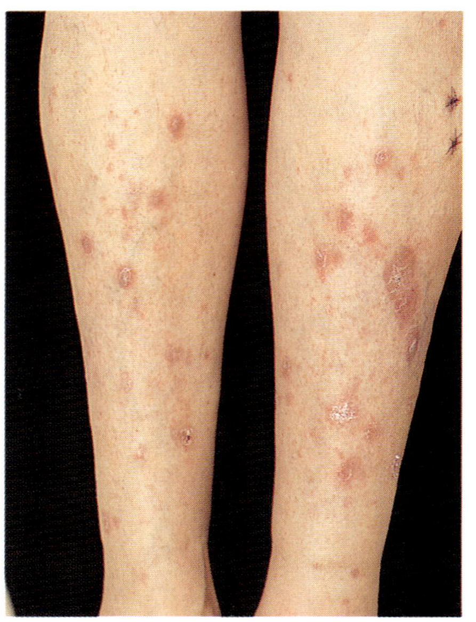

(a)

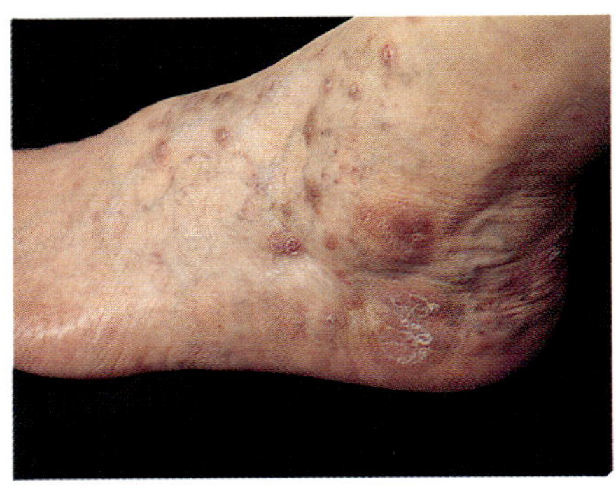

(b)

Fig 5.4 Papules and plaques of lichen planus on (a) the legs and (b) foot of different patients show some morphologic similarities to psoriasis.

induce psoriasis or aggravate preexisting disease in some cases. Flare-ups of psoriasis may be associated with streptococcal tonsillitis or pharyngitis and upper respiratory viral infections. Acute guttate psoriasis is frequently the initial episode of chronic psoriasis.

GENETICS

There is no doubt that heredity plays a role in the development of psoriasis. Early age of onset of psoriasis tends to be associated with familial aggregation and more severe disease. For example, in 40% of patients with an early age of onset immediate family members were also affected. The frequency of psoriasis in relatives of early-onset psoriatics and late-onset psoriatics in one study was 14% vs 5% of parents and 14.5% vs 2.7% of children, respectively [5]. The latter figure might be expected in the general population. Conversely, of psoriatics indicating familial aggregation, 73% had an age of onset before 30 years [1]. However, if a patient developed psoriasis after age 20 years and had no parent with psoriasis, only 3% of siblings had psoriasis. In patients with psoriasis before age 15 years and one parent with psoriasis, 50% of siblings developed psoriasis by age 60 years. Patients with severe psoriasis with an age of onset of 15 years or less were three times more likely to have siblings with psoriasis than patients with onset after age 30. Twin studies have shown two-thirds concordance for monozygotic twins compared to 18% for dizygotic twins. The lack of complete concordance in monozygotic twin pairs suggests that environmental factors are also important and supports the theory of multifactorial inheritance of psoriasis.

Two types of nonpustular psoriasis can be distinguished on the basis of family history, HLA associations, and age of onset [6]. Type I patients were those with a family history, onset during the second decade, and a close association between HLA-Cw6, B13, and Bw57 (a subtype of B17). Type II psoriasis manifests during the fifth decade, lacks parents and siblings with the disease, and is associated with HLA-Cw2 and B27 with a relative risk of developing psoriasis of 6.1 and 3.1, respectively.

Farber and Nall [1] disputed the bimodal age incidence: their peak age of incidence was in the second and third decades. They postulated that the bimodal curve reported [5] may be an artifact of an excess of HLA-B13- and B17-positive patients in the study population who tended to have an earlier onset of disease.

A study of 12 families with 15 sibling pairs with psoriasis was analyzed for haplotype sharing [7]. All sibling pairs shared at least one haplotype, and 13 of 15 were HLA identical compared to an expected frequency of four.

The development of psoriasis is related to the effects of one or more genes located near the HLA region, which are able to influence autoreactivity. However, no differences in the patients of T-cell receptor variable regions could be detected in lesional biopsies from patients with type I and type II nonpustular psoriasis [8]. The association between HLA-B13 and

B17 seems to be due to linkage dysequilibrium with the gene for Cw6. The Cw6 antigen is probably a marker for the gene determining susceptibility to psoriasis. Populations with very low prevalence of psoriasis lack HLA-B13 and/or B17.

PLAQUE-TYPE PSORIASIS

The typical fully developed clinical lesion of psoriasis is a well-demarcated red, round to oval plaque one or more centimeters across, surmounted by white silvery scales overlying bony prominences (Fig. 5.5). Indeed, plaque-type psoriasis is the most common morphologic variant encountered in practice and for this reason is called psoriasis vulgaris. Psoriasis vulgaris can assume many appearances depending on the anatomic site involved, the activity of disease (i.e., stable, progressive, or resolving), and any treatment given (Fig. 5.6). In darkly pigmented patients, the red to violet color distinction is lost and lesions appear hyperpigmented with various shades of brown to black, especially if they are scratched or rubbed (Figs 5.7–5.10). The scale may be white and powdery, micaceous and peel off in thin transparent sheets, rupioid implying a "dirty" appearance; or ostraceous, referring to a heaped-up surface like that of an oyster shell (Fig. 5.11).

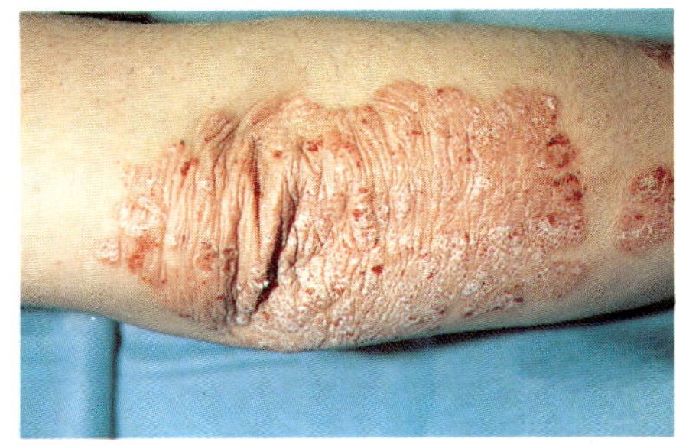

Fig 5.5 Typical plaque-type psoriasis on the elbow.

The primary lesion of all variants is probably a pinpoint erythematous macule, otherwise clinically nondiagnostic, that expands circumferentially, develops induration, and exfoliates. Some of the scales are adherent and may become heaped up over time if not physically or chemically dislodged. Such lesions may coalesce with each other to form large plaques with irregular ("geographic") outlines. The distinction between involved and uninvolved skin is usually sharp. The edge of the untreated lesion is discernibly raised by palpation unless it is very early or resolving. A ring of vasoconstriction surrounding the plaque may be observed (Woronoff ring) especially during UV light therapy (Fig. 5.12). When the psoriatic plaque attains a sufficient amount of scale, the Auspitz sign may be elicited. When the adherent scale is scraped off, pinpoint bleeding points become evident as dilated capillaries traumatized near the skin surface discharge their contents. The Auspitz sign is the clinical correlate to the histopathologic finding of a thinned epidermis overlying the dermal papillae between elongated tube-like rete pegs ("thin suprapapillary plate") [9]. Recently, the historical significance as opposed to the clinical importance of the sign has been emphasized. Bernhard [10] called attention to the lack of sensitivity and specificity of the Auspitz sign.

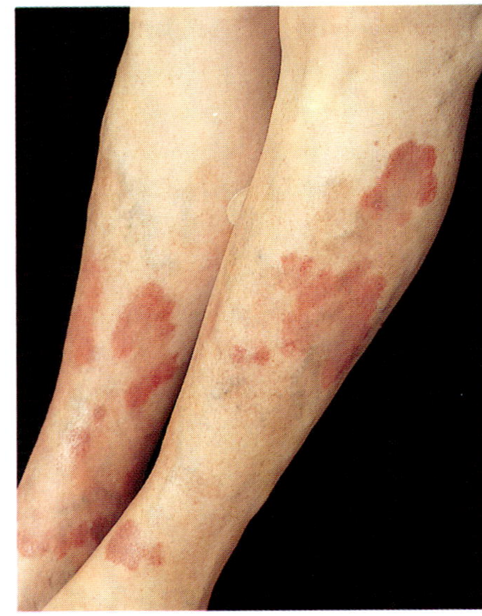

Fig 5.6 Partially treated psoriasis on the legs.

The most common areas of involvement are the elbows, knees, scalp, sacrum, umbilicus, intergluteal cleft, and genitalia (Fig. 5.13). The latter three areas are often overlooked in a cursory examination of the skin but can be very helpful for diagnosis. The involvement is more or less symmetric, for example, lesions may be present on both knees although not exactly of the same size, configuration, or location. Of course, only one knee, one elbow, or one side of the head may have psoriasis. Limited psoriasis on the

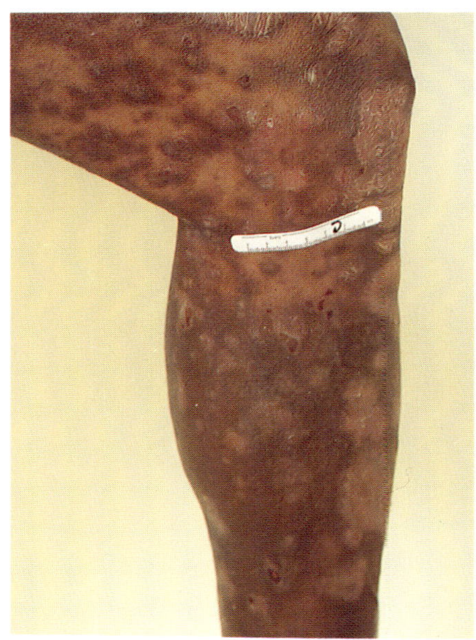

Fig 5.7 Psoriasis of the leg of a black man.

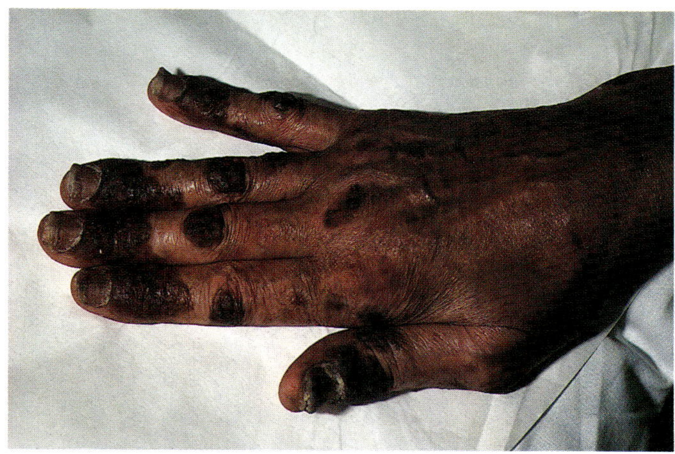

Fig 5.8 Psoriasis of the distal fingers and nails of a black man.

extremities or the nape of the neck may be difficult to distinguish from subacute or chronic nummular eczema or lichen simplex chronicus (LSC). In the former, the lesions are usually not so well defined from normal skin and the scale has a yellowish to crusted appearance. In the latter, lichenification, the accentuation of the normal skin markings, is present and this is rarely seen in psoriasis. However, pruritus may occur in eczema, LSC, and psoriasis: excoriation with fissuring can be seen in psoriasis of the scalp and the nape of the neck (Fig. 5.14).

As some plaques of psoriasis expand, they may clear centrally spontaneously or with any treatment but particularly systemic retinoids. This results in annular, arciform, or other bizarre patterns of psoriasis (Fig. 5.15) on the skin raising such differential diagnoses as tinea corporis, erythema annulare centrifugum, erythema gyratum repens, and mycosis fungoides (Fig. 5.16).

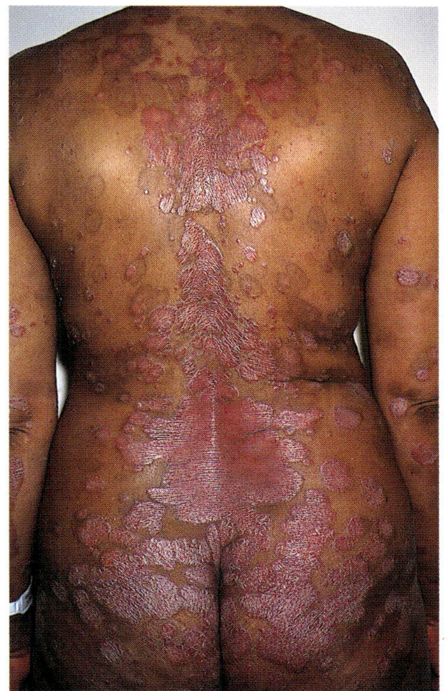

Fig 5.9 In this black woman with severe generalized psoriasis vulgaris, the active plaques retain violet color while resolving lesions are hyperpigmented.

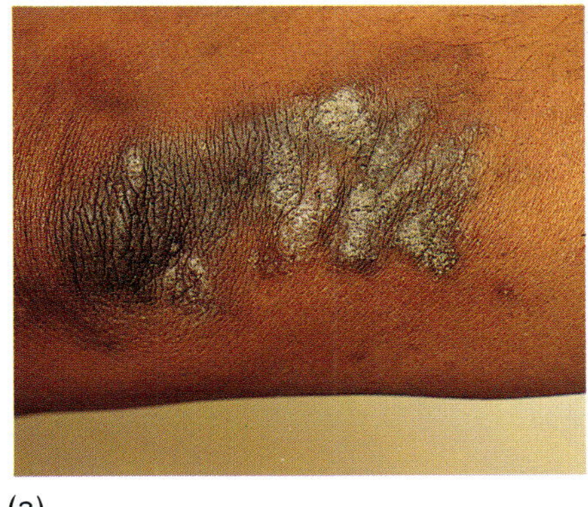

(a)

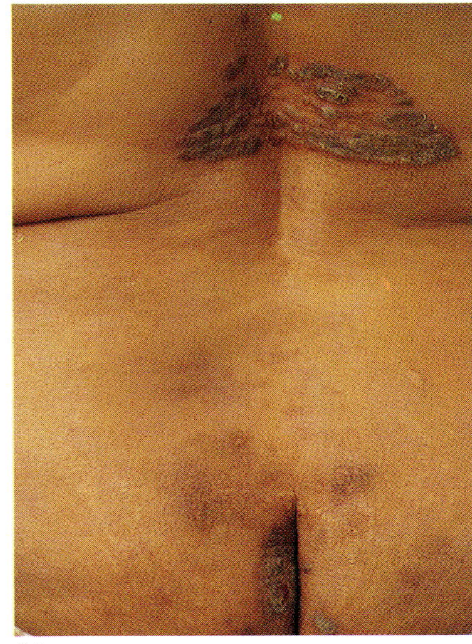

(b)

Fig 5.10 (a) Psoriasis on the elbow. (b) Plaques on the back and buttocks.

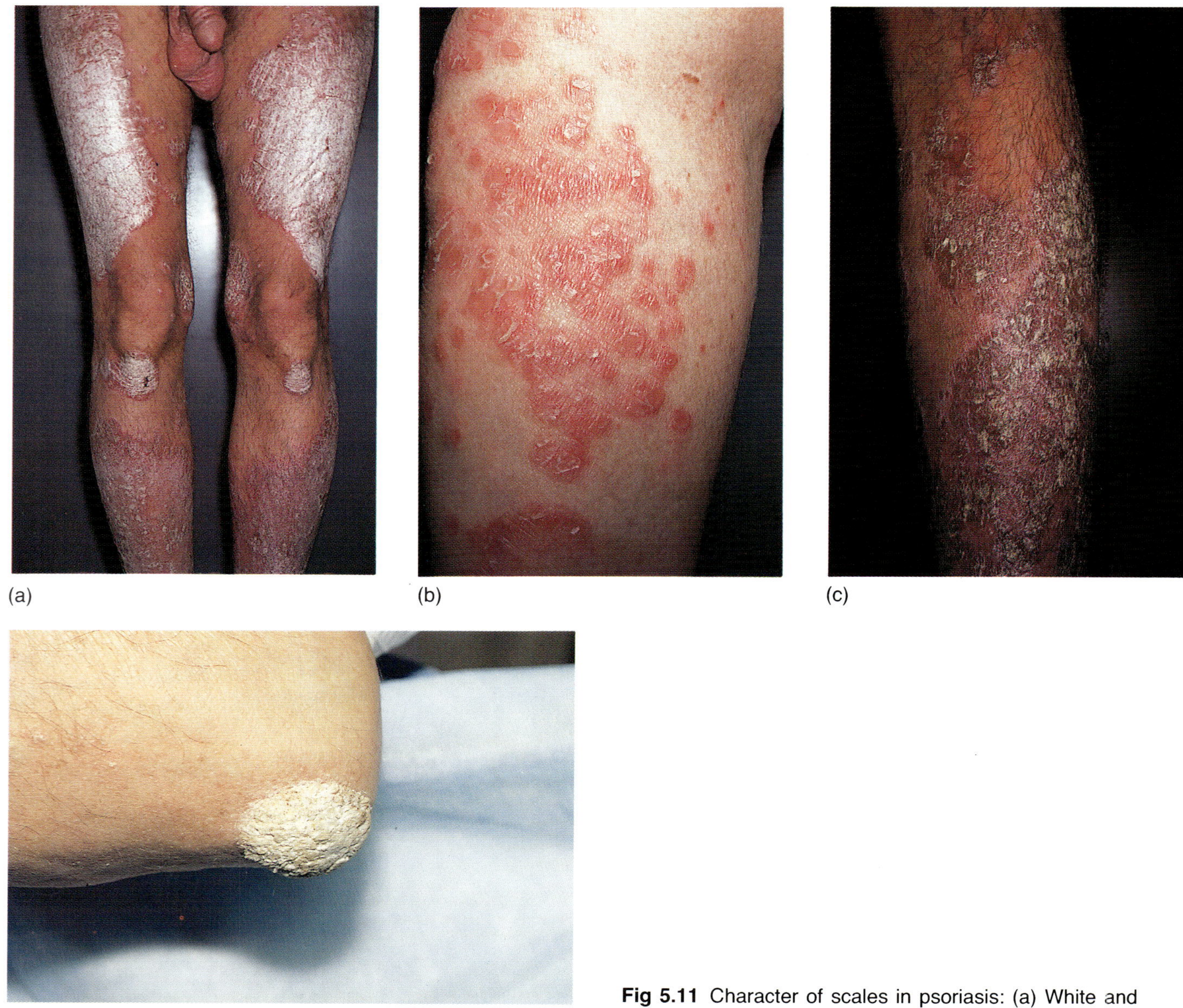

(a) (b) (c) (d)

Fig 5.11 Character of scales in psoriasis: (a) White and powdery; (b) micaceous; (c) rupioid; (d) ostraceous.

Any one of the most common sites of predilection may also be the solitary manifestation of psoriasis. While this is well-recognized for the scalp, it also typically occurs on the male genitalia, usually the glans penis. Napkin dermatitis was the first sign of psoriasis in 10 of 14 infants appearing after candidal infections or primary irritant dermatitis [11]. The Koebner phenomenon may play a role in recurrent lesions in these locations.

Genital psoriasis

Patients with penile psoriasis may fear the worst and delay presentation to their doctor. Unfortunately, some general practitioners, venereologists, and urologists are not familiar with the clinical manifestations of penile psoriasis and may heighten concerns of sexually transmitted disease or cancer. It is

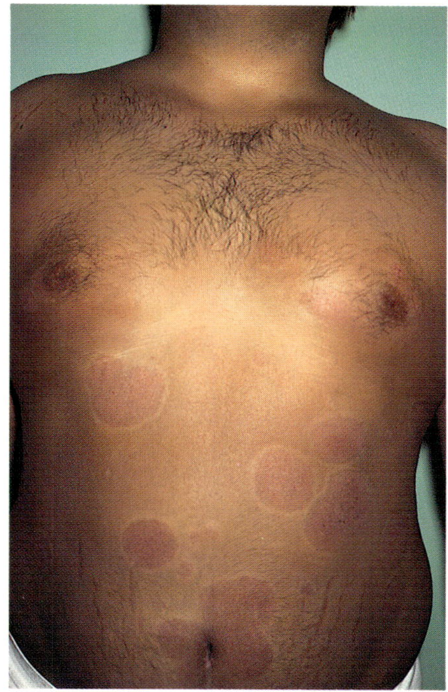

Fig 5.12 Woronoff rings are the pale zones surrounding resolving plaques in this man receiving psoralen UVA and topical steroids.

not uncommon for the doctor to prescribe a mild corticosteroid or antifungal cream. Neither of these medicaments or their combination will worsen the psoriasis and may in fact provide some temporary relief; however, the patient has still not been given a diagnosis, possibly without a complete skin examination or any education about psoriasis [12].

The clinical history of penile psoriasis is usually one of a mild chronic dry, peeling process that becomes redder and more apparent after sexual intercourse (Fig. 5.17). It does not itch. A differential diagnosis of papulosquamous disorders that can affect the penis must be considered: LP, seborrheic dermatitis, chronic eczema (irritant or contact allergic), secondary syphilis, and dermatomycosis. The latter two can be eliminated easily with serologic testing and potassium hydroxide examination of skin scrapings or fungal culture. Seborrheic dermatitis typically involves the hairy areas of the face, nasolabial folds, scalp (dandruff), mid-chest, axillae, and groin but still may be difficult to differentiate from psoriasis clinically (and histologically). The eczematous dermatoses usually itch and may be temporally related to the use of lubricants, spermicides, and latex in condoms or diaphragms. LP of the glans penis tends to be more violaceous and less scaly than psoriasis; it may be annular or have the distinctive morphology of Wickham's striae. Surprisingly, LP of the penis is usually not pruritic. The typical distribution of LP on the skin, nails, and oral mucous membranes clinches the diagnosis. When there are no other signs to help clarify the diagnosis, and serology and cultures are negative, biopsy and/or allergy patch testing may be the next logical step.

Penile psoriasis responds very well to twice daily applications of a medium potency corticosteroid ointment such as triamcinolone acetonide

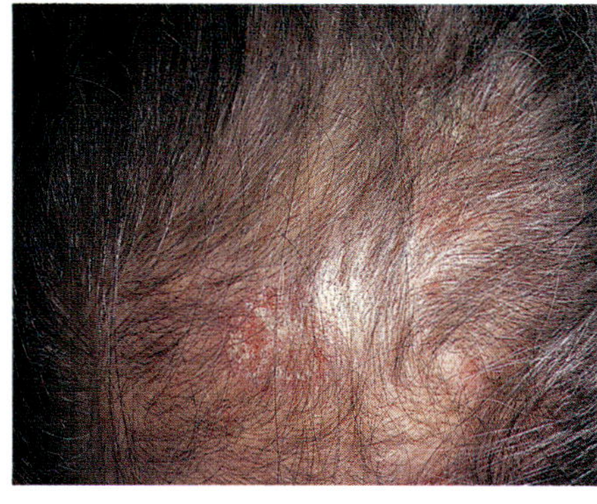

(a)

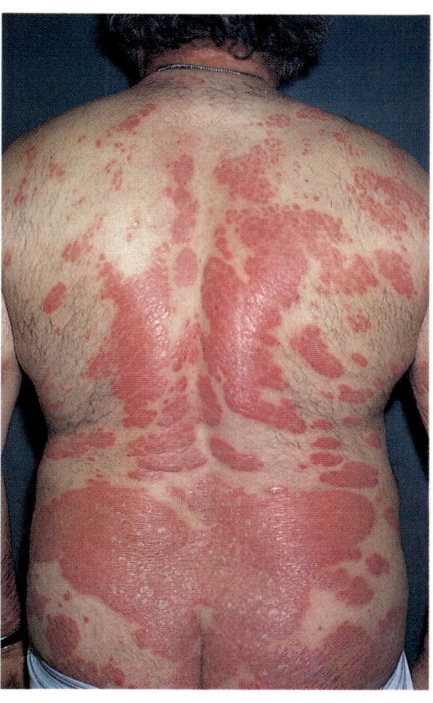

(b)

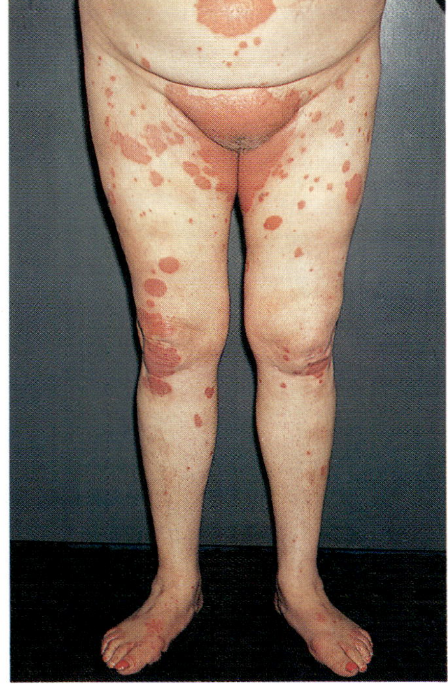

(c)

Fig 5.13 Common areas of psoriasis involvement: (a) the scalp; (b) sacrum and intergluteal cleft; (c) umbilicus and genitalia.

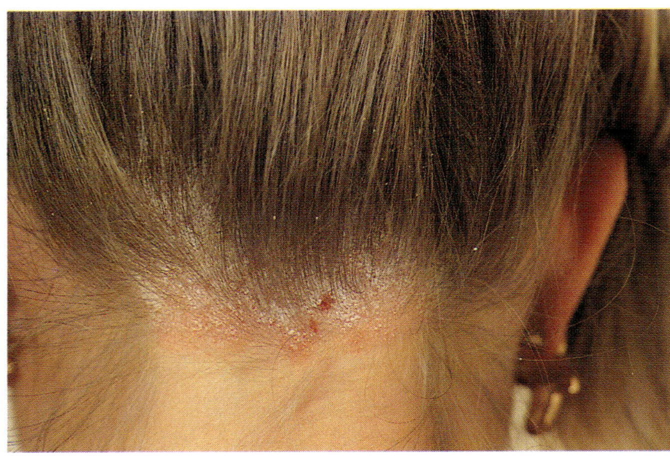

Fig 5.14 Scalp and nape of neck psoriasis with excoriations.

0.1%, fluocinolone acetonide 0.025%, or hydrocortisone valerate 0.2% for 1–2 weeks. Thereafter, a single application following intercourse after washing the penis with soap and water usually prevents aggravation of the condition by the Koebner phenomenon. While employing this treatment, I have not encountered problems such as atrophy, striae, or sexual dysfunction. Anthralin or coal tar products are irritants and should not be applied to the genitalia, which must also be shielded during exposure to UVB or PUVA.

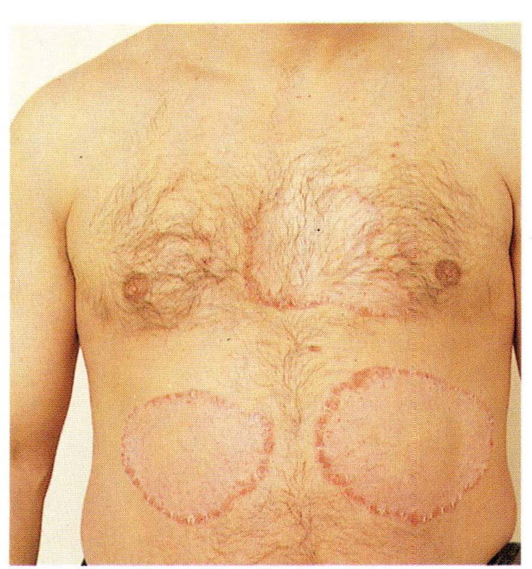

Fig 5.15 Annular psoriasis in a patient responding to the synthetic retinoid, acitretin.

Palm and sole psoriasis

Psoriasis of the palms and soles usually begins on the pressure-bearing areas and may not be as well demarcated as plaques on the rest of the body. They usually have a reddish brown color and may not be symmetric owing to differences in use of the dominant hand or foot (Fig. 5.18). Involvement may extend to the entire volar surface with paronychial and nail disease (Fig. 5.19). Fissures may occur on fingertips and skin folds (Fig. 5.20). Confusion with hand dermatitis of other causes is possible unless there are more typical psoriasis lesions on the elbows, knees, or scalp. Thick inveterate ("elephantine") plaques may develop gradually in some patients who neglect their skin on the sacrum and extremities (Fig. 5.21) [13].

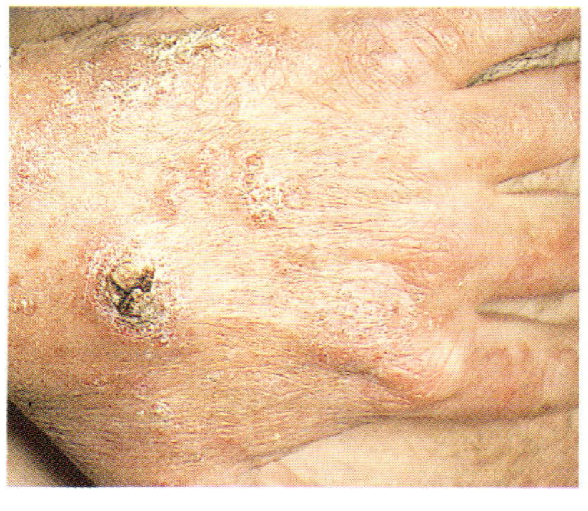

(a)

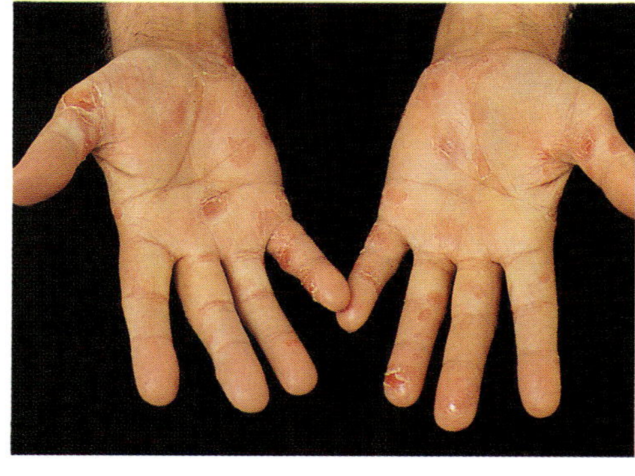

(b)

Fig 5.16 Cutaneous T-cell lymphoma (mycosis fungoides type) originally misdiagnosed as psoriasis on (a) the back of the hand and (b) palms of different patients.

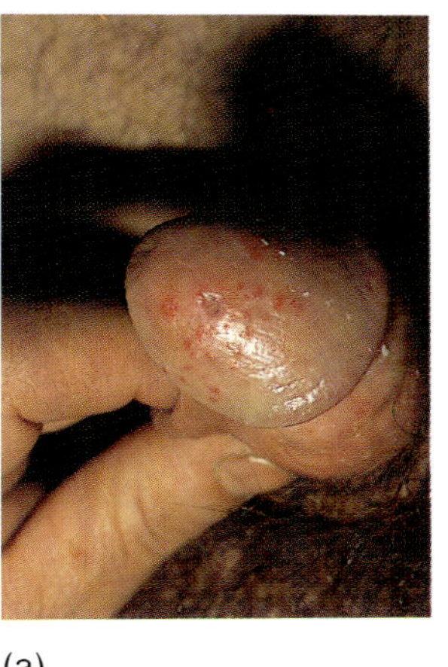

(a)

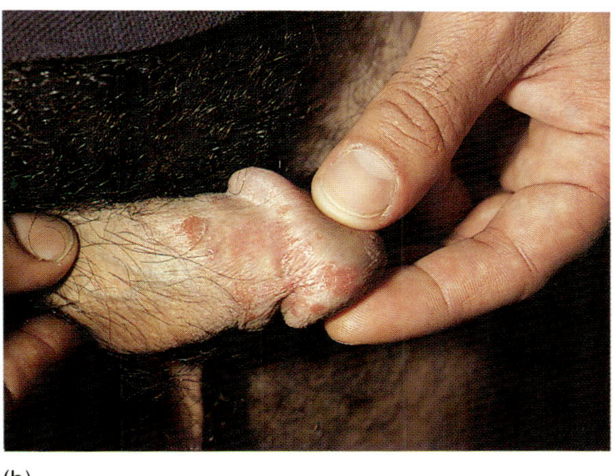

(b)

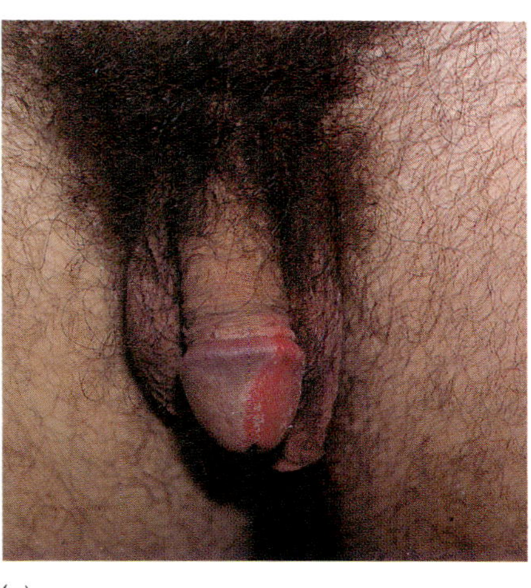

(c)

Fig 5.17 Psoriasis of the penis: (a) discrete papules on glans resemble lichen planus; (b) erythema and scaling of the preputial skin resembles seborrheic dermatitis; (c) red plaque on glans penis suggests the diagnosis of squamous cell carcinoma *in situ* or extramammary Paget's disease.

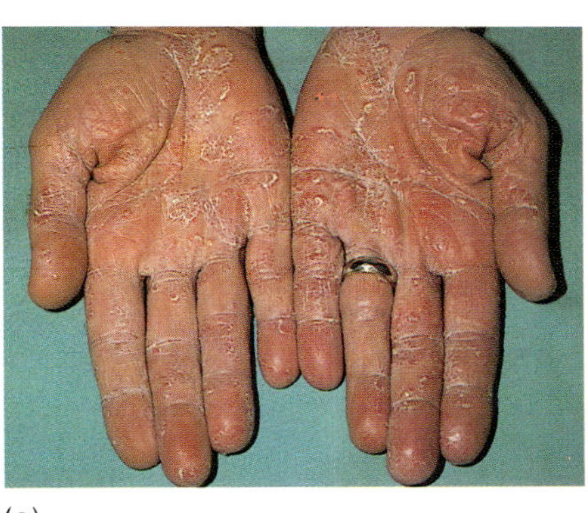

(a)

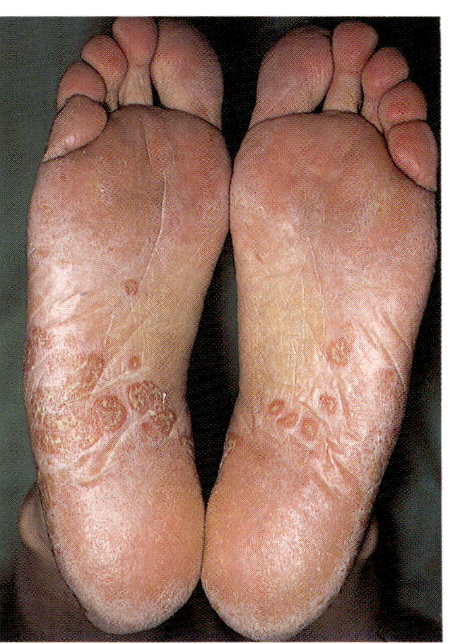

(b)

Fig 5.18 (a) Psoriasis of the palms. (b) Psoriasis of the soles (same patient).

Fig 5.19 Severe paronychial and nail involvement.

Facial psoriasis

Facial lesions usually represent the extension of psoriasis from the scalp on to the forehead, sideburn area, ears, and postauricular area where fissuring may occur (Fig. 5.22). The external auditory canal may also be affected by psoriasis especially in erythrodermic states and enough scale rapidly accumulates in this tight space to reduce significantly the air conduction of sound (Fig. 5.23). The desquamated skin must be irrigated and debrided as often as once per month when the disease is active in order to maintain normal hearing in elderly patients with a preexisting deficit. Facial psoriasis has been considered to be a sign of severe or extensive disease (Fig. 5.24). In erythrodermic psoriasis, the face may be completely covered. A few small guttate lesions may occur on the face during an acute guttate flare. Small patches of psoriasis, more white scales than erythema, may be seen on the upper eyelids of mild to moderate cases of psoriasis vulgaris. The temptation is to incorrectly invoke the diagnosis of eczematous dermatitis or seborrheic blepharitis. When only the head is involved, the presentation may be very similar to seborrheic dermatitis. In the latter, the lessions are less discrete and the scale is more yellowish and greasy rather than silvery and dry. Involvement of the nasolabial fold is typical for seborrheic dermatitis. In cases where it is not possible to distinguish between the two, the contracted terms "sebopsoriasis" or "seborrhiasis" are appropriate.

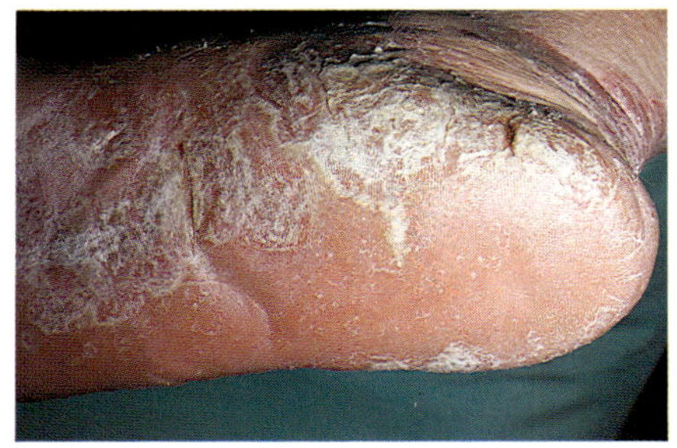

Fig 5.20 Fissuring of psoriasis of sole at pressure points and natural folds.

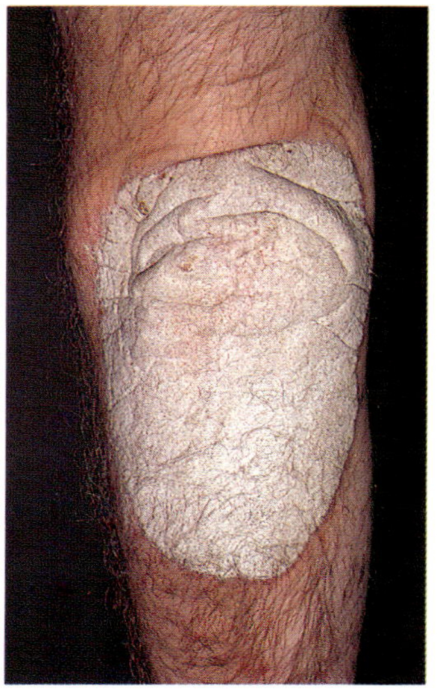

Fig 5.21 Neglected "inveterate" or "elephantine" plaque of psoriasis on an elbow.

Flexural or inverse psoriasis

Flexural or inverse psoriasis may also mimic seborrheic dermatitis. By definition, it occurs in the intertriginous areas: axillae, inframammary areas, groins, natal cleft, antecubital, and popliteal fossae (Fig. 5.25). Obese persons are particularly prone to flexural psoriasis. The appearance is that of a smooth well-demarcated salmon-colored macular patch. It is usually devoid of scale, is moist, and superficially eroded with fissuring right at the "hinge" of the body fold (Fig. 5.26). Dry areas have a "glazed-over" appearance and are frequently colonized with *Candida albicans*, staphylococci, and streptococci. Inverse psoriasis may occur alone but is more frequently accompanied by plaque psoriasis elsewhere. Scraping and culture is recommended here followed by the appropriate oral antibiotic coverage. Astringent compresses, allowing to air dry, topical antifungal creams, and nonfluorinated corticosteroids such as hydrocortisone with iodoquinol or iodochlorhydroxyquin are palliative. The venerable dyes, Castellani paint and gentian violet, are still excellent for drying fissures and erosions in intertriginous areas [see reference 14 for formulations]. The lesions may not clear without significant weight reduction and systemic antipsoriatic therapy.

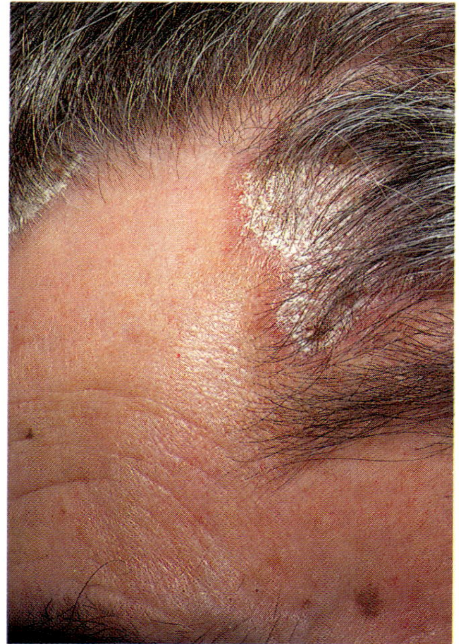

Fig 5.22 Psoriasis of the scalp extends onto the forehead and temple.

Treatment

The treatments of ordinary plaque-type psoriasis are selected from the

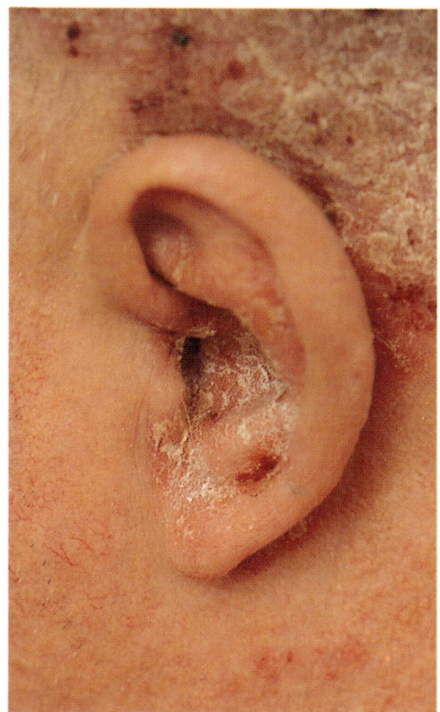

Fig 5.23 Severe psoriasis of the external ear and auditory canal.

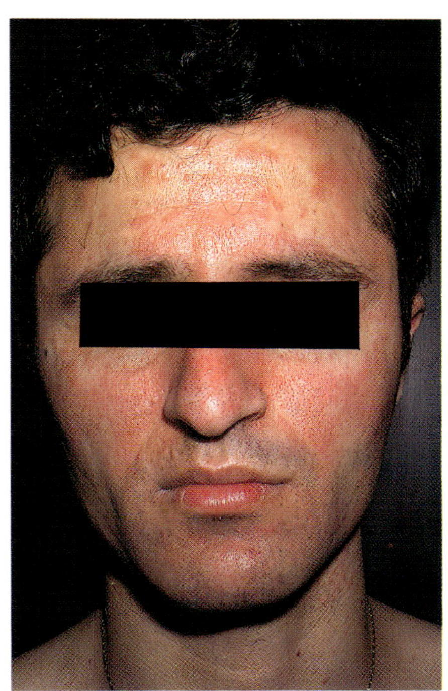

Fig 5.24 Psoriasis of the face indicates severe psoriasis elsewhere on the body.

"lines" shown in Table 5.1 based on criteria covered in their respective chapters. The lines of therapy are arranged in the most likely order of adoption for a case of moderate severity. Topical therapies are less toxic than light therapy, which is less toxic than systemic therapies. Line III comprises the most efficacious treatments having the greatest potential toxicity. Line IV drugs are weakly to moderately effective but have a low toxic potential. It is usually acceptable to combine treatments from different lines.

Table 5.1 Lines of therapy for psoriasis

I Topical therapy
Emollients
Keratolytics
Salicylic acid
Lactic acid
Urea
Calcipotriol*
Anthralin (usually short contact)
Corticosteroids
Topical
Hydrocolloid occlusive dressing
Intralesional injections
Coal tar
II Light therapy
Natural sunlight
UVB
UVB + coal tar (Goeckerman regimen)
UVB + anthralin (Ingram regimen)
III Systemic therapy (high efficacy, high toxicity)
Photochemotherapy (PUVA)
Retinoids (may be combined with UVB or PUVA)
Etretinate
Acitretin*
Isotretinoin†
Methotrexate
Cyclosporine†
IV Systemic therapy† (modest efficacy, low toxicity)
Sulfasalazine
Hydroxyurea
Calcitriol
Antibiotics
Fish oil

* Not available in USA.
† Not Food and Drug Administration-approved for psoriasis.

GUTTATE PSORIASIS

The clinical appearance of guttate psoriasis may be likened to splashing a pail of water on a naked body from a distance and every drop of water that alights on the skin becomes a lesion (Fig. 5.27). This form of psoriasis most often affects children and young adults. A recent epidemiologic survey of 112 children with psoriasis showed that only 26% had the guttate type and the majority had plaque type [15]. The prevalence of guttate psoriasis in the psoriatic population in general is about 18%. There is frequently a prior history of upper respiratory infection, pharyngitis, or tonsillitis. Streptococcal infection has been implicated in the pathogenesis of guttate psoriasis, particularly β-hemolytic streptococcus, Lancefield Group A [16]. Cases of acute guttate flares of psoriasis have recently been reported, which were believed to be precipitated by skin infections with Lancefield Groups C and G streptococci. Elevation of streptococcal antibodies in serum, antistreptolysin O and anti-DNAse, which are used for the presumptive diagnosis of previous streptococcal infections, are not specific for any Lancefield Group [17].

The clinical lesions range in diameter from 0.1 to 1.0 cm and are not as indurated or scaly as plaque-type psoriasis. They predominate on the trunk and proximal extremities and are likely to involve the face. The eruption becomes more symmetric with time. Guttate psoriasis may be the initial manifestation of psoriasis or it may represent an acute flare of preexisting chronic plaque-type psoriasis (Fig. 5.28). In the latter instance, the diagnosis is secure, and a prior streptococcal infection may be suspected. In the new case, however, differential points must be raised. In the young child, confirmation of a streptococcal infection by culture or serology may be most helpful. A history of psoriasis in one or both parents increases the likelihood of early onset psoriasis, especially in females. In the older child or young adult, the differential diagnosis includes pityriasis rosea, secondary syphilis, and guttate parapsoriasis.

Telfer and coworkers [18] confirmed the association of recent streptococcal infection with guttate psoriasis. Serologic evidence of a recent infection was present in 19 of 33 (58%) patients with acute guttate and seven of 27

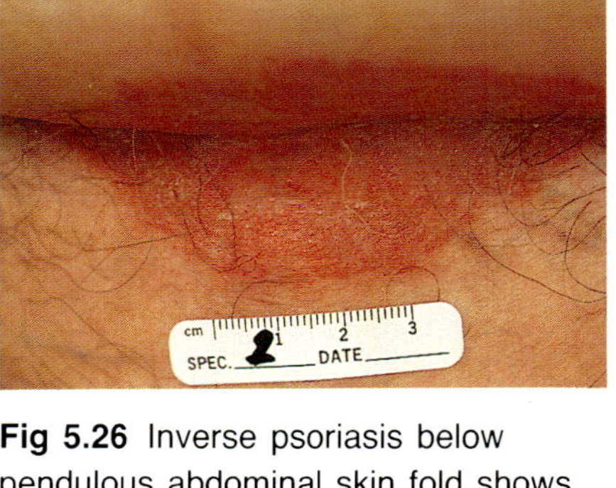

Fig 5.26 Inverse psoriasis below pendulous abdominal skin fold shows superficially eroded glazed-over surface.

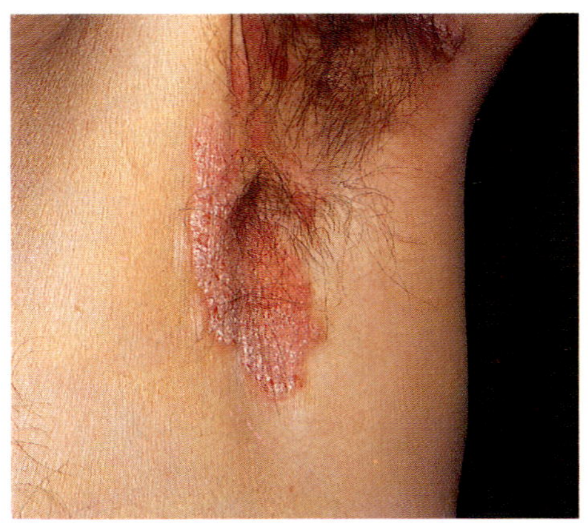

(a)

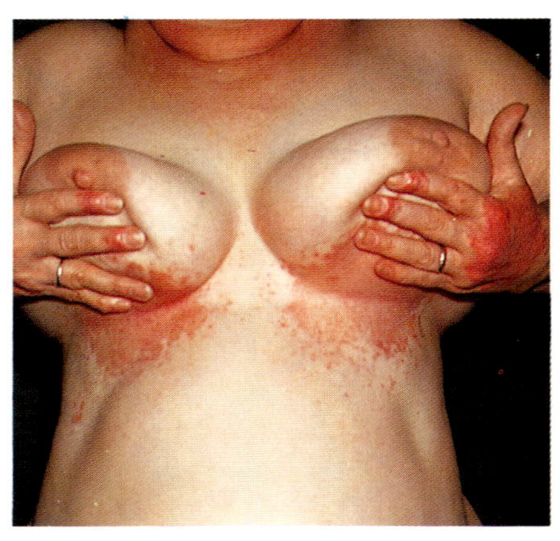

(b)

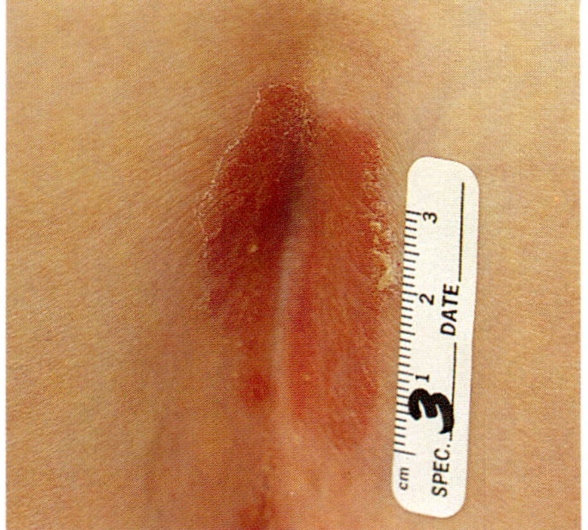

(c)

Fig 5.25 Flexural or inverse psoriasis: (a) axilla; (b) inframammary; (c) natal or intergluteal cleft.

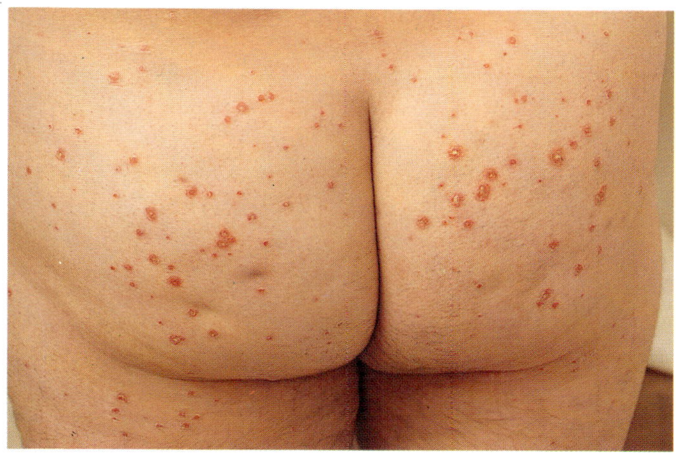

Fig 5.27 Eruptive guttate psoriasis on the buttocks.

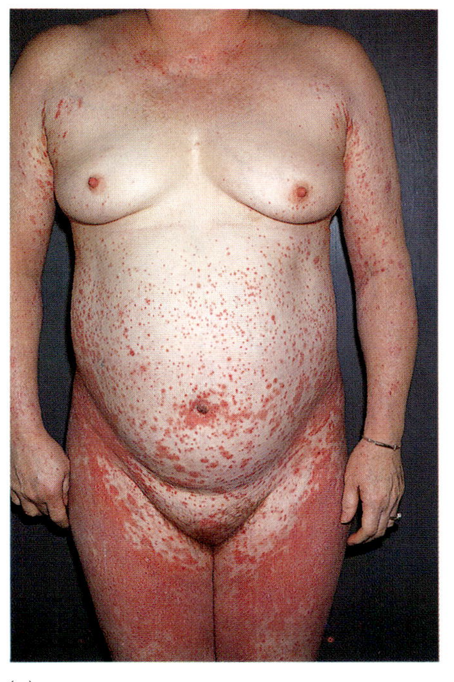

(a)

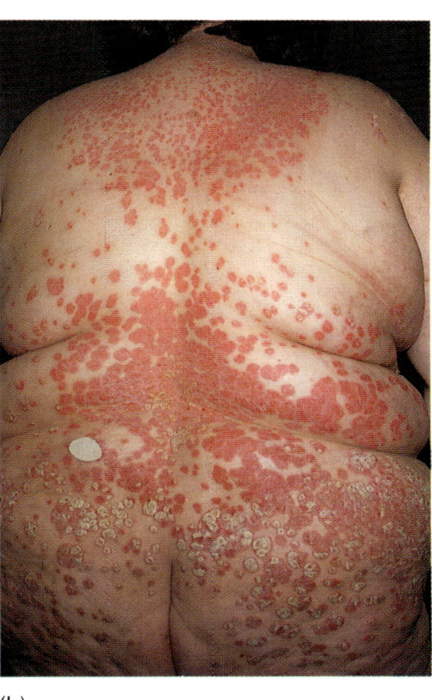

(b)

Fig 5.28 (a) and (b) Guttate flare of preexisting plaque-type psoriasis.

(26%) patients with guttate flares of chronic psoriasis. Cultures for *Streptococcus pyogenes* were positive in 26 and 13% of the cases, respectively. The 13 streptococcal isolates obtained comprised 10 different serotypes indicating that the ability of streptococci to trigger psoriasis is not serotype-specific. Other Lancefield Groups were found with equal frequency in the study group and control population (101 patients with warts).

The pathogenesis of guttate psoriasis triggered or aggravated after hemolytic streptococcal infections is unknown. Hypotheses include activation of the alternative complement pathway and cross-reactivity between streptococcal M protein surface antigens and human epidermis. McFadden and colleagues [19] confirmed that one M protein (M6) showed the closest homology with 50 kDa keratin type I out of 4721 ubiquitous human peptides analyzed. Moreover, the homology involved the α-helical "coiled-coil" structure found in both M6 and 50 kDa keratin. Antisera raised to M proteins stained the stratum corneum of normal and psoriatic epidermis (to a variable extent). While circulating antistratum corneum antibodies are found in most normal individuals, psoriatic skin almost always shows *in vivo* deposition of immunoglobulin in the stratum corneum lending additional support to the cross-reactivity hypothesis.

Treatment

Nine patients with streptococcal-associated psoriasis, on the basis of positive cultures for β-hemolytic streptococci from throats or skin folds or elevated serologic tests for streptococcal antibodies, were treated with penicillin or erythromycin 250 mg q.i.d. for 10–14 days and rifampin 600 mg daily for the final 5 days of therapy. Only five of nine patients had guttate psoriasis. All patients achieved 80–100% clearing of their skin lesions [20]. A subsequent study randomized 10 similar patients each to receive the same antibiotics plus rifampin or placebo. Nineteen of 20 patients had guttate psoriasis. Only three of 20 patients (the normal carriage rate) were colonized with group A β-hemolytic streptococci. The rest were diagnosed on the basis of serology. No clinical improvement was detected in any treatment group up to 6 weeks after treatment [21].

In general, new onset guttate psoriasis related to streptococcal infection involutes rapidly within a 4-week period with antibiotic treatment. In patients who are genetically predisposed to psoriasis, that is, there is familial aggregation of the disease, guttate psoriasis may evolve into localized or extensive chronic plaque-type psoriasis. In patients with chronic psoriasis who develop a guttate exacerbation, empiric treatment with antibiotics is indicated. It should be noted that a 10-day course of penicillin V or erythromycin is safe and less costly than either the culture or the antistreptococcal serology.

If guttate psoriasis does not improve within a 4-week period, if it progresses, or is associated with preexisting moderately severe psoriasis, outpatient UVB or natural sunlight if available is almost always indicated. It is difficult to justify a full Goeckerman regimen for new guttate psoriasis; however, this may be appropriate for long-standing guttate or flaring psoriasis. The prognosis is good with outpatient therapy consisting of white petrolatum or coal tar gels applied prior to suberythemogenic UVB administered three to five times weekly.

The importance of streptococcal antigens in psoriasis cannot be denied, but the association with guttate psoriasis may be exaggerated. Baker and colleagues [22] found that the lymphocyte transformation response to sonicated group A β-hemolytic streptococci was significantly higher in 42 patients with chronic plaque-type psoriasis compared with nonpsoriatic controls. Interestingly, it was not elevated in the patients with guttate psoriasis. No correlations between the degree of lymphocyte proliferation to streptococcal antigens and either the antistreptolysin O titer or the extent and activity of disease were observed.

PUSTULAR PSORIASIS

History

The pustular variants of psoriasis bring to life the most controversial nosology, colorful eponyms, and difficult treatment problems known to the clinician. The patients with generalized disease are often among the most seriously ill requiring hospitalization [2]. The pustuloses can be separated into localized and generalized forms (Table 5.2). Palmoplantar pustulosis (PPP) is by far the most common pustular variant. It accounted for 1.7% of cases of psoriasis in a survey of 401 Irish patients, only one of whom had generalized pustular psoriasis (GPP) [23].

The various forms have been recognized, reported, and embellished in the dermatologic literature spanning nearly 100 years [24]. In 1872 Hebra described impetigo herpetiformis as a fatal generalized pustular eruption in pregnant women. In 1898 Hallopeau reported an inflammatory pustular condition of the fingers and hands related to trauma and a tendency for local destruction and generalization called acrodermatitis continua. GPP of von Zumbusch was first reported in 1910 in a patient with preexisting psoriasis vulgaris. In 1956, Sneddon and Wilkinson [25] described a chronic benign sterile pustular disease called "subcorneal pustular dermatosis" based on the typical histology lacking spongiosis, acantholysis, bacteria, and a deeper epidermal pustule. This condition is now considered a variant of subacute annular psoriasis by some [26], but enough clinical differences exist to consider subcorneal pustular dermatosis an entity *sui generis*. In a series of publications between 1968 and 1971, Ryan and Baker [27–29] reported the characteristics of 155 patients with GPP. They recognized the recurrent spreading annular variant of pustular psoriasis and the eruptive or exanthematic forms. They showed conclusively that GPP of von Zumbusch could be the final common denominator of all pustular variants especially if the patients received systemic steroids for preexisting psoriasis.

Table 5.2 Pustular psoriasis variants

I Localized
One or more plaques with pustules
Palmoplantar pustulosis
Annular (?subcorneal pustular dermatosis of Sneddon and Wilkinson)
Acropustulosis (Acrodermatitis continua of Hallopeau)
?Keratoderma blennorrhagicum (Reiter's syndrome)
II Generalized
Von Zumbusch-type
Impetigo herpetiformis
Acute generalized exanthematous pustulosis

PALMOPLANTAR PUSTULOSIS

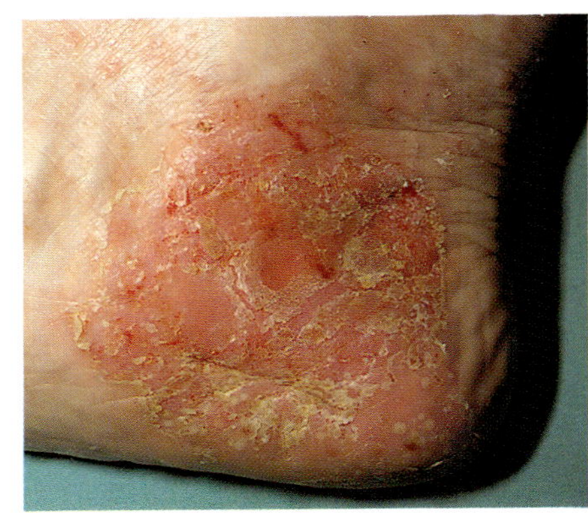

Fig 5.30 Note pustules at the periphery of a well-defined plaque on the heel and ankle.

PPP is a chronic recurring eruption consisting of yellowish pustules on a background of redness and scaling on the thenar and hypothenar eminences and/or the instep of the sole and sides of the heel. Lesions are typically observed in all stages of development from vesicles to vesicopustules to frank pustules to dried brown maculopapules (Fig. 5.29). Lakes of pus are usually not seen unless the condition generalizes (Fig. 5.30). In a large series of GPP, 7.9–13.5% of patients had preexisting PPP [26,29]. As many as 20–30% of patients with PPP have ordinary psoriasis plaques elsewhere on the body.

Despite the reported associations with psoriasis vulgaris and GPP, some authors still consider PPP to be a separate dermatologic disorder. Evidence supports both points of view in a survey of 170 patients with PPP [30]. The authors identified 25 patients (15%) with seronegative spondyloarthropathies similar to psoriatic arthritis. Eight of the patients were HLA-B27-positive associated with sacroiliitis and ankylosing spondylytis, but none of the patients was positive for HLA-B13, B17, B37, and Cw6 which have been associated with psoriasis vulgaris.

Treatment

Recalcitrance to therapy is the rule for PPP, a testament to the numerous inconsistently effective treatments which have been reported. Topical keratolytics, steroids, tars, and UVB are generally ineffective. Systemic agents used have included dapsone, sulfapyridine, colchicine, tetracyclines, trimethoprim-sulfamethoxazole, clofazimine, and methotrexate (MTX). Grenz-ray treatment gives a modest temporary response [31]. Studies in

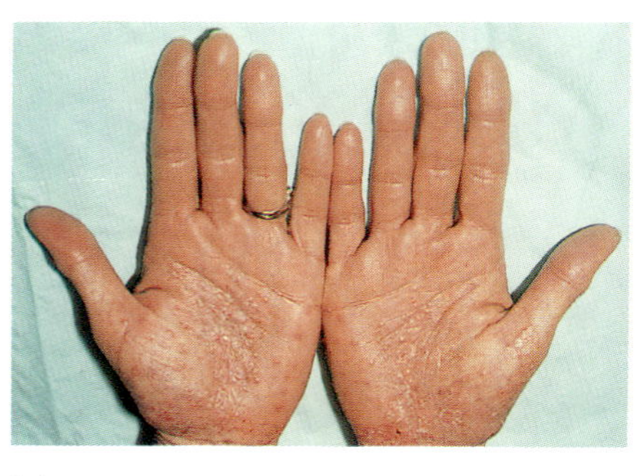

(a)

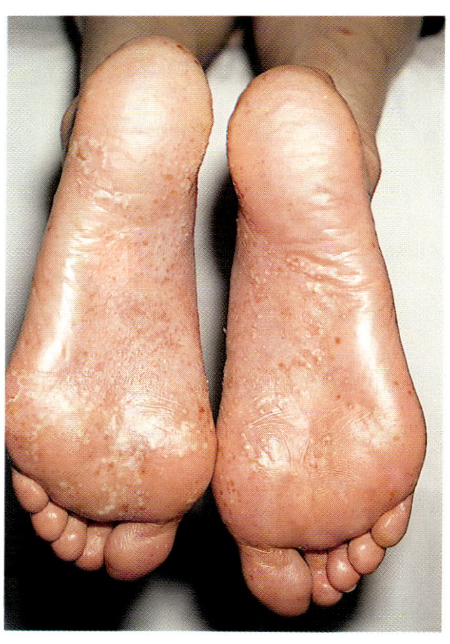

(b)

Fig 5.29 (a) and (b) Palmoplantar pustulosis demonstrates lesions in all stages of development: vesicles, pustules, and dried brown scaly macules and papules (same patient).

progress indicate that low-dose cyclosporine (1.25–2.5 mg/kg per day) is significantly more effective than placebo at suppressing the formation of new pustules [32].

The most effective treatments reported to date with the largest numbers of patients are the aromatic retinoids, etretinate [33], or acitretin [34,35] 30–50 mg/day alone or combined with psoralen UVA (PUVA). Re-PUVA (retinoid plus PUVA) with etretinate 0.6 mg/kg per day was significantly more effective than either treatment alone [36]. Chronic maintenance therapy is required to prevent relapse. A case of PPP generalizing after the withdrawal of etretinate has been reported [37]. Bathwater PUVA is effective and avoids the nausea or pruritus of oral 8-methoxypsoralen, systemic photosensitivity, and long-term toxicity of retinoids. Modifications of topical steroid therapy have been successful in remitting PPP. Goette and colleagues [38] injected triamcinolone acetonide 3.5–5.0 mg/ml intralesionally using a "fanning" technique. The procedure was painful but preferred by patients because clearing lasted for 3–6 months without additional treatment. Clobetasol propionate 0.05% lotion applied weekly under Duoderm extra-thin hydrocolloid dressings cleared 18 of 19 PPP cases in 1–7 weeks [39]. Two-thirds remained clear for 2–8 months after discontinuation of therapy.

GENERALIZED PUSTULAR PSORIASIS OF VON ZUMBUSCH

The evolution of GPP, whether *de novo* or from a preexisting psoriatic state, consists of fiery red, irregular patches with round, arcuate, serpiginous borders surmounted by myriads of 1–2-mm superficial pustules. There is a predilection for flexural areas but any site may be involved. The pustules coalesce forming lakes of pus, desquamate, and form new pustules as the border moves in waves every 27–72 hours (Figs 5.31, 5.32). Patients are usually prostrate and febrile. The laboratory shows leukocytosis, hypocalcemia, and hypoalbuminemia. The ionized serum calcium is usually within normal limits, but cases with postsurgical hypoparathyroidism, hypocalcemia, and tetany have been reported that clearly responded to correction of serum calcium [40,41].

The average of age of onset is about 50 years and the sex incidence is approximately equal. From the earlier series, the most striking finding was that one-fourth of patients had their attack of GPP within 1 month of first receiving or withdrawal of systemic steroids [29]. These cases were considered to be steroid-provoked. Other precipitating factors identified included preceding infections and drugs. Some of these patients had the exanthematous type of pustular psoriasis.

Treatment

Among the steroid-treated patients, 67% had preexisting ordinary psoriasis compared to 56% of the entire group of 155 patients. Thirty-four of 106

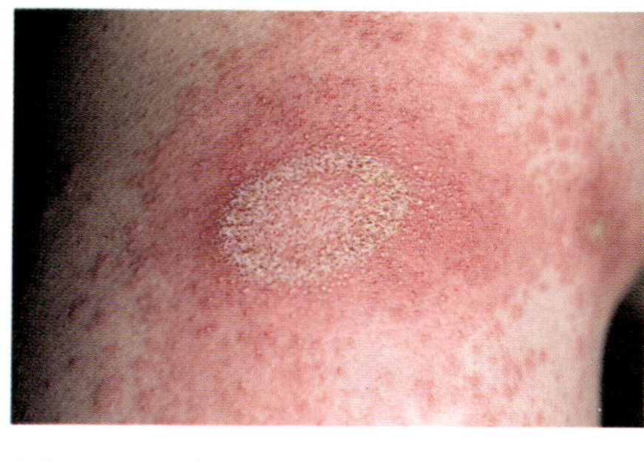

(a)

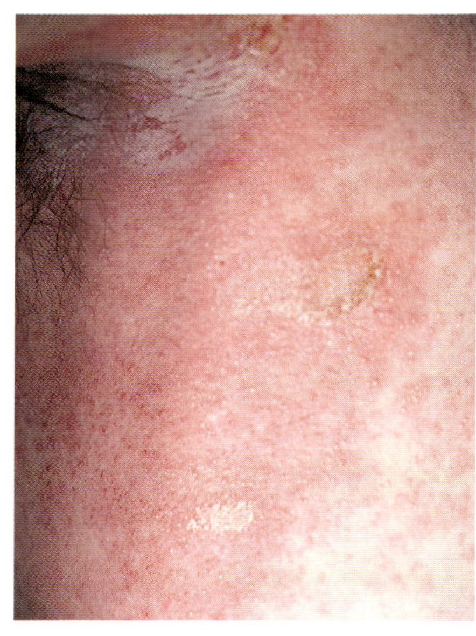

(b)

Fig 5.31 Generalized pustular psoriasis (same patient): (a) coalescence, central desquamation, and centrifugal spread of tiny pustules; (b) demonstrates "lake" of pus in axilla.

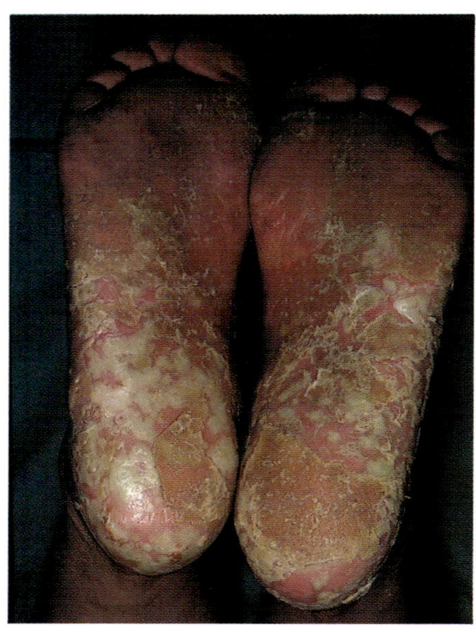

(a)

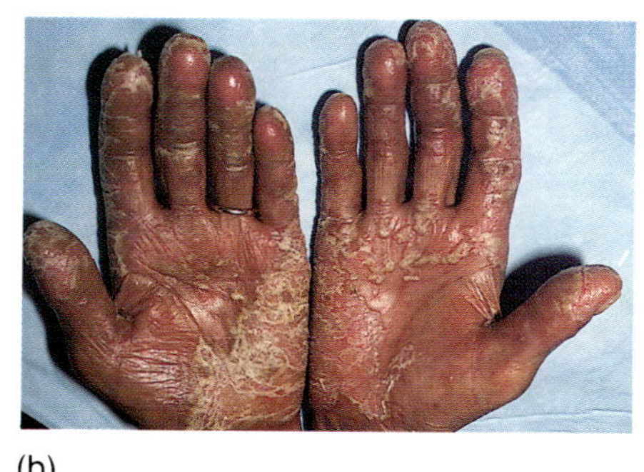

(b)

Fig 5.32 Generalized pustular psoriasis of palms and soles showing (a) "lakes" of pus and (b) desquamation. Same patient.

patients followed up died, eight from uncontrollable GPP and nine as a complication of therapy — seven from steroids, two from MTX. GPP developing from acrodermatitis continua had the worst prognosis in this series [29]. GPP evolving from PPP or atypical flexural forms of psoriasis was likely to have spontaneous remission of the GPP with continuation of the original problem. GPP in 73 of 104 patients was treated with systemic steroids, but these patients tended to suffer from increasingly severe GPP relapses upon withdrawal of steroids. Moreover, MTX was less efficacious in patients previously treated with steroids. The rebound relapse after steroid withdrawal was not always controllable with MTX. Because spontaneous remission was common in untreated patients and the morbidity and mortality associated with steroid or MTX treatment was high (daily MTX was used at the time), the authors advocated a conservative approach to therapy: von Zumbusch's original patient suffered nine episodes of GPP over 10 years. His most recent episodes had become milder. "Would he have survived so long had his physician been armed with corticosteroids and folic acid antagonists?" [28].

Success is achieved with tapwater or mild antiseptic wet dressings in hospital with topical steroids [26]. A variety of systemic agents (steroids, MTX, dapsone, sulfapyridine, and etretinate) or 2% crude coal tar with and without UV were needed as adjunctive therapy of the more severe relapsing recalcitrant GPP cases. In contrast to Ryan and Baker [29], the seven patients with GPP after acrodermatitis continua (Fig. 5.33) resolved with few complications, although more aggressive systemic therapy was needed including cyclosporine in one case. The most common complication of GPP was secondary infection including septicemia resulting in one death. Another patient died of Guillain–Barré syndrome. One patient developed a bleeding duodenal ulcer secondary to systemic steroid treatment. Hypocalcemia was found in 17 of 63 (27%) but 10 cases could be explained by hypoalbuminemia. The most common precipitating factors were believed to be upper respiratory infections (16%) and decreasing the dose of steroids.

With the advent of systemic retinoid therapy which can rapidly halt pustulation and decrease systemic symptoms, etretinate for men and post-menopausal women or isotretinoin for women of childbearing potential are the treatments of choice [42]. The past complications of systemic steroids should be avoided. If conversion to MTX or PUVA for long-term maintenance is desired, the retinoid can be gradually tapered to prevent a relapse of GPP. Cyclosporine should be reserved for those patients unresponsive to retinoids [32,43]. Low ionized calcium can be corrected rapidly by calcium infusion. Antibiotics are usually not effective for GPP *per se*, but septicemia can occur as a complication and appropriate antibiotics might be life-saving in such a situation. In one study, seven consecutive patients with GPP and coagulase positive staphylococcal septicemia were treated with a 6-week course of antibiotics which terminated the pustular phase in all but one patient [44]. One patient died due to infection by antibiotic-resistant bacteria. Corticosteroids or MTX were not used. The GPP in these cases may have remitted spontaneously after 6 weeks in hospital, but the bottom line is to perform blood cultures upon admission and treat empirically if sepsis is suspected.

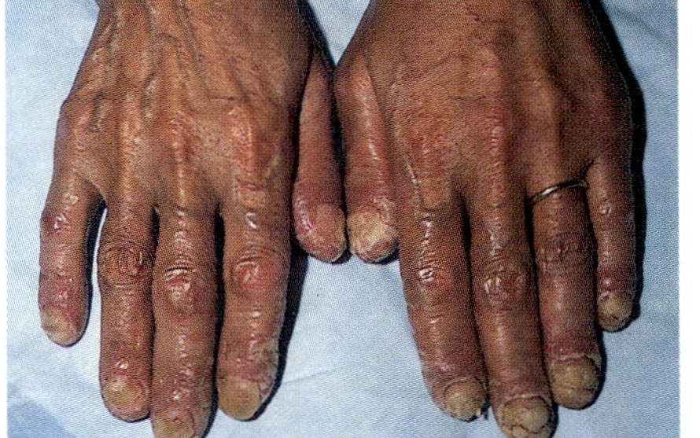

Fig 5.33 Acrodermatitis continua of Hallopeau or chronic acropustulosis.

Juvenile pustular psoriasis

GPP in children is rare. These patients usually do not have preceding psoriasis vulgaris but a previous diagnosis of napkin dermatitis [45] or seborrheic dermatitis is common. The morphology and systemic signs of GPP in children are the same as for adult-onset GPP. The most common precipitating factors included infections, coal tar, and sun exposure. GPP occurred during the first year of life in seven of 13 children reported by Zelickson and Muller [46].

The condition was well-controlled in most cases by the conservative regimen of hospitalization, wet dressings, and topical steroids. When they were used, systemic steroids, dapsone, and sulfapyridine were relatively ineffective. When systemic therapy is needed, etretinate (for males) and isotretinoin are safe in the short term for children. There were no deaths, but three of 13 patients developed Gram-positive septicemia. In adult life, one of the patients subsequently experienced flares of pustular psoriasis during each of two pregnancies. Hubler [24] reported a similar patient with GPP at age 5 who later developed GPP when she was 6 months pregnant. She had two brothers with recurrent GPP who had the onset during the first year of life. All three siblings in this very rare example of familial GPP settled into chronic acropustulosis (Fig. 5.33) requiring long-term MTX maintenance.

Tonsillectomy had no effect on the number of attacks or pustulation in one identicle twin compared with his counterpart: both patients developed GPP at 48 days of life [47].

Impetigo herpetiformis

As originally described, impetigo herpetiformis refers to GPP in a pregnant woman without a prior history of psoriasis. The clinical morphology is similar to GPP: there are round, arcuate, polycyclic patches covered with tiny pustules in a concentric array. Lesions expand by peripheral extension. The old pustules break down, crust over, and may become vegetative in flexural areas [48]. Lesions typically heal with hyperpigmentation. Constitutional signs and symptoms are common as is leukocytosis, hypocalcemia, and hypoalbuminemia. Most cases occur during the third trimester, but it can occur earlier. Impetigo herpetiformis recurs with each successive pregnancy.

Cases have been reported in men and elderly women with hypocalcemia [41], but to call such cases "impetigo herpetiformis" obviates the need for the term. These patients have GPP. Pregnancy is a precipitating factor for GPP; therefore, patients with a prior history of psoriasis vulgaris or pustular psoriasis who flare during pregnancy should not be considered to have impetigo herpetiformis [49]. Impetigo herpetiformis recurs with successive pregnancies with increasing morbidity and promptly remits postpartum.

Prednisone 20–60 mg daily has been used to decrease pustulation and improve constitutional symptoms related to intense inflammation, but this treatment is unsatisfactory and contradicts the negative experience with steroids in GPP. MTX, sulfones, and retinoids would ordinarily not be given to pregnant women. Serum calcium levels must be restored and any superinfection treated with antibiotics. Fetal morbidity and mortality are increased. Termination of pregnancy is the definitive treatment of impetigo herpetiformis. Depending on gestation dates, vaginal delivery by induced labor, Cesarean section, or therapeutic abortion should be considered.

Pathomechanisms in pustular psoriasis

As to be expected, aberrations in the function of various leukocyte types have been sought and found in many cases of pustular psoriasis. In one study, 20 patients with pustular psoriasis (including GPP, PPP, and acrodermatitis continua) had significantly higher polymorphonuclear leukocyte (PMNL) chemotaxis than patients with psoriasis vulgaris [50]. By contrast, monocyte chemotaxis was lower in pustular psoriasis than psoriasis vulgaris and not different than normal controls. Different directed migration responses of leukocytes in pustular vs common psoriasis supports the hypothesis of a different etiopathogenesis. On the other hand, phagocytosis of immunoglobulin G (IgG)-coated latex particles by PMNLs was significantly enhanced in patients with either psoriasis vulgaris or PPP [51]. Natural killer cells play an important role in host defense. Natural killer cell cytotoxicity of mononuclear cells isolated from peripheral blood of four patients with GPP was significantly reduced compared to psoriasis vulgaris and healthy controls [52]. A rapid decline in the absolute number of lymphocytes in 10 patients 1 day prior to a generalized pustular flare of psoriasis in the face of fever and leukocytosis has been seen [53]. Nine of the patients had received systemic steroids within 1 month of the flare confirming the precipitating role of these drugs. The authors proposed that steroid-induced stability of lysosomal membranes may have led to reactive lability when the steroids were withdrawn.

A 12 kDa PMNL chemotactic factor, thought to be a C5-cleavage product, was identified in the stratum corneum of psoriasis vulgaris, pustular psoriasis, PPP, and subcorneal pustular dermatosis [54]. Recently, a few cases of GPP complicated by pulmonary capillary leak syndrome have been reported, suggesting the involvement of cytokines, i.e., interleukin-1 and tumor necrosis factor [55].

Exanthematous psoriasis

An eruptive variant of GPP called "exanthematic pustular psoriasis" because it arose rapidly in the absence of preexisting psoriasis, was usually precipitated by infection or drugs, and tended to spontaneous resolution, has been observed by Ryan and Baker [29]. Similar cases have probably been reported in the literature as GPP precipitated by drugs [56,57]. A consortium of French investigators analyzed 63 cases of so-called acute generalized exanthematous pustulosis (AGEP) [58]. They found that 55 (80%) could be attributed to drugs, particularly antibiotics of the penicillin and macrolide families. Skin contact with mercury and enterovirus infection were also considered important causes.

The clinical appearance of AGEP is very similar to GPP with the abrupt onset of fever, pustulation, leukocytosis, and hypocalcemia within 5 days (< 24 hours in half the cases) of taking the drug. Polymorphous skin lesions (facial edema, purpura, vesicles, targetoid lesions) and erosions of the oral mucous membranes were recorded in about half the cases. The histology of lesions showed subcorneal and intraepidermal spongiform pustules. There were some other subtle pathologic differences from GPP. Clinical differences that helped the authors to distinguish AGEP from GPP, even in the 11 patients with preexisting psoriasis, included recent drug intake, higher fever, greater leukocytosis and eosinophilia, lack of arthritis, and spontaneous resolution within 15 days. They suggested that AGEP may be a drug-induced reaction pattern, which is more likely to occur in persons with a psoriatic diathesis.

ERYTHRODERMIC PSORIASIS

The least common form of psoriasis is exfoliative dermatitis or psoriatic erythroderma representing 1–2% of all cases. Erythroderma in general is a scaling inflammatory process of the skin that involves all or almost all of the skin surface (Fig. 5.34). Psoriasis comprises 16–25% of cases in series of erythroderma [59,60]. The remainder include a variety of causes: eczematous dermatitis, seborrheic dermatitis, pityriasis rubra pilaris, drug-induced, lymphoma and leukemia (Fig. 5.35). Erythrodermic psoriasis usually develops gradually or acutely during the course of chronic psoriasis, but it may be the initial manifestation of psoriasis, even in children. The mean age of patients at the onset of erythroderma is 48–55 years, and males outnumber females.

As the psoriatic erythroderma evolves, the original psoriasis plaques gradually lose their distinct outlines and surface characteristics blending into a background of bright erythema with generalized exfoliation. Sterile

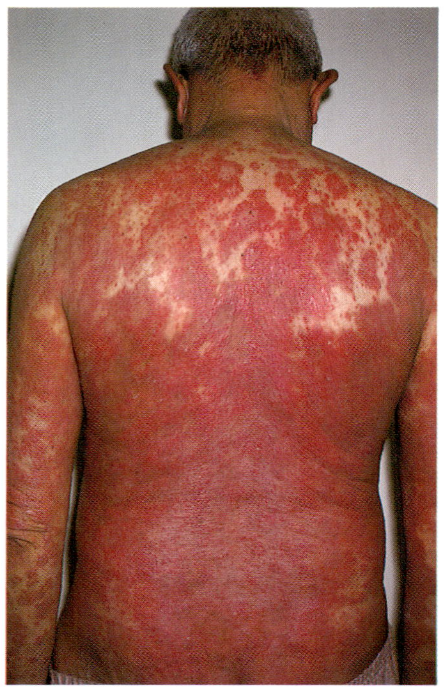
(a)

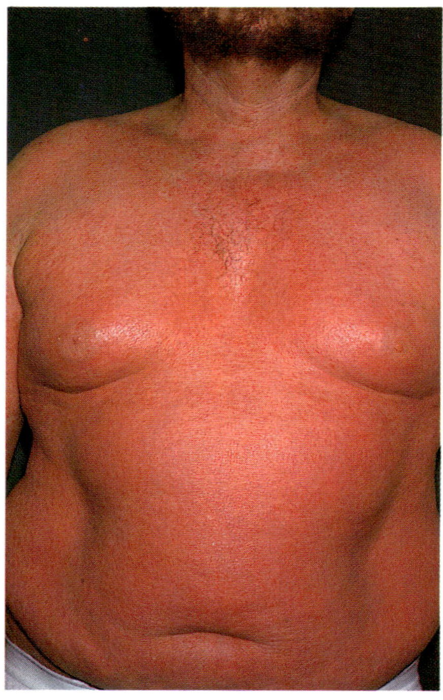
(b)

Fig 5.34 Psoriatic erythroderma: (a) almost all of the skin surface is affected; (b) the entire body skin is involved.

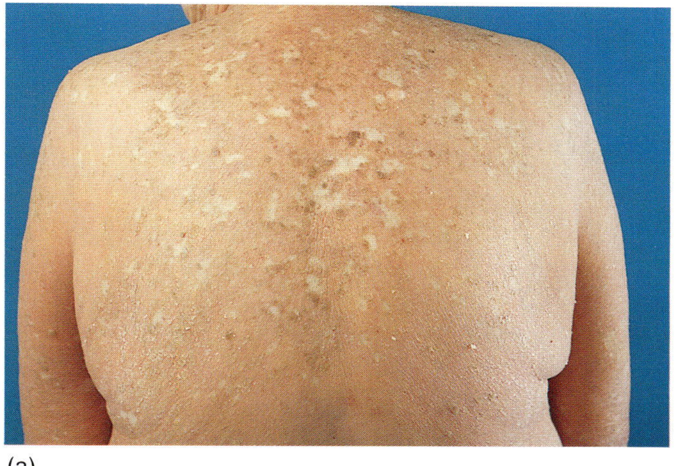

(a)

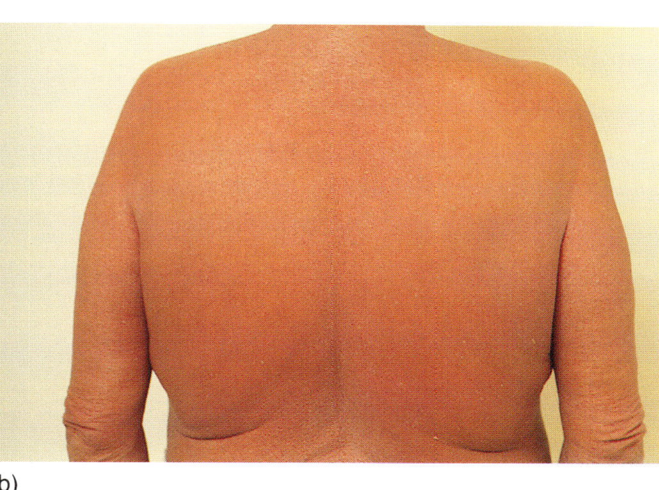

(b)

Fig 5.35 The differential diagnosis of erythroderma: (a) pityriasis rubra pilaris; (b) Sézary syndrome.

pustules may develop in some areas; in the most unstable cases, GPP may develop (Fig. 5.36). Concomitant psoriatic arthropathy is common.

Precipitating factors for erythroderma include systemic illnesses, emotional stress, and alcoholism, but the most important ones seem to be treatment-related and therefore preventable, especially the inappropriate use of potent topical, oral, and intramuscular corticosteroids (Table 5.3) [61].

Fig 5.36 In the most severe cases, the distinction between erythrodermic and pustular psoriasis is lost.

Complications of psoriatic erythroderma

Patients with acute erythroderma are uncomfortable, complain of chills, and may have low grade fever. Thermoregulation is compromised because while radiant and convective heat loss from the skin surface is increased, the erythrodermic skin sweats less than normal. There is increased water loss by diffusion. Protein (keratin), iron, and folic acid are lost during the profuse scaling. Resulting laboratory abnormalities may include hypovolemia, hypoalbuminemia, anemia, folic acid deficiency, and leukocytosis.

Table 5.3 Treatment-related precipitating factors for erythrodermic psoriasis

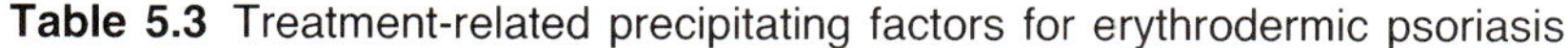

Treatments for psoriasis
Systemic steroids
Topical steroid excess
Tar sensitivity
Methotrexate withdrawal
Etretinate
PUVA burn
PUVA + phototoxic drug
UVB burn
Allergic reaction to medications for other ailments
Penicillin
Gold injection
Chloroquine
Hydroxychloroquine

In patients with a compromised cardiovascular system (the typical patient is an older male), high output cardiac failure, although uncommon, is a risk. Lower-extremity edema is common resulting from a combination of dependence, local inflammatory mediators, hypoalbuminemia, and cardiac failure. Hyperuricemia was reported in 25% of patients with psoriatic erythrodermas tested [61]. Patients with psoriatic arthritis may be incorrectly diagnosed as having gout because of these elevated uric acid levels [62]. A single case report suggested that hypophosphatemia may be another metabolic complication [63].

Sixty-two percent of patients with psoriatic erythroderma had elevated serum lactic dehydrogenase (LDH) [61]. LDH is a ubiquitous cytosolic enzyme which consists of five isozymes [64]. Elevation of LDH in patients with extensive inflammatory skin diseases is probably a nonspecific measure of epidermal injury because LDH5 predominates in muscle and epidermis. In a survey of consecutive admissions to a university inpatient dermatology service, three of eight patients with extensive plaque-type psoriasis and four of seven patients with various other severe dermatoses had elevated LDH levels (A.B. Hessel, C. Camisa, unpublished data).

Treatment

Patients who have been withdrawn abruptly from systemic steroids, excessive potent topical steroids, or MTX have the most unstable psoriasis and may develop erythroderma and/or pustular psoriasis. We admit such patients to hospital and treat them conservatively (Table 5.4) until the patient is stable enough to receive more aggressive therapy. If the patient is not known to have a prior diagnosis of psoriasis, we perform several representative skin biopsies. A surveillance blood culture is performed. If there are any pustules, a culture is taken. A blood smear for circulating Sézary cells is ordered along with the complete blood count.

Psoriatic erythroderma can be controlled eventually in most patients with the standard Goeckerman regimen, PUVA, etretinate, MTX, or cyclosporine. It reverts back to the preerythrodermic status. Systemic steroids and potent topical steroids are eschewed. A minority of patients remain unstable and have repeated episodes of erythroderma during their lifetime.

Table 5.4 Conservative care of erythroderma

Hospitalization
Bedrest with leg elevation
Colloidal oatmeal in whirlpool bath twice daily
Rehydration if necessary
Antibiotics if necessary
Vitamin and iron supplementation
Compresses to face and flexural areas if there are fissures or exudation
Liberal emolliation with Aquaphor
1% hydrocortisone in Aquaphor 1–2 times daily

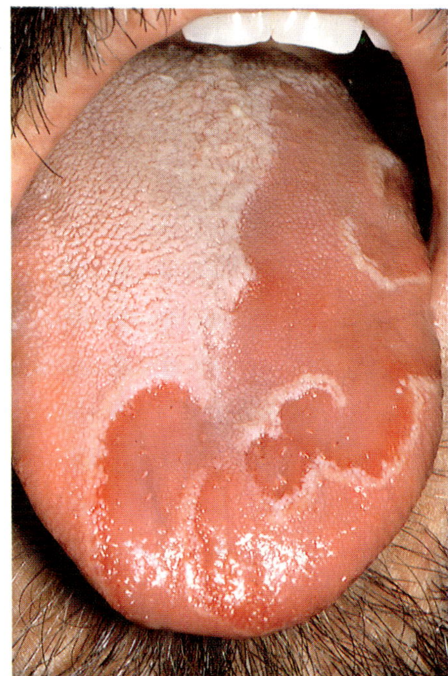

Fig 5.37 Benign migratory glossitis or geographic tongue.

ORAL LESIONS

Oral lesions of psoriasis are very uncommon. Pindborg [65] believes there are four types of psoriatic oral lesion: (i) minute round or oval whitish lesions that can be scraped off leaving a bleeding surface; (ii) whitish plaques with red areas that parallel activity of skin lesions; (iii) bright red areas in pustular and erythrodermic psoriasis and Reiter's syndrome; and (iv) benign migratory glossitis (BMG).

BMG, also known as geographic tongue, is a common inflammatory disorder of unknown etiology that affects about 2% of normal persons in the USA. The clinical lesions are distinctive showing well-demarcated red depapillated areas of the dorsal tongue delineated along its periphery by a slightly elevated whitish-yellow arc or annulus (Fig. 5.37). Similar lesions also affect the lateral and ventral tongue and can extend onto the labial, buccal, and soft palatal mucosa. In such cases, the lesion may be called stomatitis areata migrans (SAM) (Fig. 5.38). Synonyms include "ectopic geographic tongue," geographic mucositis, and erythema migrans. Geographic tongue and mucositis are usually asymptomatic and do not require any treatment. Histopathology may be indistinguishable from psoriasis with epithelial hyperplasia, spongiosis, and exocytosis of neutrophils and lymphocytes. Parakeratosis and psoriasiform hyperplasia are normal findings for the dorsal tongue, however.

Fissured tongue (FT), also called lingua plicata and scrotal tongue, is a normal variant consisting of a deep anteroposteriorly-oriented groove from which smaller fissures radiate laterally. The incidence of FT increases with age. The prevalence is estimated to be 3–5%. There is a high association of FT with BMG (up to 20%) (Fig. 5.39) [65]. Surveys of consecutive psoriatic patients have revealed a range of prevalences of BMG (1–6%) and FT (9.5–14%). In one study BMG was found in 11 of 63 (17.5%) of patients with GPP [26]. Pogrel and Cram [66] observed SAM (15 on the hard palate and four on the buccal mucosa) in 19 of 100 patients admitted

Fig 5.38 Stomatitis areata migrans: (a) ventral tongue; (b) buccal mucosa.

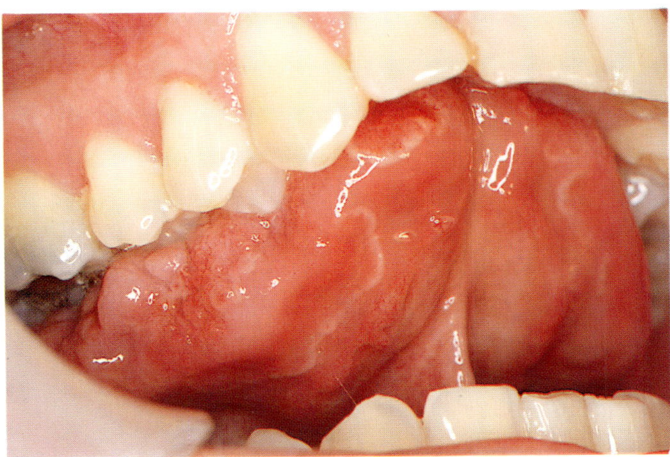

(a)

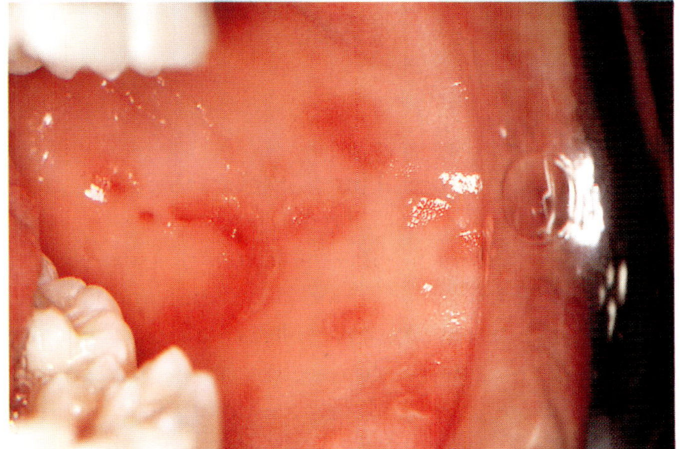

(b)

to a psoriasis day-care center for an acute exacerbation of psoriasis. In general, the course of SAM followed that of psoriasis. Eight cases resolved after 3 weeks of intensive psoriasis treatment. We performed intraoral examinations of 75 consecutive psoriatic patients in a 4-month period in 1992 for this chapter. The prevalence of FT was 21.3%, BMG 14.7%, and SAM 1.3%. FT and BMG coexisted in four of 75 patients. The only patient with SAM also had FT, BMG, and generalized plaque-type psoriasis, which was flaring at the time of his first oral examination. His psoriasis was cleared by outpatient UVB thrice weekly, and the SAM resolved.

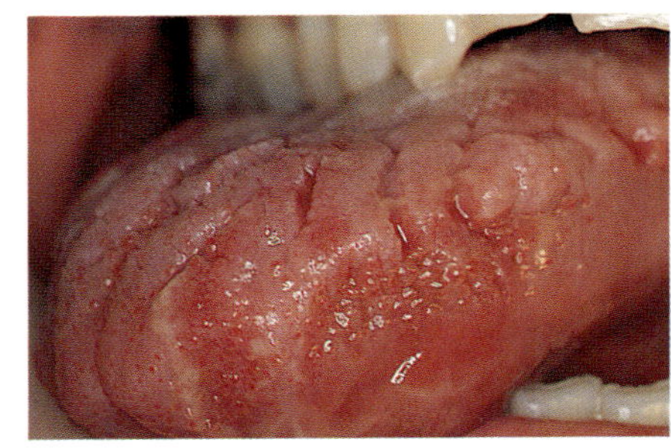

Fig 5.39 Association of benign migratory glossitis and fissured tongue.

In a group of 200 patients with psoriasis vulgaris compared to age- and sex-matched controls attending a dental clinic, the incidence of BMG and SAM was 10.3 and 5.4%, respectively, compared to 2.5 and 1.0% [67]. The differences were statistically significant by χ^2 analysis. There was no difference in the incidence of FT (16.7% vs 20.3%) despite the known association between FT and BMG. The prevalence of FT and BMG in psoriasis was similar in our series. There was no particular association of BMG or SAM with either stable or progressive disease or correlation with the extent of body surface area involved. In a study of 19 specimens with biopsy-proven SAM from a university oral pathology laboratory, the only two patients who also had cutaneous psoriasis showed involvement of the palate or gingiva [68].

It is not surprising for two common conditions, psoriasis and migratory mucositis, to occasionally coexist. The prevalence of BMG seems to be higher in psoriatics than the general population and SAM is more likely to occur in severe active psoriasis. If SAM is indeed intraoral psoriasis, then it apparently has a greater tendency to involve the bound keratinized tissues of the gingiva and hard palate than SAM in nonpsoriatics. In a report of six cases of SAM, the only patient with gingival and hard palate lesions also had pustular psoriasis and arthritis [69]. The clinical courses of the oral lesions and psoriasis paralleled each other.

It is moot whether BMG or SAM represent incidental inflammatory lesions unrelated to psoriasis or specific oral manifestations of psoriasis. Most cases are not symptomatic and are not associated with skin lesions. When they are associated, the oral lesions may or may not correlate with activity or severity of the skin disease and do not require specific treatment.

HISTOPATHOLOGY

Histopathology is useful but not invaluable in the diagnosis of psoriasis. In the overwhelming majority of cases, it is preferable to make a clinical diagnosis. The clinician has the luxury of knowing the family and personal history, anatomic distribution of lesions, and the varying morphology of lesions of different ages as well as nail changes. The pathologist is at a disadvantage as he or she receives only a miniscule sample of a dynamic process frozen at a random time point. The classic histology of psoriasis may only be seen in a lesion that is 1 week to 1 month old [70]. Unfortunately, it may not be possible to distinguish histologically with confidence

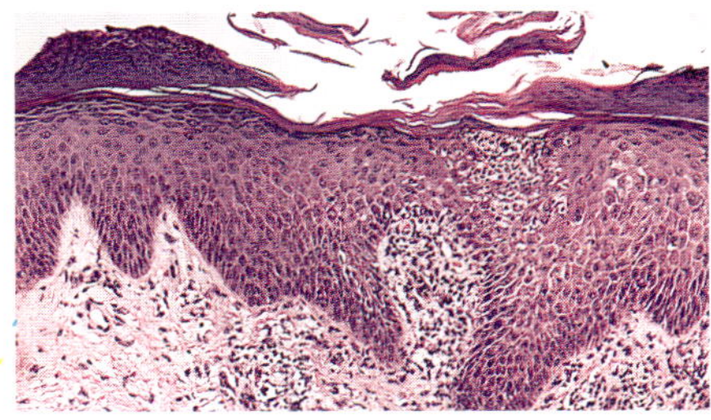

Fig 5.40 Biopsy of psoriasis shows epidermal hyperplasia, mounds of parakeratosis containing neutrophils, and early spongiform pustule.

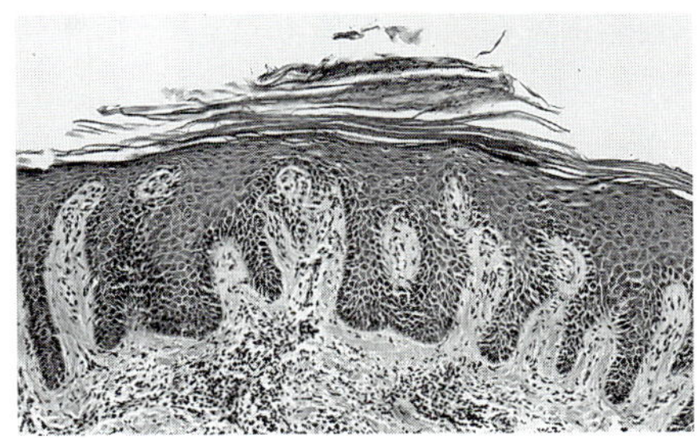

Fig 5.41 Psoriasiform hyperplasia. Some of the rete ridges are bulbous with a tendency to coalesce.

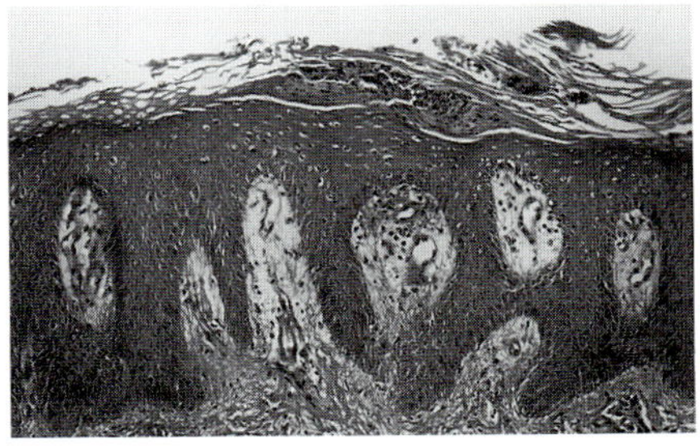

Fig 5.42 This biopsy specimen demonstrates hyperkeratosis, neutrophils in the stratum corneum, and edematous dermal papillae.

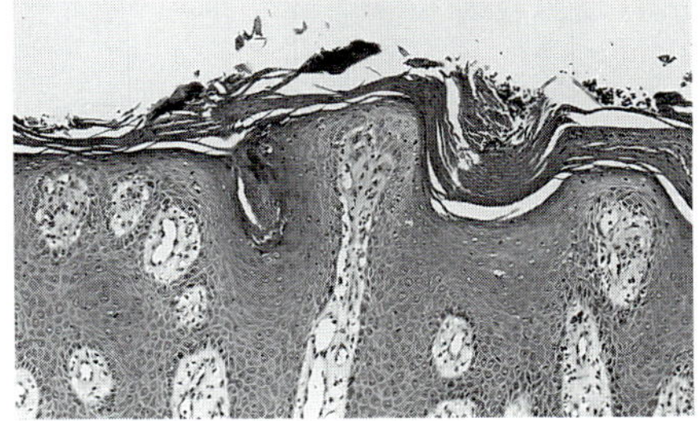

Fig 5.43 Dilated tortuous capillaries in the dermal papillae with thinning of the "suprapapillary plate."

a clinically typical lesion of psoriasis from "chronic dermatitis" or "psoriasiform dermatitis" in a substantial proportion of cases.

Dermatopathology textbooks [70,71] have emphasized the rapidly evolving nature of the psoriatic lesion and the changing histologic picture. For example, the earliest pinhead-sized macule shows nonspecific findings: slight epidermal hyperplasia, erythrocytes packed in dilated capillaries and exravasated in dermal papillae, and a sparse perivascular lymphocytic infiltrate [72].

It is not until neutrophils enter the picture, however, that a specific diagnosis can be made. The neutrophils move rapidly because the earliest diagnostic lesion, a small smooth-surfaced papule, shows mounds of parakeratosis-containing neutrophils, the earliest manifestation of Munro microabscesses. The older scaly lesions show aggregations of neutrophils in the upper stratum spinosum, which form small spongiform pustules of Kogoj while mononuclear cells remain confined to the lower epidermis (Fig. 5.40). Meanwhile, the epithelium becomes increasingly hyperplastic, more mitotic figures are seen, and the epidermis develops the classic "psoriasiform" appearance. "Psoriasiform" implies elongated regular rete ridges that are thin with bulbous tips and a tendency to coalesce (Fig. 5.41). The dermal papillae are correspondingly widened at their summits, appear edematous (Fig. 5.42), and contain dilated tortuous capillaries (Fig. 5.43). Extravasated erythrocytes may be seen here. The suprapapillary epidermis is thinned. A fully developed lesion may show confluent parakeratosis, but many biopsies show orthokeratosis admixed with parakeratosis, either in a focal vertical column or in alternating layers attesting to the episodic nature of the psoriatic process. Where there is parakeratosis there is usually a reduction of keratohyaline granules and a diminished or absent stratum granulosum underlying it (Fig. 5.44) [73]. A resolving plaque of psoriasis shows compact orthokeratosis and return of the granular layer.

Without the presence of spongiform pustules or Munro microabscesses, the diagnosis of psoriasis cannot be made with certainty [71]. Exocytosis of neutrophils is found in 95% of biopsies and aggregations of neutrophils in 31% of biopsies of active psoriatic plaques on the back (Fig. 5.45) [74]. Munro microabscesses were found in 75% of specimens (Fig. 5.46). Griffin and colleagues [75] advanced the concept of "hot spots" of activity showing neutrophil infiltration and other acute histologic changes within a chronic plaque. The acute areas were described as 1–6-mm "islands" that are more elevated, erythematous, and with a more yellowish scale than the surrounding "sea" of chronic psoriasis. The clinical relevance of the hot spots is that a histologic diagnosis is more likely if they are sought for biopsy, they are less responsive to superpotent topical steroids, and they illustrate how the psoriagenic stimulus varies within a single plaque.

SUMMARY

In summary, a fully developed lesion of psoriasis when sampled at the active margin of an enlarging plaque may show these characteristic features:

1 psoriasiform hyperplasia;
2 elongation and edema of dermal papillae;
3 thinned suprapapillary plates with occasional spongiform pustule;
4 absence of the granular layer;
5 continuous parakeratosis;
6 neutrophils in the stratum corneum (Munro microabscesses).

When erythrodermic psoriasis is acute, it usually shows enough of these characteristics to allow the diagnosis to be established [59]. However, exfoliative dermatitis due to any cause including psoriasis frequently shows "chronic dermatitis" or "psoriasiform dermatitis."

In the pustular variants of psoriasis, GPP of von Zumbusch, acrodermatitis continua of Hallopeau, impetigo herpetiformis, and possibly even Reiter's disease the microscopic spongiform pustule of Kogoj enlarges to form a macropustule. The neutrophils aggregate within the interstices of a sponge-like network formed by degenerated and thinned epidermal cells. As the neutrophils move up into the horny layer they become pyknotic and assume the appearance of large Munro abscesses. The epidermal changes are similar to those seen in common psoriasis. In some patients with GPP or annular pustular psoriasis and AGEP the macropustules may assume a subcorneal position, causing some investigators to consider subcorneal pustular dermatosis to be variant of or else highly associated with pustular psoriasis [76]. Older lesions of keratoderma blennorrhagicum may be differentiated from pustular psoriasis by the presence of a greatly thickened horny layer [71].

In patients with localized PPP, some of whom have ordinary psoriasis elsewhere, the fully developed lesion is a large intraepidermal unilocular pustule that is rounded on both sides. Spongiform pustules may be seen in the epidermal walls of the macropustule [70]. The earliest lesion shows spongiosis with mononuclear cells in the lower epidermis and tips of the dermal papillae, followed by an intraepidermal vesicle containing primarily mononuclear cells [77]. As the cavity expands, the stratum corneum becomes the roof, neutrophils invade and transform the vesicopustule into a pustule [78].

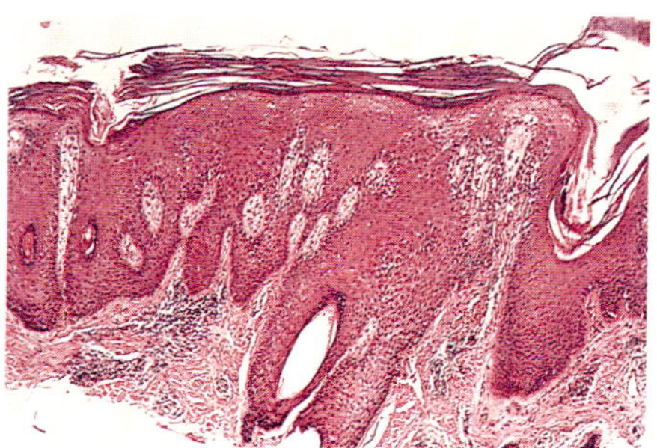

Fig 5.44 Diminution or absence of the stratum granulosum.

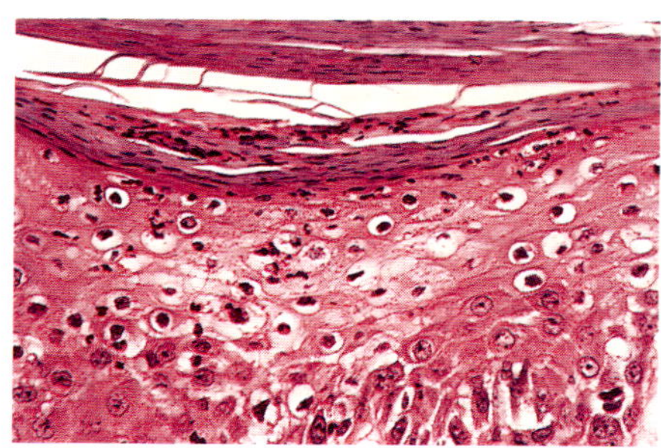

Fig 5.45 Exocytosis of neutrophils and formation of Munro microabscess.

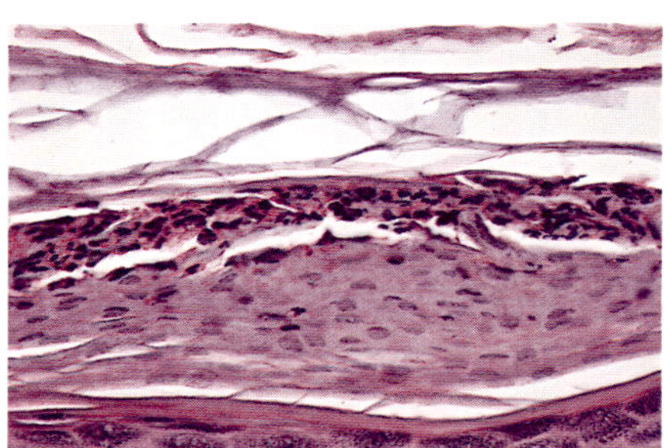

Fig 5.46 High-power view of Munro microabscess.

REFERENCES

1 Farber EM, Nall L. Epidemiology: natural history and genetics. In Roenigk HH Jr, Maibach HI, eds. *Psoriasis*, 2nd edn. New York: Marcel Dekker, Inc., 1991:209–58.

2 Bohm M, Voorhees J, and the Committee on Psoriasis. White paper on hospitalization for psoriasis care. *J Am Acad Dermatol* 1984;10:842–51.

3 Boyd AS, Neldner KH. The isomorphic response of Koebner. *Int J Dermatol* 1990;29:401–10.

4 Heng MCY, Allen SG, Haberfelde G, Song MK. Electron microscopic and immunocytochemical studies of the sequence of events in psoriatic plaque formation following tape-stripping. *Br J Dermatol* 1991;125:548–56.

5 Christophers E, Henseler T. Psoriasis type I and type II as subtypes of nonpustular psoriasis. In Roenigk HH Jr, Maibach HI, eds. *Psoriasis*, 2nd edn. New York: Marcel Dekker, Inc., 1991:15–21.

6 Christophers E, Henseler T. Patient subgroups and the inflammatory pattern in psoriasis. *Acta Derm Venereol* 1989;69(Suppl. 151):88–92.
7 Suarez-Almazor ME, Russell AS. The genetics of psoriasis. *Arch Dermatol* 1990;126:1040–2.
8 Schmitt-Egenolf M, Boehncke WH, Christophers E, *et al.* Type I and Type II psoriasis show a similar usage of T-cell receptor variable regions. *J Invest Dermatol* 1991;97:1053–6.
9 Farber EM. The language of psoriasis. *Int J Dermatol* 1991;30:295–302.
10 Bernhard J. Auspitz sign is not sensitive or specific for psoriasis. *J Am Acad Dermatol* 1990;22:1079–81.
11 Farber EM, Nall L. Perianal and intergluteal psoriasis. *Cutis* 1992;50:336–8.
12 Farber EM, Nall L. Genital psoriasis. *Cutis* 1992;50:263–6.
13 Baker H, Wilkinson DS. Psoriasis. In Rook A, Wilkinson DS, Ebling FJG, eds. *Textbook of Dermatology*, 3rd edn. Oxford: Blackwell Scientific Publications, 1979:1328.
14 Shupack JL, Gold JA, Stiller MJ, Orbuch P. *Dermatologic Formulary Skin and Cancer Unit New York University*. New York: McGraw-Hill, 1989.
15 Nanda A, Kaur S, Kaur I, Kumar B. Childhood psoriasis: an epidemiologic survey of 112 patients. *Pediatr Dermatol* 1990;7:19–21.
16 Barker JNWN. The pathophysiology of psoriasis. *Lancet* 1991;338:227–30.
17 Henderson CA, Highet AS. Acute psoriasis associated with Lancefield group C and group G cutaneous streptococcal infections. *Br J Dermatol* 1988;118:559–62.
18 Telfer NR, Chalmers RJ, Whale K, Colman G. The role of streptococcal infection in the initiation of guttate psoriasis. *Arch Dermatol* 1992;128:39–42.
19 McFadden J, Valdimarsson H, Fry L. Cross-reactivity between streptococcal M surface antigen and human skin. *Br J Dermatol* 1991;125:443–7.
20 Rosenberg EW, Noah PW, Zanolli MD, *et al.* Use of rifampin with penicillin and erythromycin in the treatment of psoriasis. Preliminary report. *J Am Acad Dermatol* 1986;14:761–4.
21 Vincent F, Ross JB, Dalton M, Wort AJ. A therapeutic trial of the use of penicillin V or erythromycin with or without rifampin in the treatment of psoriasis. *J Am Acad Dermatol* 1992;26:458–61.
22 Baker BS, Powles AV, Malkani AK, *et al.* Altered cell-mediated immunity to group A haemoloytic streptococcal antigens in chronic plaque psoriasis. *Br J Dermatol* 1991;125:38–42.
23 Powell F, Young M, Barnes J. Psoriasis in Ireland. *Ir J Med Sci* 1982;151:109–13.
24 Hubler WR Jr. Familial juvenile generalized pustular psoriasis. *Arch Dermatol* 1984;120:1174–8.
25 Sneddon IB, Wilkinson DS. Subcorneal pustulosis dermatosis. *Br J Dermatol* 1956;68:385–94.
26 Zelickson BD, Muller SA. Generalized pustular psoriasis. A review of 63 cases. *Arch Dermatol* 1991;127:1339–45.
27 Baker H, Ryan TJ. Generalized pustular psoriasis: a clinical and epidemiologic study of 104 cases. *Br J Dermatol* 1968;80:771–93.
28 Ryan TJ, Baker H. Systemic corticosteroids and folic acid antagonists in the treatment of generalized pustular psoriasis. Evaluation and prognosis based on the study of 104 cases. *Br J Dermatol* 1969;81:134–45.
29 Ryan TJ, Baker H. The prognosis of generalized pustular psoriasis. *Br J Dermatol* 1971;85:407–11.
30 Szanto E, Linse U. Arthropathy associated with palmoplantar pustulosis. *Clin Rheumatol* 1991;10:130–5.
31 Lindelof B, Beitner H. The effect of grenz ray therapy on pustulosis palmoplantaris. A double-blind bilateral trial. *Acta Derm Venereol* 1990;70:529–31.
32 Reitamo S, Erkko P, Remitz A. Cyclosporin for palmoplantar pustulosis. *J Autoimmun* 1992;5(Suppl. A):285–7.

33 White SI, Puttick L, Marks JM. Low-dose etretinate in the maintenance of remission of palmoplantar pustular psoriasis. *Br J Dermatol* 1986;115:577–82.
34 Schroder K, Zaun H, Holzmann H, *et al.* Pustulosis palmo-plantaris. Clinical and histological changes during etretin (acitretin) therapy. *Acta Derm Venereol* 1989; Suppl. 146:111–6.
35 Lassus A, Geiger J-M. Acitretin and etretinate in the treatment of palmoplantar pustulosis: a double-blind comparative trial. *Br J Dermatol* 1988;119:755–9.
36 Rosen, K, Mobacken H, Swanbeck G. PUVA, etretinate, and PUVA-etretinate therapy for pustulosis palmoplantaris. *Arch Dermatol* 1987;123:885–9.
37 Miyagawa S, Muramatsu T, Shirai T. Generalization of palmoplantar pustulosis after withdrawal of etretinate. *J Am Acad Dermatol* 1991;24:305–6.
38 Goette DK, Morgan AM, Fox BJ, Horn RT. Treatment of palmoplantar pustulosis with intralesional triamcinolone injections. *Arch Dermatol* 1984;120:319–23.
39 Volden G. Successful treatment of chronic skin diseases with clobetasol propionate on a hydrocolloid occlusive dressing. *Acta Derm Venereol* 1992;72:69–71.
40 Stewart AF, Battaglini-Sabetta J, Millstone L. Hypocalcemia-induced pustular psoriasis of von Zumbusch. *Ann Intern Med* 1984;100:677–80.
41 Moynihan GD, Ruppe JP Jr. Impetigo herpetiformis and hypoparathyroidism. *Arch Dermatol* 1985;121:1330–1.
42 Moy RL, Kingston TP, Lowe NJ. Isotretinoin vs etretinate therapy in generalized pustular and chronic psoriasis. *Arch Dermatol* 1985;121:1297–301.
43 Dlugosz A. Pustular psoriasis and cyclosporin. *Int J Dermatol* 1988;27:205.
44 McFadyen, Lyell A. Successful treatment of generalized pustular psoriasis (von Zumbusch) by systemic antibiotics controlled by blood culture. *Br J Dermatol* 1971;85:274–6.
45 Judge MR, McDonald A, Black MM. Pustular psoriasis in childhood. *Clin Exp Dermatol* 1993;18:97–9.
46 Zelickson BD, Muller SA. Generalized pustular psoriasis in childhood. Report of thirteen cases. *J Am Acad Dermatol* 1991;24:186–94.
47 Takematsu H, Rokugo M, Takahashik, Tagami H. Juvenile generalized pustular psoriasis in a pair of monozygotic twins presenting strikingly similar clinical courses. *Acta Derm Venereol* 1992;72:443–4.
48 Winton GB, Lewis CW. Dermatoses of pregnancy. *J Am Acad Dermatol* 1983;6:977–98.
49 Lotem M, Katzenelson V, Rtoem A, *et al.* Impetigo herpetiformis: a variant of pustular psoriasis or a separate entity? *J Am Acad Dermatol* 1989;20:338–41.
50 Ternowitz T. Monocyte and neutrophil chemotaxis in psoriasis. Relation to the clinical status and the type of psoriasis. *J Am Acad Dermatol* 1986;15:1191–9.
51 Lundin A, Hakansson L, Hallgren R, *et al.* Studies on the phagocytic activity of the granulocytes in psoriasis and palmoplantar pustulosis. *Br J Dermatol* 1983;109:539–74.
52 Kaminski M, Szmurlo A, Pawinska M, Jablonska S. Decreased natural killer cell activity in generalized pustular psoriasis (von Zumbusch type). *Br J Dermatol* 1984;110:565–8.
53 Sauder DN, Steck WD, Bailin PB, Krakauer RS. Lymphocyte kinetics in pustular psoriasis. *J Am Acad Dermatol* 1981;4:458–60.
54 Tagami H, Juatsuki K, Iwase Y, Yamada M. Subcorneal pustular dermatosis with vesiculobullous eruption. Demonstration of subcorneal IgA deposits and a leukocyte chemotactic factor. *Br J Dermatol* 1983;109:581–7.
55 McGregor JM, Barker JN, MacDonald DM. Pulmonary capillary leak syndrome complicating generalized pustular psoriasis: possible role of cytokines. *Br J Dermatol* 1991;125:472–4.
56 Murphy FR, Stolman LP. Generalized pustular psoriasis. *Arch Dermatol* 1979;115:1215–6.
57 Matsumura N, Takematsu H, Saijo S, *et al.* Exanthematic type of pustular psoriasis

consisting of two types of pustular lesion. *Acta Derm Venereol* 1991;71:442–4.

58 Roujeau J-C, Bioulac-Sage P, Bourseau C, *et al.* Acute generalized exanthematous pustulosis. Analysis of 63 cases. *Arch Dermatol* 1991;127:1333–8.

59 Abrahams J, McCarthy JT, Sanders SL. 101 cases of exfoliative dermatitis. *Arch Dermatol* 1963;87:96–101.

60 Hurley HJ. Papulosquamous eruptions and exfoliative dermatitis. In Moschella SL, Pillsbury DM, Hurley HJ, eds. *Dermatology*. Philadelphia: WB Saunders, 1975:449.

61 Boyd AS, Menter A. Erythrodermic psoriasis. Precipitating factors, course, and prognosis in 50 patients. *J Am Acad Dermatol* 1989;21:985–91.

62 Wolfe F, Cathey MA. The misdiagnosis of gout and hyperuricemia. *J Rheumatol* 1991;18:1232–4.

63 McElhenny BE, Todd DJ, McCance D, *et al.* Erythrodermic psoriasis. Report of a case associated with symptomatic hypophosphatemia. *Clin Exp Dermatol* 1993; 18:167–8.

64 Takayasu S, Fujiwara S, Waki T. Hereditary lactate dehydrogenase M-subunit deficiency: lactate dehydrogenase activity in skin lesions and in hair follicles. *J Am Acad Dermatol* 1991;24:339–42.

65 Pindborg JJ. *Atlas of Diseases of the Oral Mucosa*, 4th edn. Philadelphia: WB Saunders, 1985.

66 Pogrel MA, Cram D. Intraoral findings in patients with psoriasis with a special reference to ectopic geographic tongue (erythema circinata). *Oral Surg* 1988;66:184–9.

67 Morris LF, Phillips CM, Binnie WH, *et al.* Oral lesions in patients with psoriasis: a controlled study. *Cutis* 1992;49:339–44.

68 Zunt SL, Tomich CE. Erythema migrans–a psoriasiform lesion of the oral mucosa. *J Dermatol Surg Oncol* 1989;15:1067–70.

69 Espelid M, Bang G, Johannessen AC, *et al.* Geographic stomatitis: report of 6 cases. *J Oral Pathol Med* 1991;20:425–8.

70 Ackerman AB. *Histologic Diagnosis of Inflammatory Skin Diseases*. Philadelphia: Lea & Febiger, 1978.

71 Lever WF, Schaumburg-Lever G. *Histopathology of the Skin*, 6th edn. Philadelphia: JB Lippincott, 1983.

72 Ackerman AB, Ragaz A. *The Lives of Lesions. Chronology in Dermatopathology*. New York: Masson, 1984.

73 Cox AJ, Watson W. Histologic variations in lesions of psoriasis. *Arch Dermatol* 1972;106:503–6.

74 Gordon M, Johnson WC. Histopathology and histochemistry of psoriasis. I. The active lesion and clinically normal skin. *Arch Dermatol* 1967;95:402–7.

75 Griffin TD, Lattanand A, Van Scott EJ. Clinical heterogeneity of psoriatic plaques. Therapeutic relevance. *Arch Dermatol* 1988;124:216–20.

76 Sanchez NP, Perry HO, Muller SA, Winkelmann PK. Subcorneal pustular dermatosis: a clinico-pathologic correlation. *Arch Dermatol* 1983;119:715–21.

77 Uehara M, Ofuji S. The morphogenesis of pustulosis palmaris et plantaris. *Arch Dermatol* 1974;109:518–20.

78 Pierard J, Kint A. La pustulose palmo-plantaire chronique et recidivante. Etude histologique. *Ann Dermatol Venereol* 1978;105:681–8.

six

Psoriasis of the Scalp

Thomas N. Helm and Charles Camisa

INTRODUCTION

Psoriasis of the scalp may occur with or without cutaneous involvement elsewhere. Although scalp psoriasis may be concealed by the hair in mild cases, severe cases can cause discomfort, embarrassment, and emotional distress to patients. Concomitant pruritus, hair loss, or secondary infection may prompt patients to seek medical attention. This chapter will address the clinical manifestations of scalp psoriasis and its treatment.

EPIDEMIOLOGY

Although it is difficult to ascertain exact figures, most patients with generalized plaque-type psoriasis will develop scalp involvement at some time during their lives. Scalp involvement may be less common in guttate psoriasis, but pustular and erythrodermic psoriasis may have a higher incidence of scalp involvement. Only rarely does scalp psoriasis occur in the absence of other cutaneous findings. Overall, it has been estimated that scalp involvement occurs in at least 50% of patients with psoriasis [1].

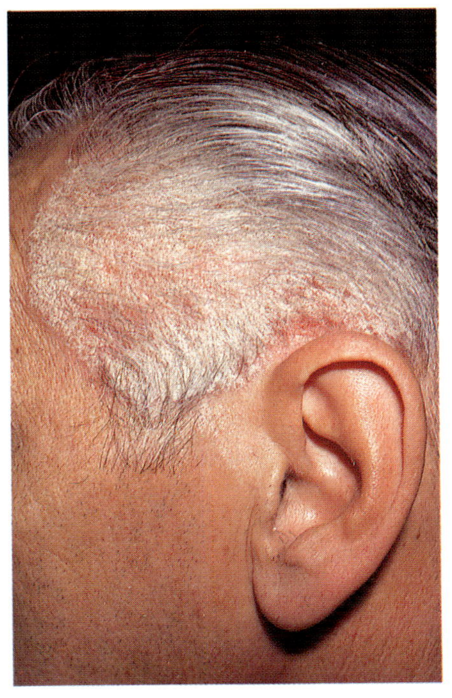

Fig 6.1 Typical psoriasis of the scalp sharply limited to the hair-bearing area.

CLINICAL FINDINGS

The cutaneous changes of scalp psoriasis range from thick adherent micaceous scale, which demonstrates Auspitz's sign on manipulation, to fine furfuraceous scale (Fig. 6.1). Scalp psoriasis may extend beyond the hairline on to the forehead (Fig. 6.2). This finding may be useful in differentiating scalp psoriasis from severe seborrheic dermatitis, which is typically limited by the hairline (Fig. 6.3). The scale of psoriasis often has a powdery consistency and silvery sheen (Fig. 6.4) whereas the scale of seborrheic dermatitis typically appears yellow and greasy. Involvement of the posterior auricular crease with scaling and fissuring is common in psoriasis (Fig. 6.5), although involvement in this location may also occur in other dermatoses, especially seborrheic dermatitis. The morphologic entity known as pityriasis (tinea) amiantacea consists of asbestos-like scales adhering to

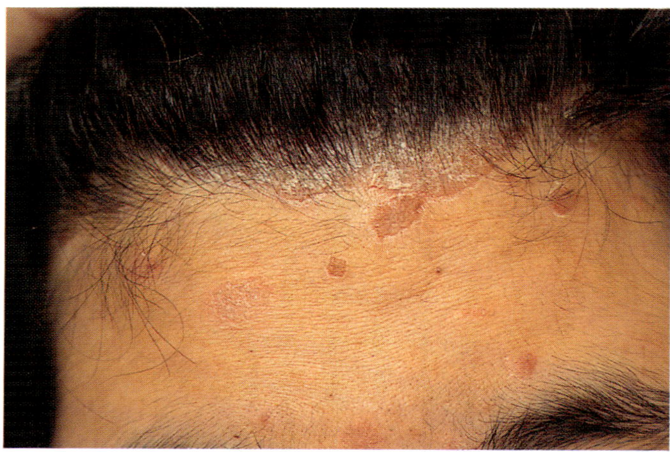

Fig 6.2 Psoriasis extends beyond hairline on to the forehead.

the scalp and hair shafts and may be an early manifestation of psoriasis (Fig. 6.6).

The differential diagnosis of scaling plaques on the scalp includes: (i) papulosquamous disorders such as lichen planus, allergic or irritant eczema, atopic dermatitis; (ii) infectious or granulomatous causes such as tinea capitis, tertiary syphilis, deep fungal diseases, and sarcoidosis; (iii) neoplastic diseases such as mycosis fungoides, B-cell lymphoma, and histiocytosis-X; and (iv) connective tissue diseases such as lupus erythematosus. Usually, associated cutaneous findings or a history of prior skin disease allow for ready differentiation among these entities. Scalp psoriasis may be accompanied by nail pitting or onycholysis, which are valuable clues to the correct diagnosis. If scaling of the scalp is diffuse, seborrheic dermatitis is more likely. Microscopic examination of scale digested by 10% potassium hydroxide is useful to exclude dermatophyte infection, and culture for fungal organisms, and serologic testing for syphilis may also be useful adjunctive tests in certain situations. Psoriasis of the scalp is frequently accompanied by pruritus, but this is true for most of the other disorders which may mimic psoriasis. Occasionally, a biopsy must be performed to confirm the diagnosis of scalp psoriasis, especially in cases where there is

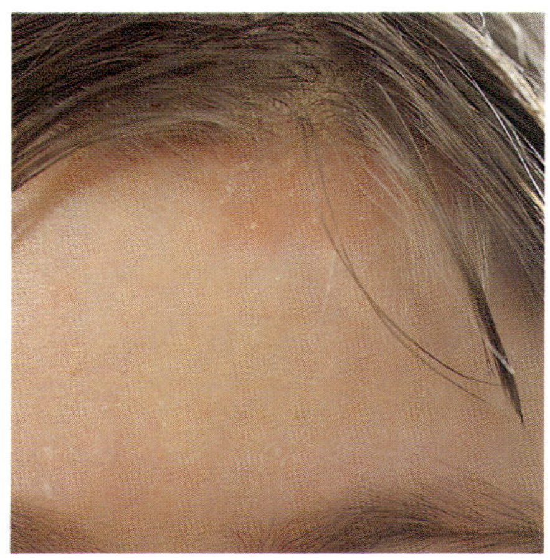

Fig 6.3 Scalp psoriasis in a child. The scale appears yellowish but the lesion extends well on to the forehead.

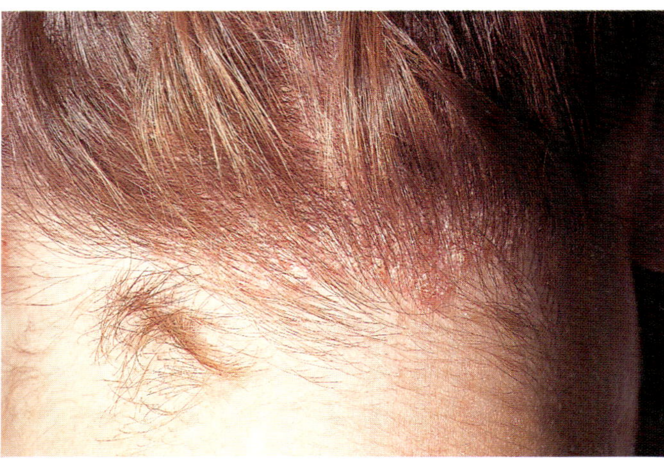

Fig 6.4 The silvery scales of psoriasis.

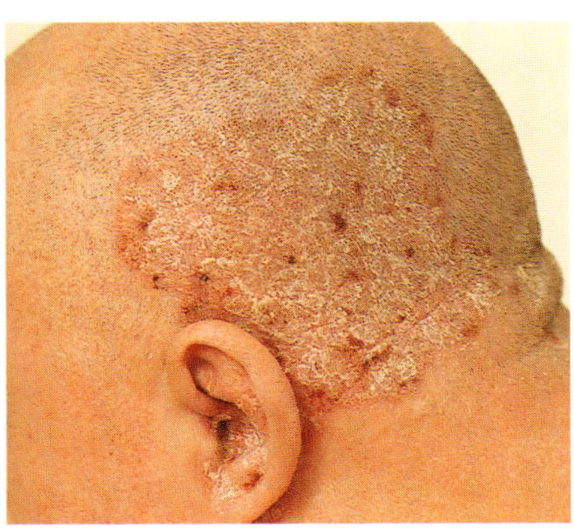

Fig 6.5 Psoriasis of the scalp involves ear and posterior auricular area. The patient shaved his head in order that natural sunlight could improve his skin.

significant hair loss, scarring, or when malignant infiltrations are diagnostic possibilities.

Biopsy of the scalp is readily achieved by the punch biopsy technique. A 4 mm specimen will usually suffice, so long as care has been taken to orient the punch parallel to the hairs exiting the scalp. Although epidermal changes are diagnostic for psoriasis, excision of the biopsy material with iris scissors at the level of the deep subcutaneous fat underneath the hair bulbs will ensure that an adequate specimen has been obtained so that other possible entities can be ruled out.

HISTOPATHOLOGY

Routine histopathologic examination typically reveals acanthosis with club-shaped rete pegs and tortuous vessels in the papillary dermis. The granular layer is diminished or absent and the epidermis often appears pale. Parakeratosis is confluent and neutrophils are often present in focal collections in the stratum corneum. Spongiform pustules with neutrophils may also be found in the epidermis. Although mounds of parakeratosis are seen in psoriasis, mounds of parakeratosis flanking follicular openings are suggestive of seborrheic dermatitis, especially when associated with spongiosis of the infundibulum. Atypical lymphocytes and histiocytic cells (Langerhans cells) are seen infiltrating the dermis and epidermis in mycosis fungoides and histiocytosis-X, respectively.

A new approach to scalp biopsy involves processing of tissue by horizontal sections, thereby increasing the number of hair follicles studied. A study of involved and uninvolved scalp in 28 psoriatic patients was performed by this method, and revealed no evidence of alopecia in involved scalp [2]; however, hair follicles may have been smaller with a decreased hair shaft size. Sebaceous glands were also decreased in size.

Light microscopy of hair bulbs obtained by hair plucks in 22 patients and normal controls revealed increased percentages of telogen and catagen hairs in psoriatic plaques compared to uninvolved areas and normal controls [3]. These results suggest that a localized or diffuse telogen effluvium may occur in some patients with scalp psoriasis. Another study of 47

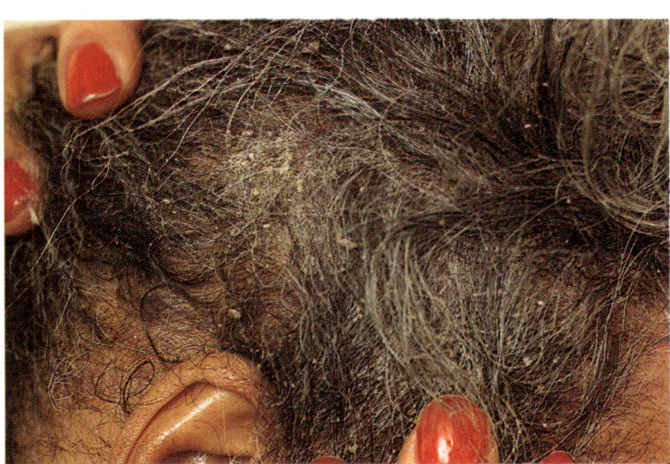

Fig 6.6 Adherent, thick scales suggest pityriasis amiantacea, but the patient has typical psoriasis elsewhere.

patients with scalp psoriasis and symptomatic hair loss found the telogen count to be increased by 25–86% in the florid stage [4].

While scarring alopecia is not usually a component of scalp psoriasis, studies of patients with psoriasis and alopecia suggest that scarring may at times be associated with psoriasis [4,5]. Elliptical biopsies through the borders of alopecic plaques demonstrated chronic inflammatory cells around the follicular infundibulum, and in one case also revealed acute folliculitis. The acute folliculitis may have been secondary to a staphylococcal infection. Wet mount and culture revealed no evidence of fungus. The authors conclude that psoriasis should be considered an inflammatory disease in which scarring alopecia can be seen as a nonspecific secondary finding. Another recent case report also indicates that chronic and severe scalp psoriasis may eventuate in residual scarring alopecia [6].

ETIOLOGY

The etiology of scalp psoriasis is unknown, although the condition seems to be aggravated by microbial organisms. *Pityrosporum ovale* and *Streptococcus pyogenes* have been implicated as organisms that might trigger the alternate complement pathway and stimulate the development of psoriatic plaques [7]. As in the other forms of psoriasis, HLA antigens Cw6, HLA-B16, B18, and B27 are found in a higher percentage than in the population at large. Whether these HLA antigens are associated with genes that produce an excessive inflammatory response to infectious organisms or are merely incidental findings is unclear.

Studies of follicular kinetics in psoriatic scalp have demonstrated unaltered hair growth in unaffected versus lesional skin [8]. The percentage of cells in the S-phase in nonlesional follicular infundibulum of psoriasis is increased compared to normal controls [9]. This is in keeping with cutaneous psoriasis in which the epidermal turnover time is sharply reduced. Compulsive and subconscious scratching or rubbing of scalp psoriasis may induce the isomorphic response and perpetuation of lesions.

TREATMENT

A variety of treatments may prove helpful in controlling scalp psoriasis, but no single treatment is consistently effective. The most commonly used treatments include shampoos, keratolytics, tar derivatives, antibiotics and antifungal agents, corticosteroid preparations, X-ray therapy, softening agents such as mineral oil, and systemic medications such as methotrexate, cyclosporine, PUVA, and retinoids. These agents will be reviewed in a sequential manner with reference to commonly available products. The subsections are arranged in order of decreasing popularity.

Mechanical debridement

Shampoos are liquid formulations, usually sodium or potassium salts of fatty acids, which act as anionic surfactants. Although simple soaps and mild detergents with surfactants may be used alone in the treatment of mild scalp psoriasis, formulations with additives like selenium sulfide, zinc pyrithione, chloroxine, sulfur, or salicylic acid often help speed clinical improvement (Table 6.1). Agents such as menthol may be added to combat pruritus. Coal tars are useful additives in disorders of keratinization because epidermal proliferation is inhibited [10] and because of their antipruritic effects. Selenium sulfide has substantivity, meaning it remains on the skin and hair after shampooing. Selenium sulfide inhibits mitosis of keratinocytes, thereby controlling hyperproliferation. It also inhibits the growth of *Pityrosporum* spores. Ketoconazole shampoo 2% also inhibits growth of *Pityrosporum* and has proven useful in the treatment of scalp psoriasis as well as seborrheic dermatitis. Pyrithione zinc shampoos have substantivity and inhibit proliferation of keratinocytes, but have the advantage of causing less irritation of the skin than tar or selenium sulfide products. Therapeutic shampoos are usually lathered into the scalp and left in place for 5–10 min before thorough rinsing. Tar shampoos may discolor light or gray hair.

Adjunctive treatment, with a shampoo machine may lead to rapid improvement of scalp psoriasis in the hospital or psoriasis day-care setting, while freeing up nursing time (Fig. 6.7). The machine consists of a chamber that encloses the scalp which is then exposed to a high-pressure liquid jet that contains water plus the therapeutic shampoo. It may be valuable for scale reduction. Steck [11] has found that 89% of patients preferred treatment by the Aquatura Shampoo machine, and that fewer telogen hairs were found in the machine filtrate than after ordinary hand shampooing. We have found the Aquatura Shampoo machine to be of limited benefit and use it mainly to insure thorough shampooing in noncompliant patients.

Keratolytics

Many topical agents influence the build up of scale. The most widely used keratolytic agents in dermatology include urea, propylene glycol, resorcinol, and salicylic acid (Table 6.2). Salicylic acid is added to shampoo and lotion products to help control flaking of the scalp, but may also be applied directly to the scalp. If widespread areas are treated, salicylism may result.

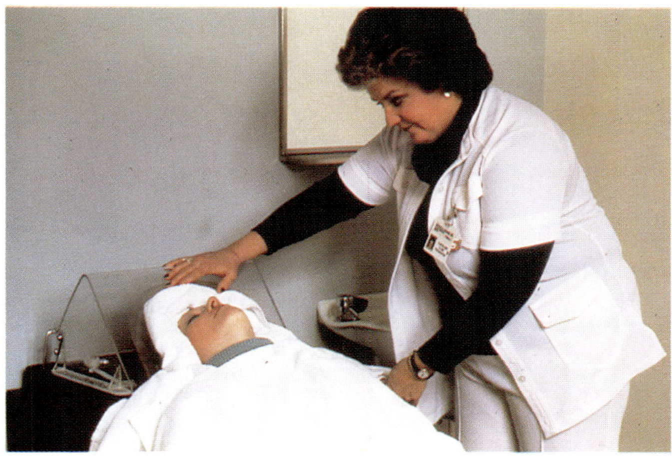

Fig 6.7 The scalp is being washed with a tar shampoo using the Aquatura shampoo machine.

Table 6.1 Common antipsoriatic shampoos

Capitrol: Chloroxine 2%, 4 oz bottle

Danex: Pyrithione zinc 1%, 4 oz bottle

Denorex (Regular and mountain fresh herbal): coal tar solution 9 and 1.5% menthol (extra strength and extra strength with conditioners); 12.55 coal tar and 1.5% menthol, 4, 8, and 12 oz bottles

DHS tar shampoo: 0.5% coal tar, 4, 8, and 16 oz bottles

DHS zinc dandruff shampoo: 2% pyrithione zinc, 6 and 12 oz bottles

Doak: 3% coal tar

Exsel: 2.5% selenium sulfide lotion, 120 ml

Head and Shoulders: 1% pyrithione zinc lotion, 4, 7, 11 and 15 oz bottles; "Normal to Dry Scalp," 7, 11, 15 oz bottles

Head and Shoulders Intensive Treatment: 1% selenium sulfide in surfactant base, 4, 7, 11 oz bottles

Ionil T Coal Tar Solution: salicylic acid; Ionil T Plus 2% Crude Coal Tar (Owentar II)

Iosel 250: selenium sulfide 2.5% lotion, 240 ml bottle

Nizoral Shampoo: 2% ketoconazole

P&S liquid: mineral oil, glycerin, and phenol, 4 and 8 oz bottles

P&S Plus Tar Gel: 8% coal tar solution (1.6% crude coal tar, 6.4% ethyl alcohol), 2% salicylic acid, 3.5 oz tube

Sebulex: 2% sulfur, 2% salicylic acid, 4 and 8 oz bottles

Sebutone: 0.5% coal tar, 2% salicylic acid, and 2% sulfur, 4 and 8 oz bottles

Selsun Blue: selenium sulfide 1% (Dry, Oily, Normal, Extra Conditioning); extramedicated also contains 0.5% menthol, 4 and 11 oz bottles

T/Gel: 2% coal tar solution

Tegrin: 5% coal tar solution, concentrated gel 2.5 oz tube, lotion 3.75 and 6.6 oz bottles

Vanseb: salicylic acid 1%, sulfur 2%, 3 oz tube or 4 oz bottle

Vanseb-T: salicylic acid 1%, sulfur 2%, coal tar solution USP 5%, 3 oz tube or 4 oz bottle

X-seb shampoo: 4% salicylic acid, 4 oz bottle

X-seb Plus: 1% pyrithione zinc, 2% salicylic acid, 4 oz bottle

X-seb T: 10% coal tar solution (2% crude coal tar, 8% ethyl alcohol), 4% salicylic acid, X-seb T Plus 10% coal tar solution (2% crude coal tar, 3% salicylic acid, 1% menthol), 4 oz bottle

Zincon: 1% pyrithione zinc, 4 and 8 oz bottles

ZNP Bar Shampoo: 2% zinc pyrithione

Table 6.2 Commonly used salicylic acid products

Hydrisalic Gel: 6% salicylic acid, 30 g
Keralyt Gel: 6% salicylic acid, 60% propylene glycol, 30 g
Saligel: 5% salicylic acid
Ureacin Lotion: 10% salicylic acid, 30, 75, 240 g

This may occur because salicylic acid is well absorbed through the skin, but renal secretion is slow.

Epilyt® has been recommended for scalp psoriasis, and leads to improvement within 2 weeks when applied under a shower cap overnight [12]. We have found Baker's P&S liquid to be quite effective when used in a similar fashion. The full regimen consists of a morning shampoo followed by the application of a corticosteroid lotion, which helps to reduce inflammation and control pruritus.

For recalcitrant heavy crusts in the scalp, the dermatologists at the Mayo Clinic advocate a preparation consisting of 20% oil of Cade (juniper wood tar), 10% sulfur, and 5% salicylic acid in a water-soluble base, thoroughly rubbing it into the scalp. Some patients find the odor of oil of Cade offensive, but the product is reportedly beneficial [13].

Topical tar

The efficacy of tar products in psoriasis has been recognized for many years (Table 6.3). The mechanism by which tar products work is not well understood. Antibacterial, antifungal, vasoconstrictive, and keratolytic effects as well as suppression of epidermal DNA synthesis have all been claimed. Use of these products may lead to folliculitis, and the odor of crude coal tar is unmistakable, making compliance with tar therapy difficult in some patients.

In one study topical tar products alone led to improvement in up to 75% of patients within 6 weeks of beginning treatment [14]. Coal tar solution in gel form (Psorigel) was applied to plaques for 5 days of the week, with only mineral oil application on the sixth day and no treatment on the seventh day. Use of a tar shampoo (Ionil T) increased the time interval between relapses.

Tar oils are also used in the Goeckerman regimen. A combination of Nivea Oil, 3% salicylic acid, and 20% liquor carbonis detergens was popular in the past, but now because of a change in Nivea Oil formulation, the mixture will not support the addition of salicylic acid. An alternative solution can be made by adding 4 ml of polysorbate 80 and 13 ml coal tar emulsion (Zetar) to each 100 ml of New Improved Nivea Oil [15]. Applied nightly under a shower cap, this product loosens scale and controls psoriatic plaques. The mixture is massaged into the scalp by parting the hair every 1 cm until the entire scalp is covered.

Table 6.3 Commonly used tar formulations

Liquid formulations
Alphosyl Lotion: 1% crude coal tar, 1.7% allantoin
Doak Tar Lotion: 5% tar distillate
Oxipor Lotion: 48.5% tar, benzocaine, salicylic acid, 30 and 60 ml
P&S Plus: 8% coal tar solution, 2% salicylic acid, 3.5 oz
T/Derm Lotion: 5% crude coal tar, 120 ml
Tegrin Lotion: 5% crude coal tar
Zetar Emulsion: 300 mg coal tar/ml, 6 oz
Gel formulations
Aquatar: 0.5% crude coal tar, 90 g tube
Estar Gel: 5% crude coal tar, 90 g tube
P&S Plus 1.6% crude coal tar, 2% salicylic acid, 105 g
Psorigel: 1.5% crude coal tar, 120 g

Anthralin

Anthralin is a derivative of the South American araroba tree [16]. It has antimitotic activity [17] but frequently causes irritation when used in concentrations higher than 0.1%. Anthralin causes a brown-red discoloration of the skin and scalp, and may cause a yellow discoloration of hair. Application to chronic scalp plaques for 8–12 hours may prove very helpful (Table 6.4), but application to acute, exudative, or highly inflamed plaques should generally be avoided.

Anthralin pomade, consisting of anthralin 0.4%, salicylic acid 0.4%, mineral oil 76%, cetyl alcohol 21.1%, and sodium lauryl sulfate 2.1% may be beneficial [18]. Shampoo can be used for removal. With this regimen, patients' scalps cleared more quickly than other areas. Anthralin is now not widely used, mainly because of irritation and discoloration of skin and light hair.

Corticosteroid preparations

Because corticosteroid products are effective, cosmetically elegant, and generally odorless, they have overtaken tar products in the treatment of scalp psoriasis (Table 6.5). If these products are used for long periods of time in an uninterrupted fashion, tachyphylaxis may occur, that is, a decreased therapeutic response is seen with the same dose of medication that was previously effective [19]. Also, newer high potency products have

Table 6.4 Anthralin or dithranol preparations

Anthra-Derm Ointment: 0.1%, 0.25%, 0.5%, 1% (42.5 g tube)
Anthranol: 0.1%, 0.2%, 0.4% (Canada)
Anthraforte: 1%, 2%, 3% (Canada)
Drithocreme: 0.1%, 0.25%, 0.5%, 1%, 50 g
Dritho Scalp: 0.25% and 0.5%, 50 g

Table 6.5 Corticosteroid scalp solutions and sprays

Aeroseb-Dex: 0.01% dexamethasone (alcohol 59%)
Barseb-HC: 1% hydrocortisone, 0.5% salicylic acid, 52 ml bottle
Cortaid/Rhulicort: 0.5% hydrocortisone acetate lotion
Cyclocort Lotion: 0.1% amcinonide, 20 and 60 ml
Decaspray (dexamethasone spray): 25 g pressurized container
Dermovate: 0.05% clobetasol propionate (Canada)
Diprolene Lotion: 0.05% betamethasone dipropionate
Elocon Lotion: 0.1% mometasone furoate, 30 and 60 ml bottles
Emo-Cort Scalp Solution: 2.5% hydrocortisone
Kenalog Lotion/Spray: 0.025% triamcinolone acetonide, 60 ml bottle, 23 and 63 g cans
Lidex: 0.05% fluocinonide solution, 20 and 60 ml bottles
Maxivate: 0.05% betamethasone dipropionate, 60 ml bottle
Penecort: 1% hydrocortisone (alcohol 57%)
Synalar Fluonid Solution: 0.01% fluocinolone acetonide, 20 and 60 ml bottles
Temovate Solution: 0.05% clobetasol propionate, 25 and 50 ml bottles
Texacort Scalp Solution: 1% hydrocortisone (alcohol 33%)
Uticort: 0.025% betamethasone benzoate

the possibility of causing hypothalamic–pituitary–adrenal suppression, even if used on only a limited part of the body [20]. Nonetheless, if used prudently, these products can quickly bring most cases of extensive scalp psoriasis under control.

High potency corticosteroids may not always offer much more clinical benefit when compared to less potent products in the Stoughton classification. When desoximetasone gel 0.05% was compared to fluocinonide gel 0.05% for the treatment of scalp psoriasis, comparable improvement was seen in both groups [21]. On the other hand, two products of the same potency classification may give differing results. Patients treated with an alcoholic solution of clobetasol propionate 0.05% had greater improvement in erythema, itching, and scaling after 2 weeks than those treated with the betamethasone-17,21 dipropionate 0.05% [22]. Folliculitis on the forehead was noted only in patients treated with betamethasone dipropionate. These studies indicate that one cannot always predict improvement in scalp psoriasis by a corticosteroid product merely by knowing its potency rating. Also, certain products within a single class may cause more side effects than others.

Initial therapy with a midpotency topical corticosteroid product seems most prudent. Patients should be advised to shampoo the hair and then apply the corticosteroid solution while the scalp is still damp, thereby enhancing absorption. Shower cap occlusion may be useful in selected cases, but is generally not necessary. Once daily application suffices in most cases. More extensive cases may require twice daily application, or application of a keratolytic gel containing salicylic acid to remove scales and improve absorption. If psoriasis is severe, many patients benefit from a regimen in which topical corticosteroids are used nightly for 1–2 weeks, and tar solutions are used on alternate weeks. One popular regimen is to use a keratolytic product (e.g., Epilyt or Baker's P&S) overnight with corticosteroid lotion in the morning until thick scale has been debrided. A combination product such as Derma-Smoothe-FS which contains peanut oil, isopropyl alcohol, and fluocinolone acetonide 0.01% can then be used nightly as needed thereafter.

In selected resistant cases where only a few, small, discrete plaques remain on the scalp, intralesional injections of triamcinolone acetonide suspension (5 mg/ml) may be extremely helpful in temporarily clearing psoriasis locally, sometimes for many months.

Antibiotics and antifungal agents

The role of microbial agents in psoriasis is uncertain. *Pityrosporum ovale* has been implicated in the etiology of scalp psoriasis, and oral ketoconazole appears to be of benefit [23]. In a randomized, double-blind study of oral ketoconazole 400 mg daily vs placebo, complete remission of the scalp lesions was reported in three of six ketoconazole-treated patients [24]. Placebo-treated patients experienced no improvement. Whether the effect of ketoconazole is due to its antifungal properties or its effect on follicular keratinization remains to be shown. Ketoconazole shampoo is now widely available and may prove to be an alternative to oral ketoconazole therapy. Unlike oral ketoconazole, hepatotoxicity would not be expected with the topical formulation.

Grenz ray therapy

Grenz ray therapy is a very effective way to control scalp psoriasis. The addition of topical corticosteroids to a course of grenz ray therapy seems to offer little additional benefit. Effective treatment may be given with the grenz ray machine set at 10 kV, 10 mA, and a half value layer of 0.3 mm aluminum, with a target skin distance of 10 cm and a half value depth of 0.5 mm [25]. Four hundred rads given weekly for 6 weeks leads to improvement. When given by experienced clinicians and recommended total doses of 1000 rads are not exceeded, this is a safe and effective alternative to cumbersome topical treatments. At higher doses of radiation or in rare disorders such as the nevoid basal cell carcinoma syndrome or xeroderma pigmentosum, carcinogenesis becomes a serious concern.

Surgery

Dellon [26] has reported improvement in one patient who underwent serial dermatomal shaving of the scalp to the level of the reticular dermis. The treated areas remained in remission 4½ years later.

Systemic therapy

Treatment with systemic agents such as methotrexate, retinoids, cyclosporine, and vitamin D_3, which are covered in separate chapters, all lead to improvement in scalp psoriasis. Transient alopecia may, however, result from some of these medications, particularly the retinoids. UVB phototherapy can control scalp psoriasis advancing beyond the frontal hairline if the hair is held or tied back during treatment. If the scalp hair is fine-textured and of decreased density as in androgenetic alopecia, both UVB or PUVA phototherapy may be of benefit in clearing scalp psoriasis. A hand-held UVA/UVB irradiation source is commercially available (Dermalight Psora-Comb, Studio City, CA) which has a removable comb for parting the hair.

SUMMARY

Scalp involvement is a very common problem which can be troubling to psoriasis patients. Although the etiology of scalp psoriasis is unclear, many effective treatments are available for its control. Judicious use of these agents can lead to remission of scalp disease with a minimum of side effects.

REFERENCES

1 Lowe NJ. Therapy of scalp psoriasis. *Dermatol Clin* 1984;2:471–6.
2 Headington JT, Gupta AK, Goldfarb M, *et al.* A morphometric and histologic study of the scalp in psoriasis. *Arch Dermatol* 1989;125:639–42.
3 Schoorl WJ, van Baar HJ, van de Kerkhof PC. The hair root pattern in psoriasis of the scalp. *Acta Derm Venereol* 1992;72:141–2.
4 Runne U, Kroneisen-Wiersma P. Psoriatic alopecia: acute and chronic hair loss in 47 patients with scale psoriasis. *Dermatology* 1992;185:82–7.
5 Wright AL, Messenger AG. Scarring alopecia in psoriasis. *Acta Derm Venereol* 1990;70:156–9.
6 Van de Kerkhof P, Chang A. Scarring alopecia and psoriasis. *Br J Dermatol* 1992;126:524–5.
7 Rosenberg EW, Belew PW. Microbial factors in psoriasis (Letter). *Arch Dermatol* 1982;118:143–4.
8 Comaish S. Autoradiographic studies of hair growth in various dermatoses: investigation of a possible circadian rhythm in human hair growth. *Br J Dermatol* 1969;81:282–3.
9 Katsuoka K, Schell H, Deinlein E, Hornstein OP. Cell kinetics in the human anagen hair follicle. *Dermatologica* 1987;174:105–9.
10 Lowe NJ, Breeding JH, Wortzman MS. New coal tar extract and coal tar shampoos: evaluation by epidermal DNA synthesis suppression assay. *Arch Dermatol* 1982; 118:487–9.
11 Steck WD. Scalp psoriasis: improved treatment with a shampoo machine. *Cutis* 1976;17:123–5.
12 Baden HP. Epilyt for scalp psoriasis (Letter). *Arch Dermatol* 1991;127:274.
13 Gibson LE, Perry HO. Goeckerman therapy. In Roenigk HH Jr, Maibach HI, eds. *Psoriasis*, 2nd edn. New York: Marcel Dekker, Inc., 1991:537.
14 Langner A, Wolska H, Hebborn P. Treatment of psoriasis of the scalp with coal tar gel and shampoo preparations. *Cutis* 1983;32:290–1, 295–6.
15 Helm TN, Ferrara RJ, Dijkstra J, Soukup J. New improved Nivea Oil cannot be used alone as vehicle for salicylic acid. *J Am Acad Dermatol* 1989;21:814.
16 Ashton RE, Lowe NJ. Anthralin use in the treatment of psoriasis. In Lowe NJ, ed. *Practical Psoriasis Therapy*. Chicago: Year Book Medical Publishers, 1986:40.

17 Lowe NJ, Breeding J. Anthralin: different concentration effects on epidermal DNA synthesis rates in mice and clinical responses in human psoriasis. *Arch Dermatol* 1981;117:698–700.

18 Farber EM, Harris DR. Hospital treatment of psoriasis: a modified anthralin program. *Arch Dermatol* 1970;101:381–9.

19 Du Vivier A, Stoughton RB. Tachyphylaxis to the action of topically applied corticosteroids. *Arch Dermatol* 1982;111:581–3.

20 Ortega E, Burdick KH, Segre EJ. Adrenal suppression by clobetasol propionate. *Lancet* 1975;i:1200.

21 Willis I, Cornell RC, Penneys NS, Zaias N. Multicenter study comparing 0.05% gel formulations of desoximetasone and fluocinonide in patients with scalp psoriasis. *Clin Ther* 1986;8:275–82.

22 Lassus A. Local treatment of psoriasis of the scalp with clobetasol propionate and betamethasone-17,21-dipropionate: a double-blind comparison. *Curr Med Res Opin* 1976;4:365–7.

23 Rosenberg EW, Belew PW. Improvement of psoriasis of the scalp with ketoconazole (Letter). *Arch Dermatol* 1982;118:370–1.

24 Farr PM, Marks JM, Krause LB, Shuster S. Response of scalp psoriasis to oral ketoconazole. *Lancet* 1985;ii:921.

25 Lindelof B, Johannesson A. Psoriasis of the scalp treated with Grenz rays or topical corticosteroid combined with Grenz rays. A comparative randomized trial. *Br J Dermatol* 1988;119:241–4.

26 Dellon AL. Long-term remission of psoriasis after dermatome shaving. *Plast Reconstr Surg* 1982;70:220–6.

seven Nail Psoriasis

EPIDEMIOLOGY

Psoriasis affecting the nails is very common, being found in 10–50% of patients. The prevalence of nail psoriasis is much higher in patients with psoriatic arthritis, occurring in over 80% of cases. The fingernails seem to be affected more often than toenails. In most cases, the changes are easier to identify in the fingernails because they are more accessible to examination, and patients are more likely to complain about changes exposed to the public eye. Many of the alterations of toenails associated with aging can be confused with psoriasis: thickening and yellowing of the nailplate, longitudinal ridges, and dystrophies (Fig. 7.1). Onycholysis may be secondary to trauma, ill-fitting shoes, bone deformities, vascular insufficiency, and dermatophytosis. The conventional wisdom is that dermatophytes are infrequently found in association with psoriatic nails, but it would be folly not to examine the scales of the palms and soles and subungual debris with potassium hydroxide and culture if the diagnosis is in doubt. Treatment of a fungal component could provide some symptomatic or cosmetic relief to the patient.

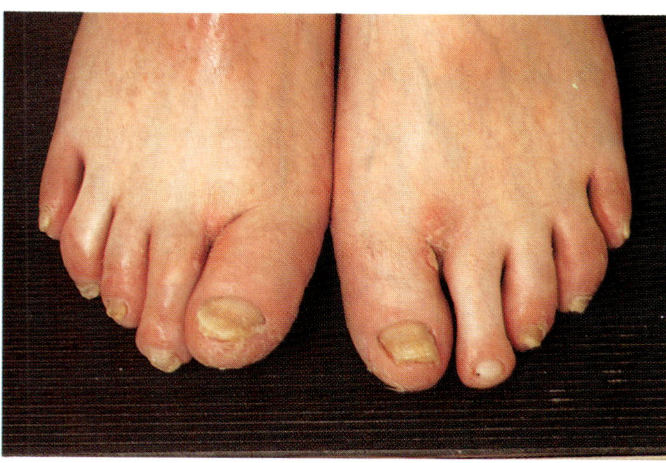

Fig 7.1 Psoriasis of the distal toes, first interdigital space, and toenails.

CLINICAL FINDINGS AND ETIOPATHOGENESIS

The morphologic alterations seen in the nail unit in psoriasis are individually not specific or diagnostic of the disease with the exception perhaps of cutaneous psoriasis of the proximal and lateral nailfolds or the volar finger pad (Fig. 7.2). The constellation of nail changes taken together, however, may be strongly suggestive of the diagnosis, even in the absence of any obvious cutaneous lesions. Such a scenario occurs in less than 5% of cases and may be seen in association with arthropathy, as a precursor to the development of skin lesions, or as the only manifestation of psoriasis seen in an individual patient.

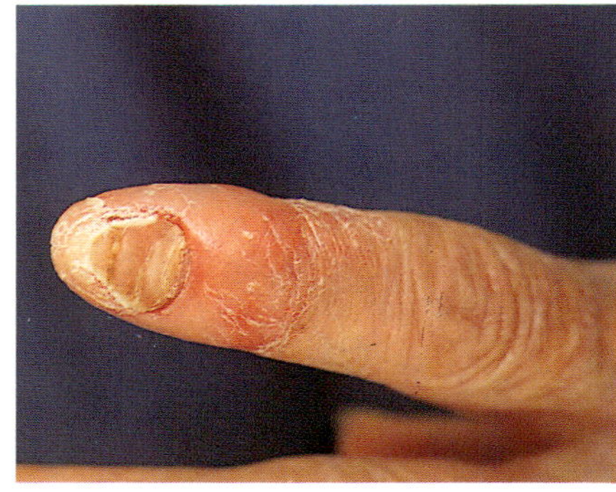

Fig 7.2 Psoriasis of fingernail, nail folds, and hyponychium.

The end result of psoriasis involving the cells of the nail matrix is usually but not always manifested in the surface texture of the nail plate, while lesions in the nailbed are generally transmitted through the plate as color changes or onycholysis. Thickening or lifting of the nail and subungual hyperkeratosis results from accumulation of scales in psoriatic lesions of the nailbed and hyponychium (Fig. 7.3).

It has been shown that there is a direct link between the linear growth rate of nails and nail matrix kinetics consistent with *in vivo* thymidine labeling studies of psoriatic epidermis. The growth rate of psoriatic nails with pitting was significantly greater than normal-appearing psoriatic nails (125 μm/day vs 109 μm/day) [1]. Both rates were significantly greater than pooled normal controls (98 μm/day). Baran and Dawber showed that systemic cytostatic drugs such as methotrexate and azathioprine markedly reduced the growth rate of nails while corticosteroids did not [1]. Etretinate therapy surprisingly increased the rate of fingernail growth in psoriasis.

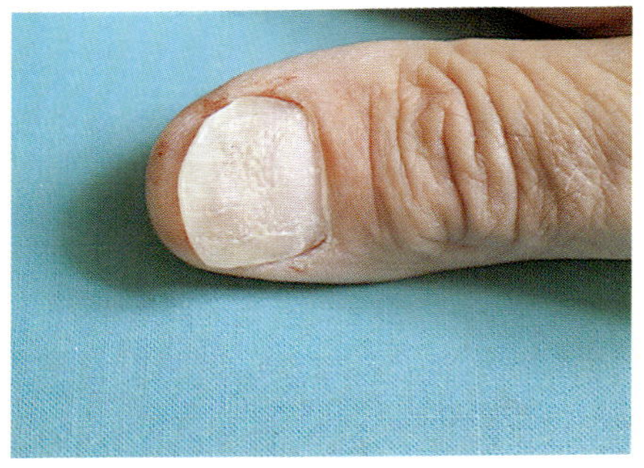

Fig 7.4 Nail pits in psoriasis.

Pitting of the nail plate is the most commonly recognized nail sign of psoriasis (Fig. 7.4). The pits are usually larger, deeper, and more randomly dispersed on the nail plate than those observed in alopecia areata. They are believed to be secondary to parakeratosis of the proximal matrix resulting in nucleated cells in the upper plate that eventually desquamate (see Fig. 7.3). Similarly, parakeratosis in an intermediate portion of the matrix

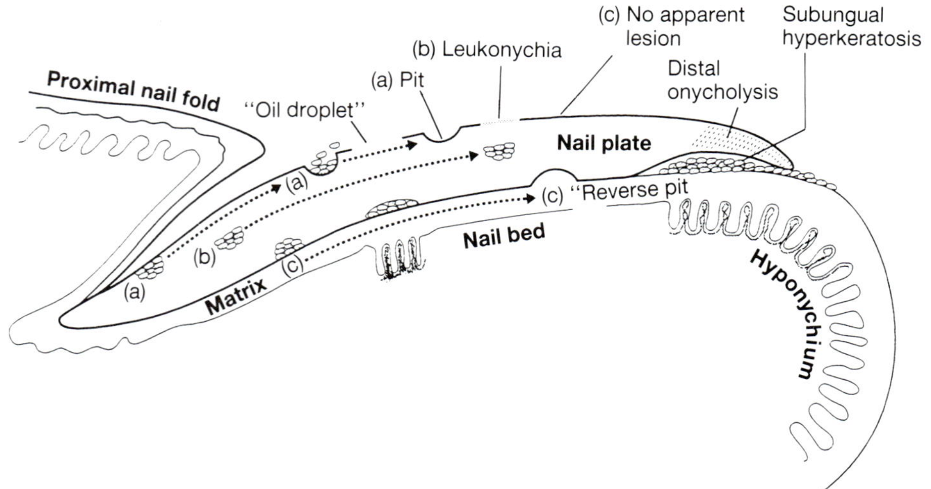

Fig 7.3 Correlation of psoriasis of the nail unit with morphologic changes.

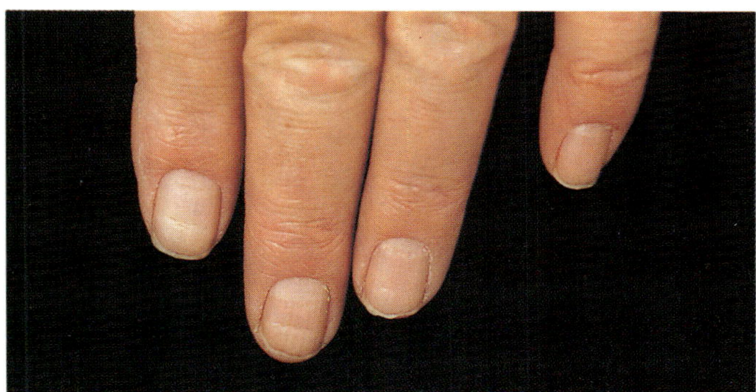

Fig 7.5 Beau's lines in psoriasis.

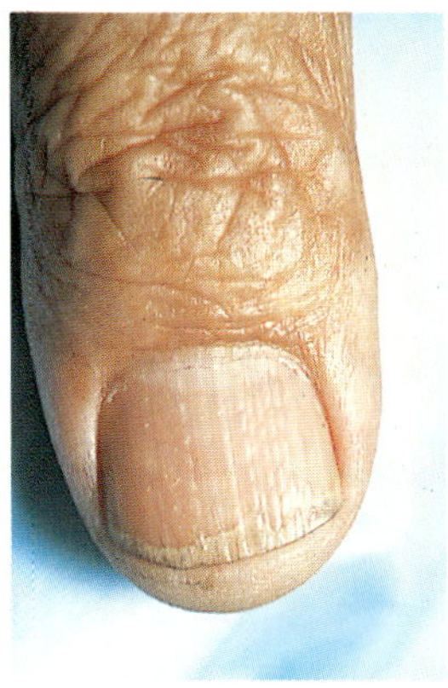

Fig 7.6 Longitudinal ridges and distal onycholysis.

may result in leukonychia. Parakeratosis in the distal matrix or lunula results in no discernible change in the plate or focal onycholysis. Small red spots in the lunula may indicate active distal matrix psoriasis, another change that is very similar to that seen in alopecia areata. Transverse ridges may represent transient matrix arrest (Beau's lines) (Fig. 7.5) or a confluence of parakeratosis in proximal matrix thereby connecting the pits. Longitudinal ridges (Fig. 7.6) result from alternating thinning and thickening of the nail plate and may correspond to psoriatic involvement focally or at regular intervals in the intermediate and distal matrix.

Splinter hemorrhages, longitudinal collections of extravasated blood under the nail plate, are very common after trauma of normal nails. Psoriatic nails are especially predisposed to these if psoriasis involves the nailbed because of the superficial location of dilated tortuous capillaries (Fig. 7.7). The oil droplet appearance of the nailbed corresponds to an early guttate lesion of psoriasis. There is a yellowish-brown spot surrounded by erythema (Fig. 7.8). The yellow greasy look is due to a serum glycoprotein which accumulates in and under the abnormal nail [2]. Large amounts of this material may be inhibitory for dermatophytes but not to yeasts. Complete crumbling of the nail plate is the result of extensive involvement of the matrix forming a nail plate of varying thicknesses with deep pits and ridging dispersed throughout (Fig. 7.9). In such an extensive case there is likely to be psoriasis of the distal nailbed and hyponychium as well, further elevating the nail plate to reveal accumulated keratinaceous debris (Fig. 7.10).

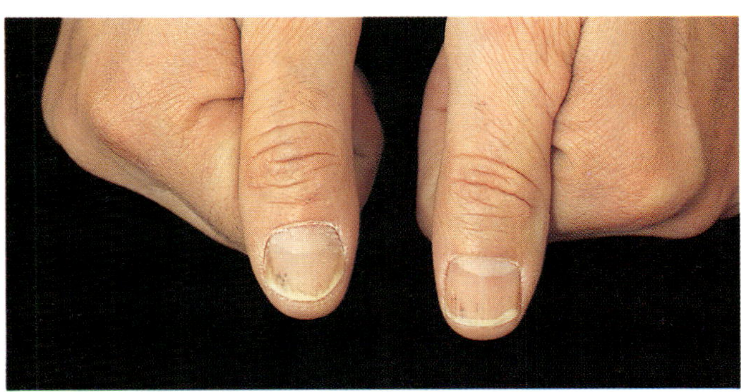

Fig 7.7 Splinter hemorrhages.

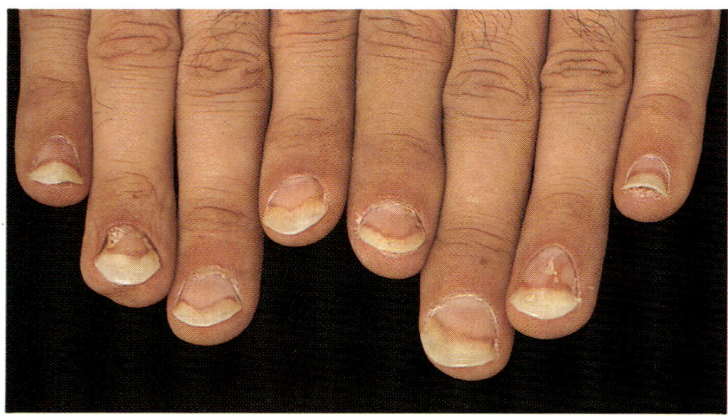

Fig 7.8 Yellowish-brown line at junction of normal nailbed and distal onycholysis. "Oil droplet" extends to lunula of left fourth finger.

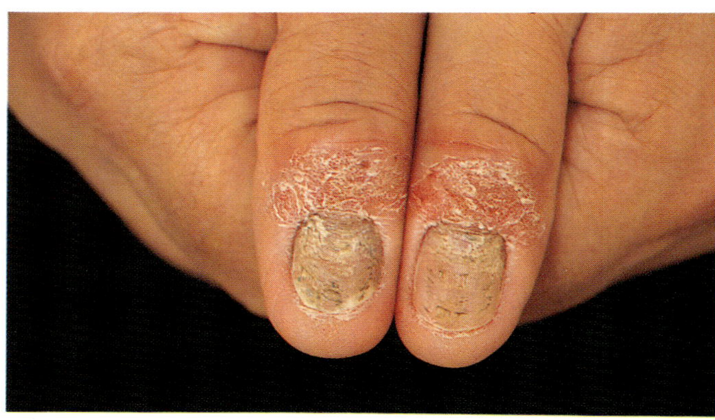

Fig 7.9 Deep pits, ridges, and yellowing of nails associated with psoriasis of proximal nail folds.

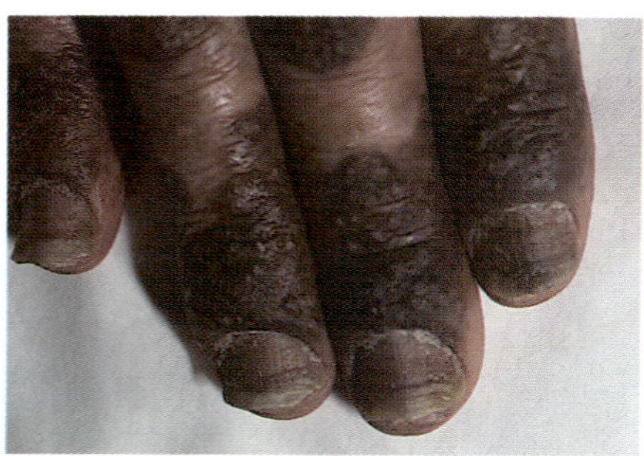

Fig 7.10

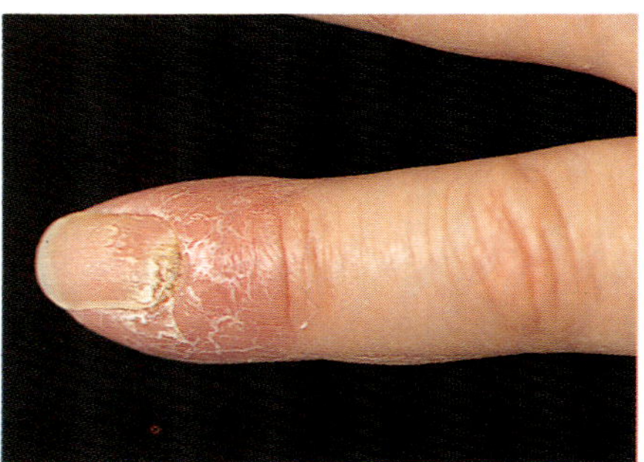

Fig 7.11

Fig 7.10 Pitting and subungual hyperkeratosis.

Fig 7.11 Chronic paronychia and nail dystrophy caused by *Candida albicans* infection resembles psoriasis.

DIFFERENTIAL DIAGNOSIS

While the oil droplet sign is very suggestive of the diagnosis of psoriasis, almost identical lesions have been noted in onychomycosis (*Candida*; Fig. 7.11) and tinea unguium (dermatophyte; Fig. 7.12).

While it is true that one or more of the features listed for psoriatic nails can be seen in the nails of alopecia areata, lichen planus, and eczema, these diseases can usually be diagnosed readily by their distinctive cutaneous lesions. There are two uncommon entities with papulosquamous skin

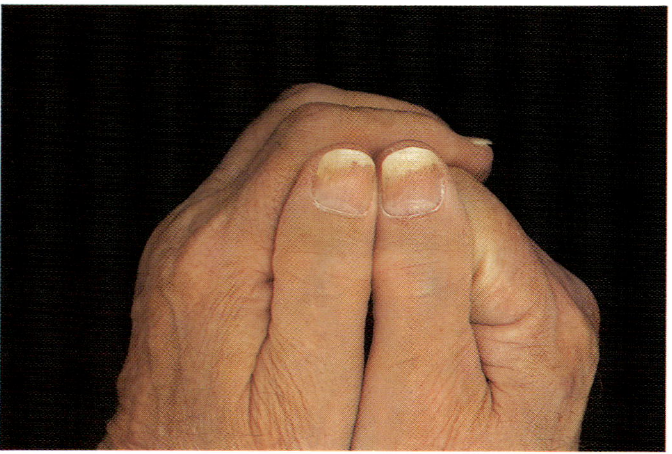

Fig 7.12 Discoloration of nail plate and distal onycholysis caused by *Trichophyton rubrum* mimics psoriasis of the nails. Compare with Fig. 7.8.

lesions and nail changes that may be referred to a dermatologic consultant. Paraneoplastic acrokeratosis or Bazex syndrome typically occurs in middle-aged men in association with a squamous cell carcinoma of the upper aerodigestive tract. Psoriasiform lesions affect the ears, nose, hands, and feet. The nail changes may be the first clue to the diagnosis of the underlying neoplasm [3]. They become thin, soft, fragile, and crumble. Subungual hyperkeratosis develops and the nail may be lost (Fig. 7.13). The skin and nail changes are reversible if the malignancy can be cured.

Another diagnostic dilemma is pityriasis rubra pilaris (PRP). In the classic adult-onset type (type I), papulosquamous lesions spread from the head (Fig. 7.14) down to the feet evolving into an erythroderma with islands of sparing (see Fig. 5.35a) [4]. The skin may have a salmon or orange hue (Fig. 7.15) with palmoplantar keratoderma (Fig. 7.16). When fully developed, the nails are thickened with subungual hyperkeratosis, distal yellow-brown discoloration. These changes are very similar to those seen in patients with the erythroderma of the Sézary syndrome [5], the leukemic phase of cutaneous T-cell lymphoma, suggesting that they may represent a nonspecific reaction pattern. The skin biopsy findings of Bazex syndrome and PRP are nonspecific, but the diagnosis of Sézary syndrome can usually be confirmed by a skin biopsy or peripheral blood smear.

Even the most severe changes of the nail in psoriasis are reversible

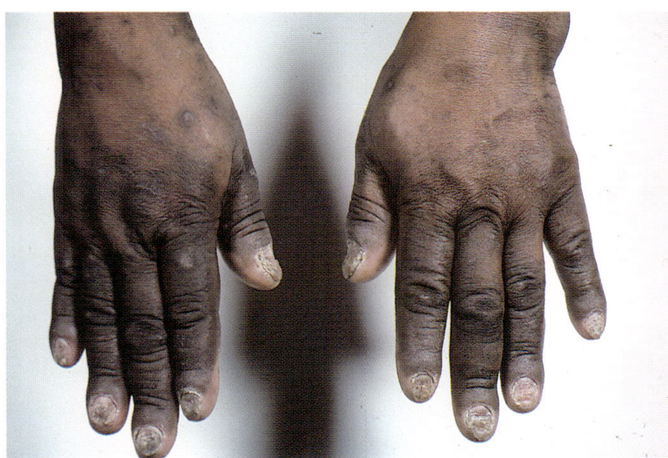

Fig 7.13 Nail changes of paraneoplastic acrokeratosis (Bazex syndrome).

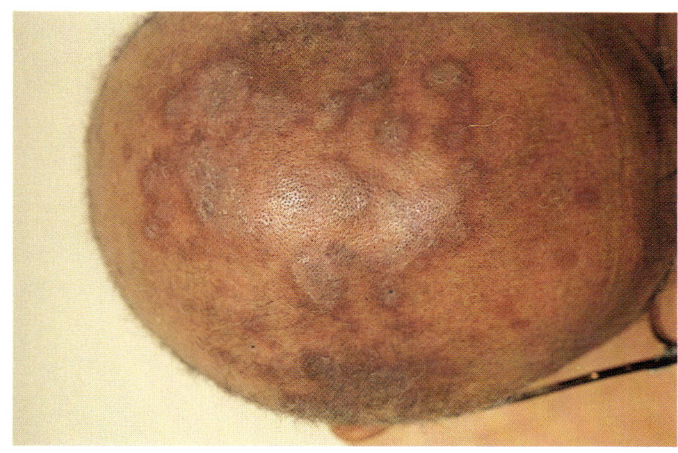

Fig 7.14 These papulosquamous lesions on the scalp of a man with pityriasis rubra pilaris were originally misdiagnosed as psoriasis.

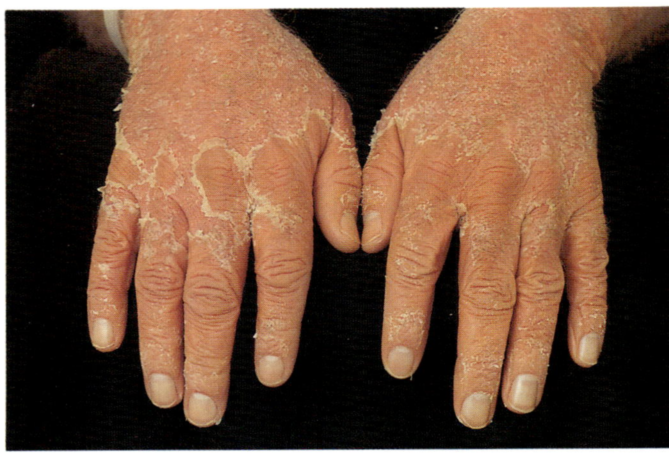

Fig 7.15 The orange or salmon hue to the skin is typical for fully evolved pityriasis rubra pilaris.

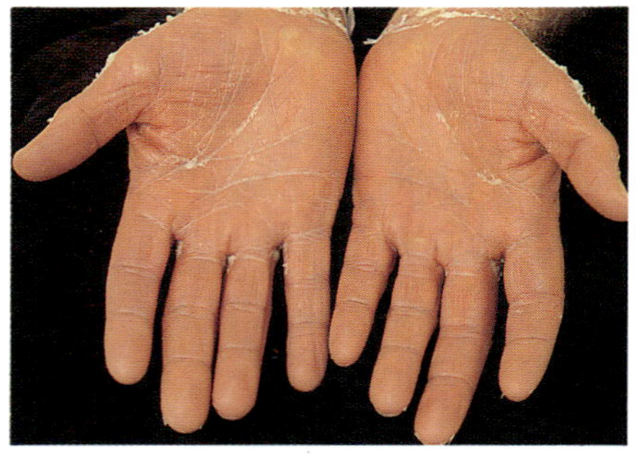

(a)

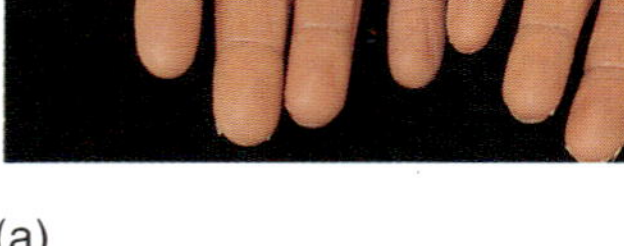

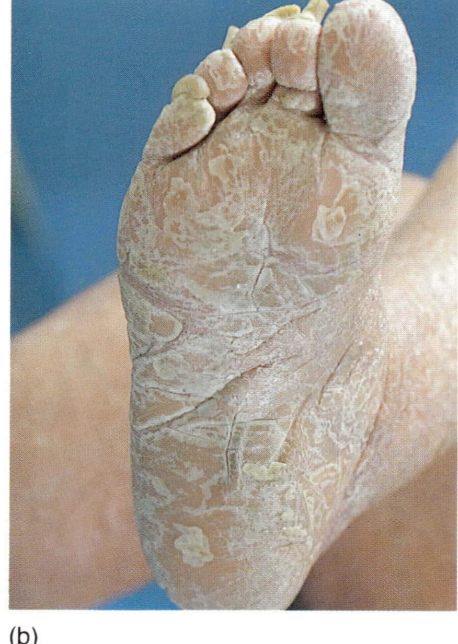

(b)

Fig 7.16 Keratoderma of the (a) palms and (b) sole seen in pityriasis rubra pilaris (different patients).

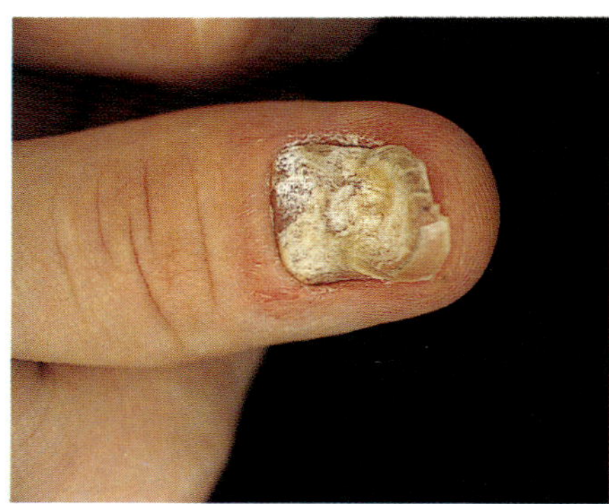

Fig 7.17 Acrodermatitis continua of Hallopeau. Note the yellowing and crumbling nail plate.

because they are due to aberrations in epidermal cell kinetics and differentiation, which usually do not result in scarring or permanent nail loss. Therefore, it is reasonable to expect that therapy will reverse the changes and induce remission if it does so for the rest of the integument. This is only partially true and difficult to obtain for several reasons. Over time, the chronic inflammatory and reparative processes may create subtle changes in the matrix or nailbed that do not allow a completely normal appearing nail plate adherent to the nailbed to regrow even after the most aggressive treatment.

In acrodermatitis continua of Hallopeau sterile pustules arise beneath the nail plate, coalescing and reforming, producing necrosis of tissue, thinning and crumbling of the nail plate, scaling and crusting of nailfold skin, and eventual shedding of the nail (Fig. 7.17). Permanent nail loss, scarring, and bone resorption may occur after years of unchecked disease. It may affect one or several digits (Fig. 7.18). Because acrodermatitis may be associated with psoriasis vulgaris, palmoplantar pustulosis, and a general-

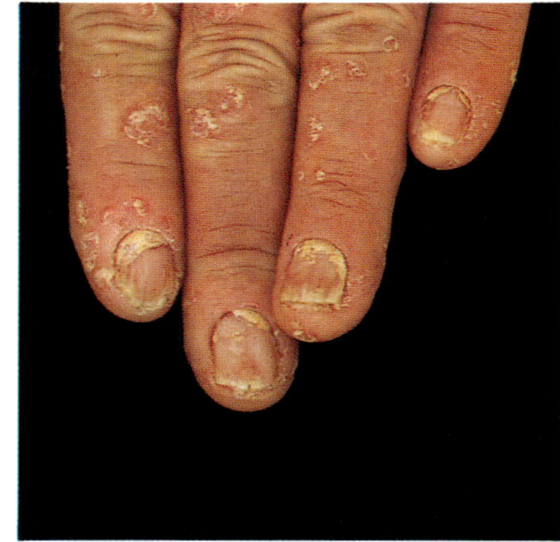

Fig 7.18 Acropustulosis affecting several digits.

ized pustular flare of von Zumbusch may be provoked, we consider it to be a localized variant of pustular psoriasis or subcorneal pustular dermatosis. Histopathologic findings (Munro microabscesses or spongiform pustules of Kogoj) and responsiveness to methotrexate tend to support this position, but it is controversial. For example, the same type of lesion can be seen in Reiter's syndrome. Perhaps it is best to lump all of these cases under the rubric of "acropustulosis." Ormsby and Montgomery wrote of acrodermatitis perstans (Hallopeau) [6]:

> The essential features are a slowly progressive dermatitis, usually of the extremities, often beginning in the region of the nail following trauma or suppurative paronychia, the initial lesions being vesicles, bullae and pustules, which in their evolution produce in the early stages a well defined slightly elevated epidermal border; in the later stages dry scaling or crusting patches with or without recurring pustules, with occasional wide dissemination through development of independent foci. The affections to be distinguished are infectious eczematoid dermatitis and pustular psoriasis.

NAIL BIOPSY

It is usually not necessary to biopsy the nail unit in psoriasis because the diagnosis can be reliably made based on the morphologic changes in the plate and/or the surrounding skin. In the case of unexplained nail dystrophy without skin lesions, particularly when there is suppurative inflammation of the nailbed, it is important to sample tissue for histology and cultures.

Small Munro abscesses are found in the parakeratotic horny layer and elongation of epidermal rete ridges in nailbed psoriasis [2]. Zaias also noted the accumulation of a PAS-positive diastase-resistant proteinaceous material in globules between cells in the horny layer within the yellowish greasy-appearing subungual keratotic lesions. In longitudinal nail biopsies of six patients clinically suspicious of psoriasis, only four could be diagnosed histologically [7]. We have had some difficulty in making a specific histologic diagnosis of psoriasis from a small nailbed biopsy. Prominent hyperkeratosis with focal parakeratosis was noted in the nailbed and hyponychium. Trapped fragments of neutrophilic nuclei were seen in parakeratotic stratum corneum overlying areas of hypogranulosis in these four cases. Serum-like proteinaceous material in the parakeratotic horny layer [2] and psoriasiform hyperplasia of the nailbed epithelium were found in only one case and were therefore considered a "minor criterion" for the histopathologic diagnosis of psoriasis. Ackerman and Ragaz [8] commented that psoriasis may be indistinguishable from onychomycosis unless fungal filaments are found.

Scher and Daniel [9] writing on nail surgery refer to: (i) longitudinal biopsy which includes the proximal nailfold, matrix, nailbed, and hyponychium; (ii) longitudinal incision of the nailbed after nail avulsion; and (iii) punch biopsy of the nailbed through the nail plate. To confirm the diagnosis of psoriasis, it is rarely ever necessary to perform a longitudinal biopsy because most of the diagnostic changes are in the nailbed and hyponychium.

It is desirable to avoid the matrix, including the lunula, when performing small biopsies that will not be sutured closed because they can produce permanent comorbidity. I recommend a modification of (ii) and (iii) above (Fig. 7.19).

After providing a digital block or a thorough ring block with local infiltration of 1% lidocaine [10], a red spot or "oil droplet" between the lunula and hyponychium should be selected for biopsy. Punch out a 4-mm cap of the nail plate; remove and place it in formalin. Next perform a 3-mm punch biopsy through the exposed nailbed (Fig. 7.19a). Because it is still often difficult to remove the cylinder of tissue without crushing or macerating it, cut away a residual triangle of distal nail plate with cuticle scissors (Fig. 7.19b). This specimen may now be submitted for fungal culture. Detach the punch biopsy specimen with gradle scissors and place in the formalin bottle containing the nail plate cap. Both should be stained with PAS, GMS, and Gram's stain for organisms. Next, using a scalpel, describe a small ellipse from the nailbed distal to the punch defect to the hyponychium for a second histopathologic specimen (Fig. 7.19c). One or more sutures may be placed here for hemostasis and to expedite healing (Fig. 7.19d). This technique is particularly useful in the diagnosis of the acropustuloses. If a vesicle or pustule is traumatically ruptured by the trephine which destroys the characteristic architecture, the second biopsy with the scalpel performed after partially cutting away the nail plate includes the hyponychium and volar skin where there is likely to be an extension of the primary disease.

TREATMENT

Topical therapy

If topical therapy is selected, the first obstacle is reaching the diseased area. As Fig. 7.3 shows, the proximal matrix is obscured by the proximal nailfold and the nail plate while the distal matrix and bed are blocked by the nail plate. The hyponychium may be covered with scales, dirt, and contaminating microorganisms. A topical corticosteroid may improve psoriasis of the surrounding skin, but has little to no effect on the appearance of the nail. Superpotent steroids under occlusion for 2 consecutive weeks may give further benefit but the need for repetitive use and incomplete improvement at best results in either noncompliance by the patient, atrophy

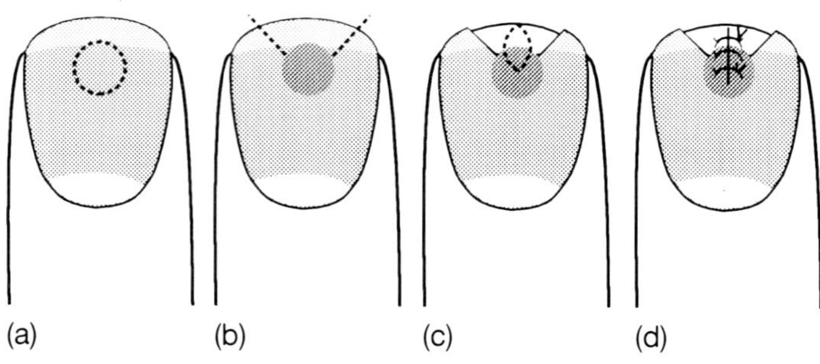

Fig 7.19 Biopsy of the nailbed and hyponychium. See text for details.

of the nailfold skin or discontinuation of this slow or failing treatment by the frustrated physician.

Getting directly at the nailbed and exposed matrix by avulsion of the nail plate may be indicated in those patients with hypertrophic crumbling nails. This can be accomplished atraumatically with the following extemporaneously compounded formulation: urea 40%, white beeswax or paraffin 5%, anhydrous lanolin 20%, white petrolatum 25%, and silica gel type H 10%, applied under plastic occlusion for 7 days [11]. A more recent modification omits the silica gel and uses 35% petrolatum [12]. After removing the dystrophic nail, South and Farber [11] recommended applying a potent corticosteroid-impregnated tape (flurandrenolide) or ointment to the denuded nailbed and proximal nailfold. They reported a 50% success rate in regrowing "normal nails" and cautioned against treating atrophic and "egg-shell type dystrophies" in this manner since they do not respond as well.

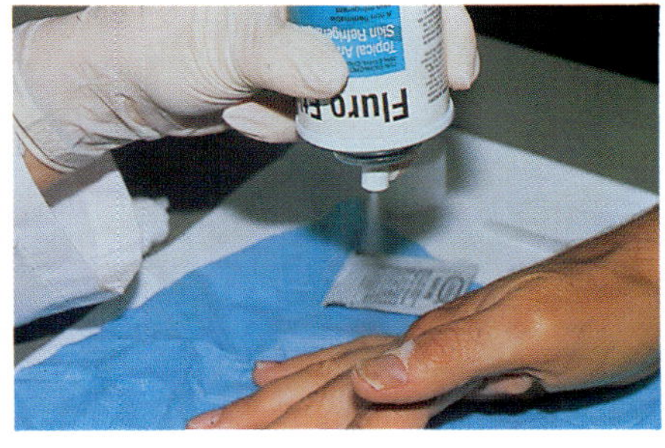

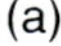

(a)

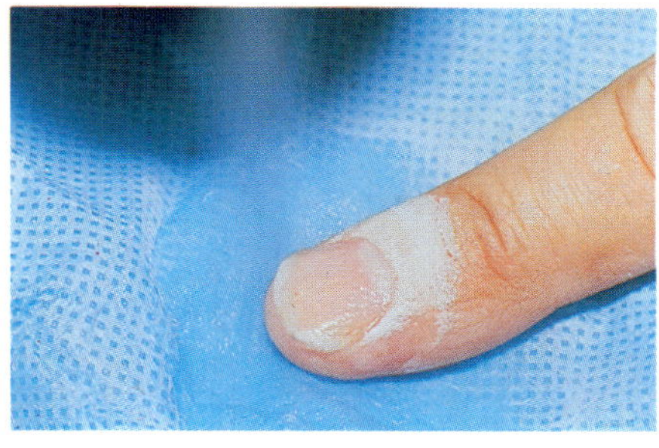

(b)

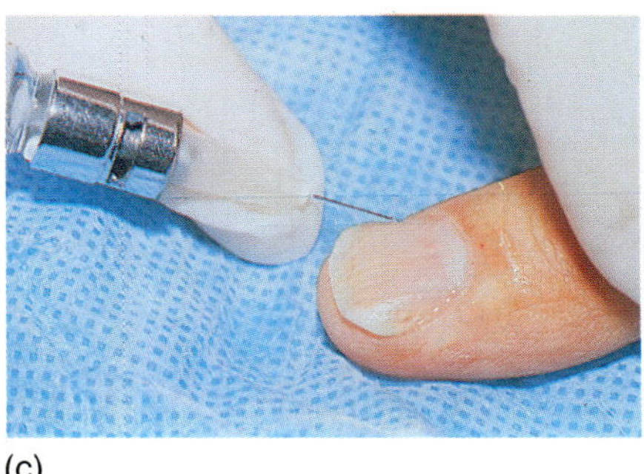

(c)

Fig 7.20 Intralesional injection of triamcinolone acetonide for psoriasis of the nail unit. (a) Spray nail fold with refrigerant. (b) Appearance of nail fold immediately prior to injection. (c) Injecting from the lateral nail fold to the lunula.

Another method of getting directly to the seat of the disease is by intralesional injection of corticosteroid. By noting the type of nail change one can deduce the location of its origin with some degree of accuracy. With highly motivated patients and skillfull operators, the results can be most satisfying. The disadvantages of the procedure are that it is painful for the patient and tedious time-consuming work for the operator. It must be repeated at monthly intervals until the desired result is obtained and maintained at some less frequent interval as new lesions appear.

We routinely use triamcinolone acetonide (TAC) suspension 10 mg/ml diluted 1 : 1 with 1% lidocaine yielding a final concentration of 5 mg/ml. The patient scrubs his or her hands with chlorhexidine cleanser. Prior to injection the area is sprayed with a refrigerant such as Flurethyl (Fig. 7.20a,b). To treat pitting, injections are given into the proximal and lateral nailfold skin extending into the proximal lunula (Fig. 7.20c). When there are oil spots, onycholysis, or subungual hyperkeratosis the 30-gauge needle is directed under the nail plate right to the affected areas. A total dose of less than 1–1.5 mg of TAC is deposited under or around a given nail unit. We have not yet observed the theoretical complication of atrophy of the nailfold skin or nail plate. Subungual hematomas and increased numbers of splinter hemorrhages do occur, however, and patients should be informed of this in advance. None of our patients has required decompression, and all hemorrhages eventually grow out. No infections have occurred.

Other topical approaches that have been tried include 5-fluorouracil (5-FU) and mechlorethamine (nitrogen mustard). One percent 5-FU solution is massaged into the nailfold areas twice daily without occlusion for 4–6 months in patients with either matrix disease or subungual hyperkeratosis [13]. Local inflammatory reactions and hyperpigmentation can occur. Distal onycholysis may be worsened by this treatment. We have found that patients generally do not comply with this regimen long enough and seek alternative treatment.

Topical nitrogen mustard, well known to dermatologists as the treatment of choice for certain forms of cutaneous T-cell lymphoma (CTCL), is also very effective at clearing psoriasis [14]. In aqueous solution, the rate of inducing delayed hypersensitivity reactions was unacceptably high [15]. It was later recognized to be a carcinogen for the skin in patients with CTCL, an acceptable risk for treating a malignancy but not for psoriasis. There are no systemic effects of topical nitrogen mustard, adverse or beneficial. In patients with acrodermatitis continua who have pustulation of the nailbed and matrix and chronic inflammation, atrophy, scarring, and anonychia can occur. In this setting it would be appropriate to try nitrogen mustard, compounded in an ointment base (10 mg mechlorethamine (Mustargen) dissolved in 95% ethyl alcohol and mixed into 100 g Aquaphor), topically applied daily to the fingertips and covered [16] for up to 6 months, the shelf life of the compound.

Physical therapy

In a double-blind study, superficial radiotherapy given as three fractionated doses of 150 cGy (90 kV, 5 mA, 1.00 mm aluminum filter) significantly improved psoriatic fingernails compared to sham-treated nails [17]. The improvement lasted for 10–15 weeks after treatment.

Marx and Scher [18] closely followed nail signs in 10 patients with generalized psoriasis receiving psoralen UVA (PUVA). They found that most changes showed 50% or more improvement after therapy (crumbling of nail plate, onycholysis, oil drop) but that pitting was unchanged by this treatment. They hypothesized that while the 8-methoxypsoralen reached the entire nail matrix via the circulation, only limited UVA radiation could penetrate the nail plate to reach the distal matrix (lunula) and nailbed to improve abnormalities there, but the proximal matrix was unpenetrable. That relatively little UVA radiation reaches the nailbed was confirmed by measuring transmission of optical radiation 600–300 nm through human toenails obtained at autopsy [19]. The investigators calculated that at 360 nm, the peak emission of most conventional lamps in PUVA units, only about 20% was transmitted through a nail of 0.5 mm thickness. For 330 nm, an order of magnitude more effective at clearing psoriasis than 360 nm, the percent transmission drops to 10% and approaches zero for thick nails (0.8–1.0 mm). They further suggested that 2.5–5 times the therapeutic dose of UVA would be needed at the surface of the nail plate to induce the same resolution of psoriasis of the surrounding glabrous skin. In other words, specific PUVA treatment directed at psoriatic nails is feasible, but would require additional dosing and protection of surrounding skin. With such high doses, PUVA-induced photoonycholysis or photohemolysis (hemorrhage followed by onycholysis) could further complicate the picture.

The investigators also showed that UVB is unlikely to help psoriatic nails because the nail, like window glass, filters out much of it, and there is a very low transmission of UVB (280–315 nm) to the nailbed.

Systemic medication

The best systemic medication for psoriasis of the nails appears to be methotrexate, but most clinicians would not use it exclusively for nail disease unless it was disabling or destructive as in the acropustuloses. In the latter case, doses of 15 mg weekly are usually sufficient. When methotrexate is used to treat severe or extensive skin involvement and/or arthropathy, the nails benefit incidentally. Oral cyclosporine 3.3 mg/kg per day combined with a superpotent topical corticosteroid has been used to control acrodermatitis continua associated with plaque psoriasis after the failure of methotrexate, retinoids, and localized superficial radiotherapy [20].

Etretinate, like methotrexate and PUVA, would likely not be used specifically to treat psoriatic nails. Patients with prominent nail involvement may experience significant improvement in crumbling of the nail plate, oil drop change, onycholysis, and subungual hyperkeratosis [21]. These beneficial changes may outweigh the unwanted effects of retinoids on nails such as thinning and fragility, onychorrhexis, onychoschizia, onychomadesis, and paronychia with granulation tissue. Acitretin may have more side effects on nails than etretinate.

The nail disease of patients with HIV-associated psoriasis responds to zidovudine along with the skin changes.

REFERENCES

1 Baran R, Dawber RPR, eds. *Diseases of the Nails and their Management*. Oxford: Blackwell Scientific Publications, 1984.

2 Zaias N. Psoriasis of the nail. A clinical-pathology study. *Arch Dermatol* 1969;99: 567–79.

3 Boudoulas O, Camisa C. Paraneoplastic acrokeratosis (Bazex Syndrome). *Cutis* 1986;37:449–53.

4 Cohen PR, Prystowsky JH. Pityriasis rubra pilaris: a review of diagnosis and treatment. *J Am Acad Dermatol* 1989;20:801–7.

5 Sonnex TS, Dawber RPR, Zachary CB, *et al*. The nails in adult type I pityriasis rubra pilaris. A comparison with Sézary syndrome and psoriasis. *J Am Acad Dermatol* 1986;15:956–60.

6 Ormsby OS, Montgomery H. *Diseases of the Skin*. Philadelphia: Lea and Febiger, 1943: 367.

7 Hanno R, Mathes BM, Krull EA. Longitudinal nail biopsy in evaluation of acquired nail dystrophies. *J Am Acad Dermatol* 1986;14:803–9.

8 Ackerman AB, Ragaz A. *The Lives of Lesions. Chronology in Dermatopathology*. New York: Masson, 1984:181.

9 Scher RK, Daniel RC. *Nails: Diagnosis, Therapy, Surgery*. Philadelphia: WB Saunders, 1990.

10 Rich P. Nail biopsy. Indications and methods. *J Dermatol Surg Oncol* 1992;18: 673–82.

11 South DA, Farber EM. Urea ointment in the nonsurgical avulsion of nail dystrophies — a reappraisal. *Cutis* 1980;25:609–12.

12 Farber EM, Nall L. Nail psoriasis. *Cutis* 1992;50:174–8.

13 Fritz K. Psoriasis of the nail: successful topical treatment with 5-fluorouracil. *Z Hautkr* 1989;64:1083–8.

14 Mandy S, Taylor JR, Halprin K. Topically applied mechlorethamine in the treatment of psoriasis. *Arch Dermatol* 1971;103:272–6.

15 Epstein E, Ugel AR. Effects of topical mechlorethamine on skin lesions of psoriasis. *Arch Dermatol* 1970;102:504–6.

16 Notowicz A, Stolz E, Heuvel NVD. Treatment of Hallopeau's acrodermatitis with topical mechlorethamine (Letter). *Arch Dermatol* 1978;114:129.

17 Yu RC, King CM. A double-blind study of superficial radiotherapy in psoriatic nail dystrophy. *Acta Derm Venereol* 1992;72:134–6.

18 Marx JL, Scher RK. Response of psoriatic nails to oral photochemotherapy. *Arch Dermatol* 1980;116:1023–4.

19 Parker SG, Diffey BL. The transmission of optical radiation through human nails. *Br J Dermatol* 1983;108:11–16.

20 Harland CC, Kilby PE, Dalziel KL. Acrodermatitis continua responding to cyclosporin therapy. *Clin Exp Dermatol* 1992;17:376–8.

21 Rabinovitz HS, Scher RK, Shupack JL. Response of psoriatic nails to the aromatic retinoid etretinate (Letter). *Arch Dermatol* 1983;119:627–8.

eight

Psoriatic Arthritis

William S. Wilke and Michael E. Sayers

INTRODUCTION

The earliest known written description which links psoriasis with inflammatory arthritis, may be the description of the co-occurrence of "leprosy" and "chronic gout" suffered for 29 years by Fray Pedro de Urrala in the seventeenth century [1]. Yet, despite its antiquity, the existence of psoriatic arthritis (PSA) as a homogeneous clinical entity, continues to be questioned [2–4]. It clearly differs from rheumatoid arthritis (RA) both in clinical presentation [5] and in radiographic appearance [6]. Although these two forms of inflammatory arthritis may share certain HLA antigen allotypes such as DR-4 [7], the occurrence of B27 and BW38 [8–11] is much higher in PSA. In addition, the incidence of inflammatory arthritis in moderate to severe psoriasis is 6–10%, considerably higher than in the general population [12–14]. Psoriatic patients with arthritis involving the distal interphalangeal joints or the axial skeleton almost surely have a musculoskeletal condition integrally related to the skin disease.

Still the question remains, especially concerning the group of patients with polyarticular asymmetric or symmetric arthritis [2–4]. Certainly some of these patients, especially those who are rheumatoid factor positive, may be experiencing the co-occurrence of two relatively common diseases. Nevertheless, whether or not this group represents a more heterogeneous population, for the purposes of this chapter, we will consider all patients with psoriasis and arthritis as part of the spectrum of PSA.

CLINICAL PICTURE

Overview of arthritis

Peripheral and axial manifestations may appear in a variety of patterns. The most widely accepted classification is that of Moll and Wright [15] in which five subsets are described [16].

1 Asymmetrical oligoarticular arthritis in which less than five joints are

involved often including the distal interphalangeal, proximal interphalangeal, and metacarpophalangeal joints of the hands and the metatarsophalangeal joints of the feet. "Sausage" digits are common (Fig. 8.1).

2 Symmetric polyarthritis involving the same joints (hands, wrists, ankles, and feet) as in RA, but differentiated from RA by the presence of distal interphalangeal involvement and the lack of nodules, vasculitis, and serologic rheumatoid factor (Figs 8.2a,b, 8.3).

3 Involvement of only the distal interphalangeal joints; a "classic" presentation of PSA which occurs in only 5% of patients. This presentation has a better prognosis than other peripheral patterns (Fig. 8.4) [17].

4 Arthritis mutilans in which proximal osteolysis, seen as the "pencil-in-cup" radiographic lesion, results in the dysfunctional "opera glass hand." This presentation is fortunately rare, occurring in only four of 118 patients in one series (Figs 8.5, 8.6) [18].

5 Ankylosing spondylitis in which the neck, thoracic and lumbosacral spine as well as the sacroiliac joints are involved, often asymmetrically in contrast to *de novo* ankylosing spondylitis [19,20], and in which severe dysfunction is rare [21]. Axial involvement alone is probably the least common presentation [22].

Most early series emphasize the preponderance of the asymmetric oligoarticular form of the disease [5,15,17,23]. More recent series, however, demonstrate that the pattern of polyarticular involvement of small to medium joints, either symmetric or asymmetric is the most common form of established disease [21,24–26]. A new clinical classification scheme has been proposed based on these changed perceptions [26]:

1 Peripheral arthritis, which includes distal interphalangeal involvement, arthritis mutilans, dactylitis, limb edema, proliferative enthesopathy as well as disease mimicking RA;

2 Sacroiliitis and spondylitis, which may be asymmetric and feature syndesmophytes with paravertebral ossifications;

3 Extraarticular osseous manifestations.

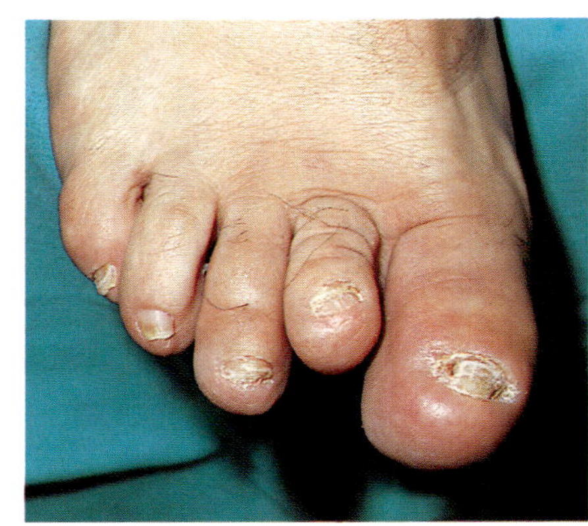

Fig 8.1 The "sausage" appearance of the first great toe with digital telescoping of the second toe, which results in the "opera glass" deformity. Note the severe nail dystrophy.

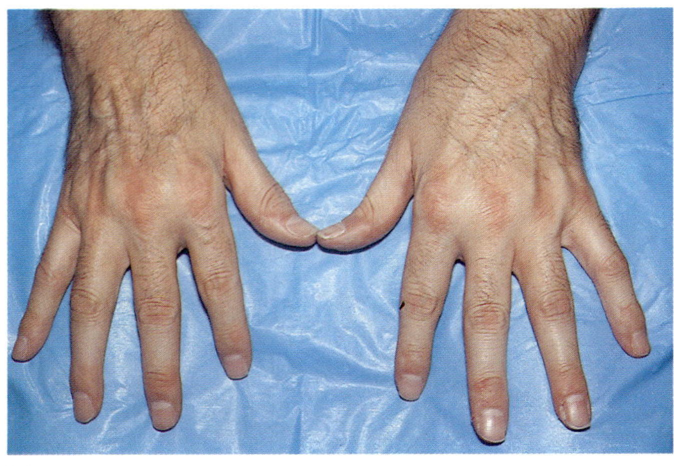

(a)

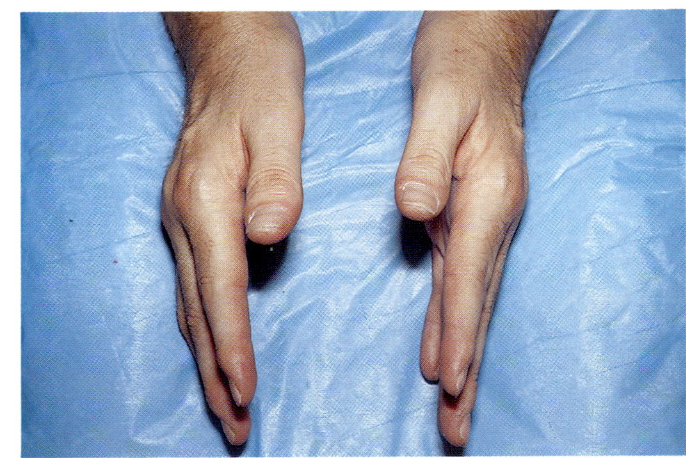

(b)

Fig 8.2 (a) Symmetric involvement of the index and middle metacarpophalangeal joints in a 24-year-old male with psoriasis and seronegative arthritis. Note the bilateral mild distal interphalangeal joint involvement of the index finger. (b) Side view of the same patient demonstrates better the metacarpophalangeal swelling and bilateral wrist swelling.

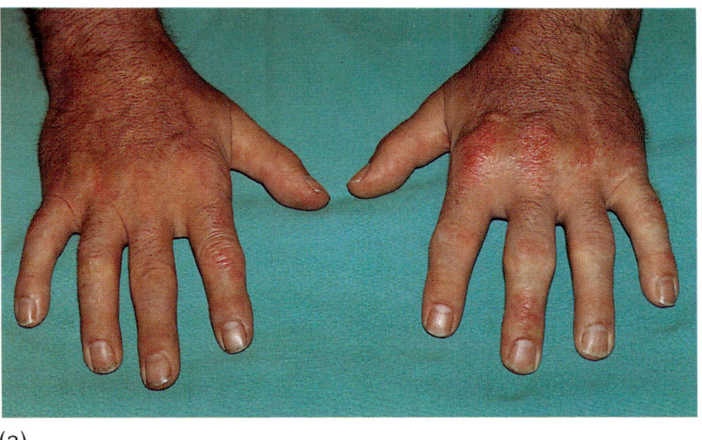

(a)

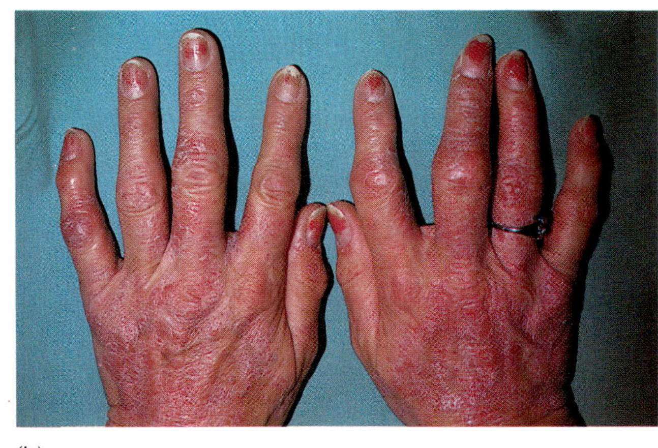

(b)

Fig 8.3 (a) Relatively symmetric swelling of the metacarpophalangeal and proximal interphalangeal joints in a 36-year-old male. Note the psoriatic skin lesions especially prominent over the dorsal aspects of the metacarpal phalangeal joints of the left hand. Also note the normal, spared nails.
(b) Different patient with marked bilateral proximal interphalangeal joints and psoriatic involvement of skin of backs of hands.

The female/male ratio varies. In series which report patients with primarily peripheral involvement, the ratio is 1 : 1 [3,22,27] or might show a slight female predominance [24,28]. Other series, in which a high frequency of axial disease is encountered, favor male predominance as high as 3 : 2 [29]. The mean age of arthritis onset for most series ranges from 32 to 45 years [17,26–28], although patients with evolving arthritis mutilans may experience onset before age 20. In fact, arthritis mutilans is three times more frequent in early onset disease than in later onset arthritis [24]. In contrast, patients with mostly oligoarticular arthritis of large joints tend to have later onset and a better prognosis [17].

The onset of articular symptoms is usually chronic and insidious but may be acute and present as monoarthritis of one digit [30]. Constitutional symptoms such as fever, fatigue, and anorexia are more frequent at the onset of arthritis mutilans [18,24].

Skin rash precedes the onset of arthritis in 64–73% of cases, and is synchronous in approximately 15% [5,24,27,31]; however, it has been reported as high as 36% in one series [23] and occurs after the onset of arthritis in 14–23% [5,24,27,31].

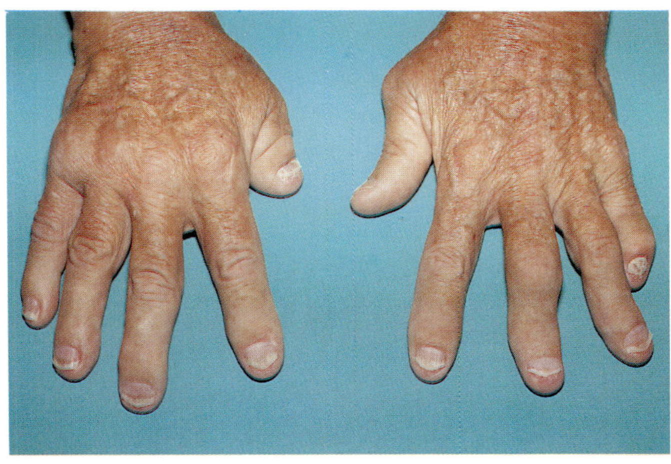

Fig 8.4 Distal interphalangeal involvement of the index and middle fingers in a 52-year-old male. Also note the boutonnière deformities of the middle and fourth finger of the left hand, telescoping of the right thumb, and onycholysis of the nails. In this case, distal interphalangeal involvement did not confer an excellent prognosis.

Peripheral arthritis

Peripheral arthritis tends to be severe in patients with the most severe cutaneous manifestations [31], such as the erythrodermic presentation [27] or in patients with psoriatic lesions on the palms and soles [32]. Parallel activity of rash and arthritis has been noted by some authors [31–33] but not by others [5,17]. Nail involvement (pitting, onycholysis, oil droplet discoloration) occurs in the vast majority of patients with peripheral arthritis; in one series correlating 100% of the time with distal interphalangeal involvement [17] and has simultaneous onset with arthritis in approximately 50% of cases (Fig. 8.7) [5,21].

Typical symmetric peripheral joint involvement includes the proximal interphalangeal, metacarpophalangeal, distal interphalangeal, knee, wrist, and ankle joints in descending order of frequency [16,17,22,31]. Distal interphalangeal involvement helps to differentiate PSA from RA. In a study which contrasted two groups of rheumatoid factor-negative patients with arthritis, 17% of those with psoriasis had distal interphalangeal involvement in contrast to 6% of those without skin disease [27]. Dactylitis, the sausage-appearance of distal interphalangeal and proximal interphalangeal joints in PSA due to periarticular enthesopathy, does not occur in RA and is therefore, a useful differential sign.

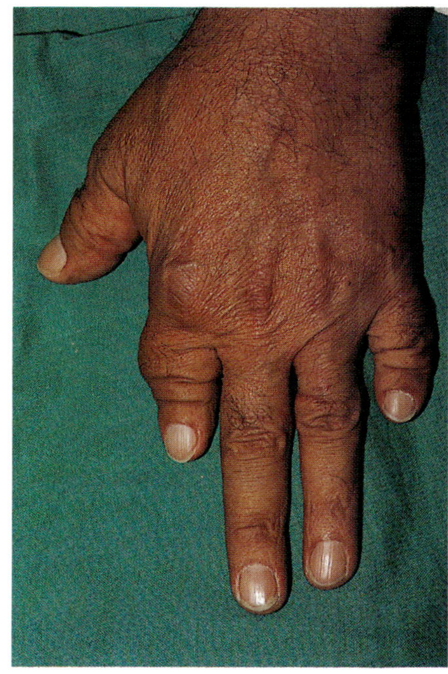

Fig 8.5 Dramatic telescoping of the index and fifth fingers in a 50-year-old male despite 10 years of methotrexate therapy. Note the sparing of the nails and the joints of the middle and fourth fingers.

Although symmetric polyarthritis is the more common form taken by established arthritis [22,30], many of these same patients may present with asymmetric arthritis at an earlier stage of disease [5,29]. Recent studies have emphasized the occurrence of manubrial sternal and foot or ankle involvement. Clinical manubrial sternal involvement was reported in 13% of 220 patients [22]. Metatarsal head and/or ankle involvement may occur in as many as 86% of some series [34]. Temporomandibular joint disease, as in RA, may occur in up to one-third of patients with PSA [35,36].

Clinical symptoms of peripheral PSA are similar to those seen in RA and include early morning stiffness, pain on motion, and joint dysfunction; these are all dependent on the severity and number of joints involved. Two early series suggested that patients with PSA complained less of pain than did patients with RA [23,28]. In one of these cohorts [28], 70% of 64 patients experienced little or no pain. A recent study of fibrositic tender points contrasted PSA patients with RA patients and showed that PSA patients experienced significantly fewer and less severely involved tender points than did RA patients [37]. Of interest, like some patients with fibromyalgia, patients with PSA have been shown to have lower levels of circulating β-endorphin than patients with other arthritides [38]. These two findings are difficult to reconcile.

The most common long-term deformities in PSA are flexion contractures of the proximal interphalangeal joints without adjacent hyperextension, which occurs in RA and results in "swan neck or boutonnière" appearance of the digits [30].

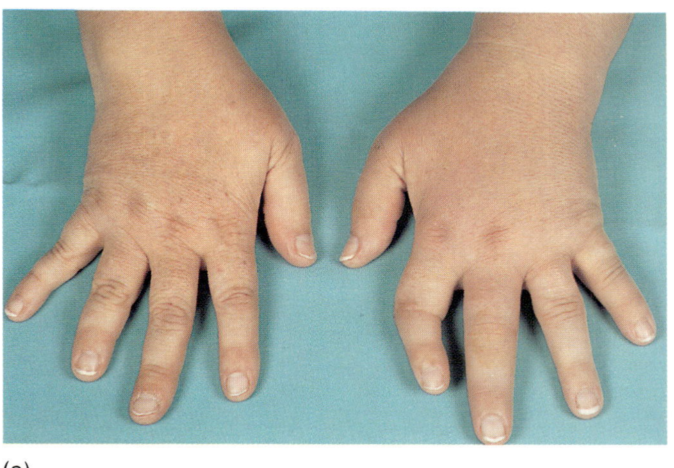

(a)

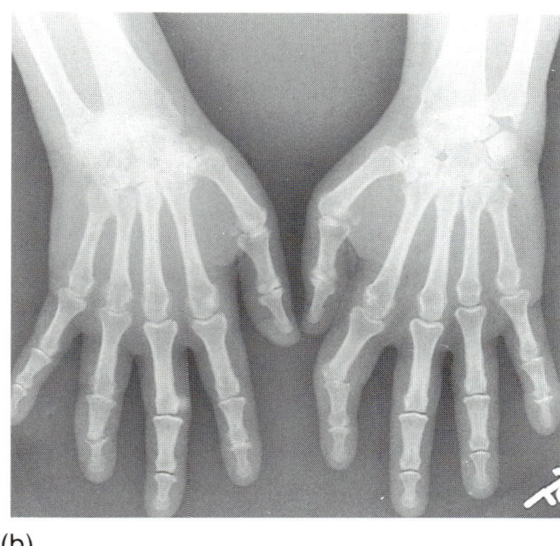

(b)

Fig 8.6 (a) Early arthritis mutilans in a 26-year-old female, which only involves the proximal interphalangeal joint of the left index finger. (b) X-rays show only mild periarticular changes with loss of joint space and erosions at the left metacarpophalangeal joint and proximal interphalangeal joint of the left index finger. Note the "pencil-in-cup" abnormality of the right fourth distal interphalangeal joint and destruction of the carpal bones in the right hand.

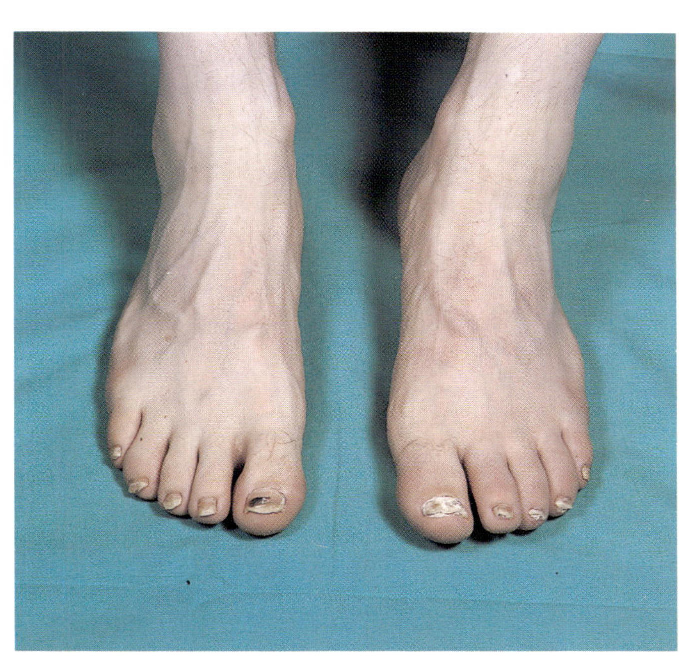

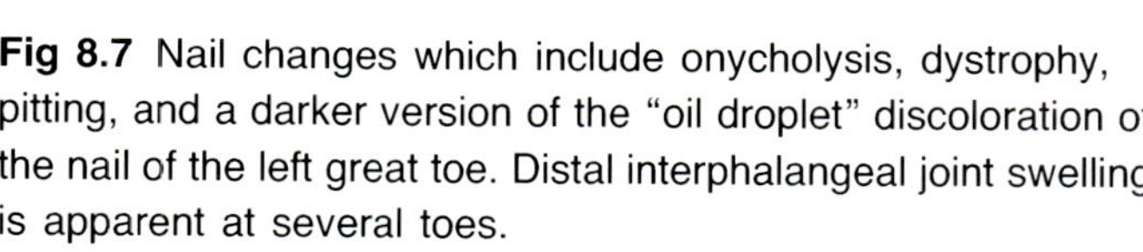

Fig 8.7 Nail changes which include onycholysis, dystrophy, pitting, and a darker version of the "oil droplet" discoloration of the nail of the left great toe. Distal interphalangeal joint swelling is apparent at several toes.

Sacroiliitis and spondylitis

Sacroiliitis occurs in 8–30% of patients with PSA [5,17,21,25,32,39–45]. In general, involvement tends to be asymmetric [27,44] although in one series of 21 patients with primarily axial involvement, 13 of 21 (62%) patients had symmetric sacroiliac erosions. Of interest, as with peripheral arthritis, symptoms are often absent despite radiographic findings. For instance, only five of 22 (23%) patients with axial involvement in one series experienced sufficient pain or stiffness to interfere with work [41].

Involvement of the spine occurs with the same frequency and generally in the same patients as does sacroiliitis [5,17,21,25,32,39–45]. Lumbosacral stiffness and dysfunction is less prominent than in ankylosing spondylitis and seems less severe than X-ray findings might predict [19,20, 40,41]. In fact, low back pain preceded any radiographic change in 14 of

22 (60%) patients in one series [41]. In another series, although both the number of syndesmophytes and the degree of sacroiliac joint involvement became more severe during a 57-month prospective followup, symptoms of pain and stiffness actually declined during the study [44].

Certain patterns of axial arthritis associations were noted in two series. Of 130 patients with PSA, those with axial involvement were more likely to be male, have iritis, and develop arthritis later in life [40]. In another series, peripheral arthritis of large joints was most often associated with sacroiliitis [45].

Juvenile psoriatic arthritis

Juvenile PSA has been estimated to be responsible for 4–8% of all inflammatory arthritis in children [46–48]. The female/male ratio is closer to that in RA at approximately 1.5 : 1 [46,49]. The age of onset is between 6 and 10 years, with knees and digits the most commonly involved joints in a pauciarticular pattern [46,50–52]. However, after onset, this disease generally pursues an asymmetric, polyarticular course [16,50]. Antinuclear antibodies have been reported in up to 63% of patients [50] and may predict a poor prognosis [48]. A polyarticular onset is also associated with poor prognosis [48,50]. Because the diagnosis may be made even in the absence of psoriasis [48,50,52], differential diagnostic difficulties abound. In order to standardize the diagnosis, certain criteria have been proposed [50]. Juvenile PSA is defined as arthritis associated but not necessarily coincident with a typical psoriatic rash or arthritis plus three of four minor criteria: dactylitis, nail pitting, psoriasis-like rash, or family history of psoriasis. Probable juvenile PSA is defined as arthritis in a patient with only two minor criteria.

Although some authors suggest a good prognosis with spontaneous remission in 40–50% of patients [16], a more recent study suggests that the course of disease has more in common with juvenile chronic arthritis [50]. At 8 months' to 13 years' followup, 23 of 35 patients (66%) in this series continued to have active disease despite the use of disease-modifying agents and/or corticosteroids in approximately 50% of patients. This finding suggests that children with polyarticular onset should be treated aggressively, as should patients with juvenile chronic arthritis.

Extra-articular manifestations

Nail involvement occurs in at least 80% of patients with PSA but in only 20% of patients with psoriasis alone [16]; it includes thickening, discoloration, subungual hyperkeratosis, transverse ridging, onycholysis, and pitting (Fig. 8.8). A combination of two or more of these abnormalities is strong evidence for the coexistence of psoriasis and may be the only clue in a patient with seronegative inflammatory arthritis [5,53]. Although some pitting of the nails occurs in 70% of the normal population [54], marked

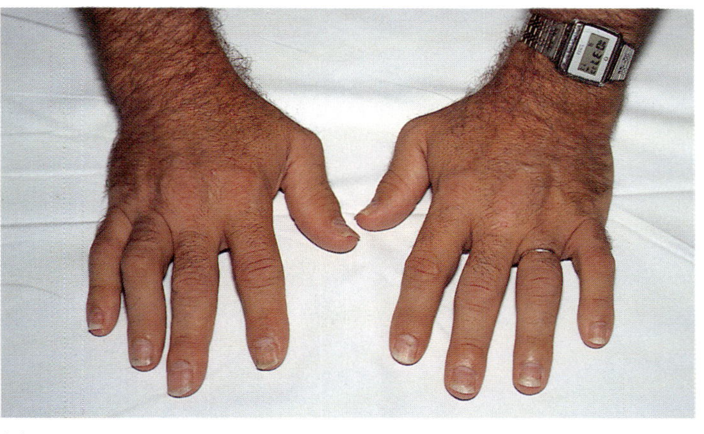

(a)

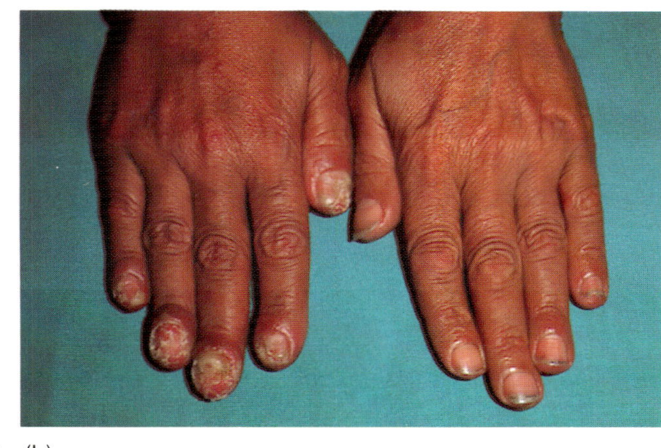

(b)

Fig 8.8 (a) Distal interphalangeal swelling which is especially prominent at the middle fingers bilaterally. Onycholysis and mild dystrophy mark this case as psoriatic arthritis.
(b) Different patient shows severe nail involvement and distal interphalangeal swelling of all fingers of right hand and sparing of the left hand.

pitting defined as more than one nail with 20 or more pits [30] is the most consistent and sensitive nail finding in PSA [55] and is associated with distal interphalangeal arthritis but does not reflect the degree of systemic arthritis or skin involvement [17].

Palmoplantar pustulosis has been reported to precede a form of inflammatory arthritis which cannot be differentiated from PSA [56] and to share immunogenetic similarities to PSA [57]. The association of arthritis and psoriasis to osteopathy due to a higher than normal rate of bone turnover has also been reported and ascribed to either vitamin D deficiency or vitamin D hormone resistance [58].

Iritis and conjunctivitis occur in 30% of patients and is seen more frequently in patients with arthritis than in patients with skin involvement alone [16]. Uveitis is more common in patients with axial involvement than in those with peripheral arthritis [17,40].

Infrequent extraarticular findings associated with PSA have been described. Glomerulonephritis with deposition of IgA, associated with elevated IgA levels and/or immune complexes has been reported in all of the spondyloarthropathies [59] and includes three patients with PSA [59–61]. Aortic regurgitation in a 60-year-old man with long-standing peripheral and axial disease and positive for HLA-B27 is probably best considered an association with genetic propensity [62]. Left ventricular abnormalities due to increased connective tissue deposition in the myocardium has been reported both in RA and PSA [63]. One case of pulmonary fibrosis in a patient with axial disease has been reported [64].

RADIOLOGY

Peripheral joint involvement

The classic and differential radiographic appearance of peripheral PSA has been described best in three series [6,54,65] and one review [16]. In two of these series [6,65] radiographic changes in PSA were contrasted to those seen in RA (Table 8.1). In both diseases bony erosion begins at the joint margin but extensive osteolysis, especially at the proximal aspects of the distal and proximal interphalangeal joints, is only seen in PSA. In some cases of PSA, bony absorption results in osteolysis of the tufts of the terminal phalanges. This same phenomenon, heralded by fluffy periosteal reaction, can be seen at the Achilles insertion of the calcaneus and is an example of the enthesiopathic nature of PSA. Bony proliferation at the distal portion of the joint, not seen in RA, completes the "pencil-in-cup" appearance of arthritis mutilans. Trabecular thickening and new bone formation at periosteal and endosteal surfaces all leading to increased bone density have been termed "ivory phalanx" (Fig. 8.9) [66]. Bony ankylosis of distal and proximal interphalangeal joints is much more common in PSA than in RA. In contrast, periosteal osteopenia and early joint space narrowing are classic changes in RA and rarely occur in PSA. Although a relatively symmetric disease (both hands or both feet involved), mirror image symmetry (both right and left 4th proximal interphalangeal joint involvement) is much more common in RA than in PSA. The lack of distal interphalangeal involvement in RA is a very helpful differential feature.

Axial involvement

The radiographic appearance of axial involvement may take two forms. In approximately 5% of psoriatic patients, the appearance is indistinguishable from ankylosing spondylitis and thought to be due to the co-occurrence of two separate diseases [16,30,40]. In most other patients (approximately 20% of patients with PSA) the appearance is different. These differences include: the occurrence of nonmarginal syndesmophytes, which arise from spinal ligaments rather than from the vertebral margin; random rather than ascending involvement; the absence of vertebral erosions, which result in "squaring" of the vertebrae in ankylosing spondylitis; limited epiphyseal joint involvement; and a low frequency of anterior ligamentous calcification (Fig. 8.10) [19,20,42,67]. In addition, sacroiliac involvement tends to be less symmetric in PSA than in ankylosing spondylitis [39,41], and cervical involvement may include subluxation (Figs 8.11, 8.12a–c) [68].

Table 8.1 Radiographic changes in psoriatic arthritis (PSA) compared to rheumatoid arthritis (RA). Adapted from Wright [6] and Avila *et al.* [65]

	DIP	MCP	Joint space narrowing	Periarticular osteolysis	Periarticular osteoporosis	Mirror image symmetry	Ankylosis
PSA	+++	+	+	+++	–	+	+++
RA	±	+++	+++	±	+++	+++	–

DIP, distal interphalangeal joint; MCP, metacarpophalangeal joint.

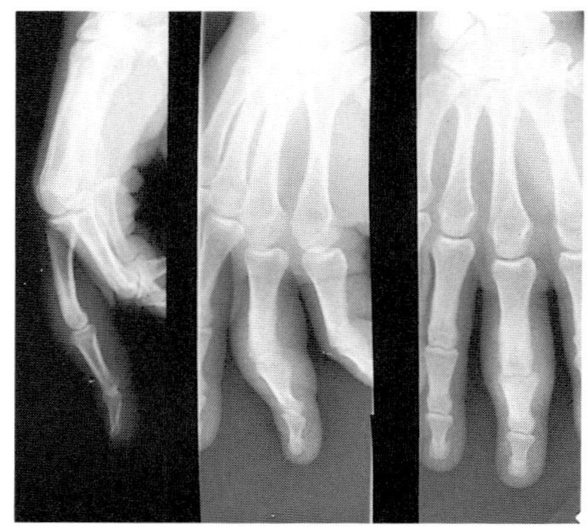

Fig 8.9 Trabecular thickening and new bone formation described as an "ivory phalanx" present in the proximal and middle phalanges of the middle finger.

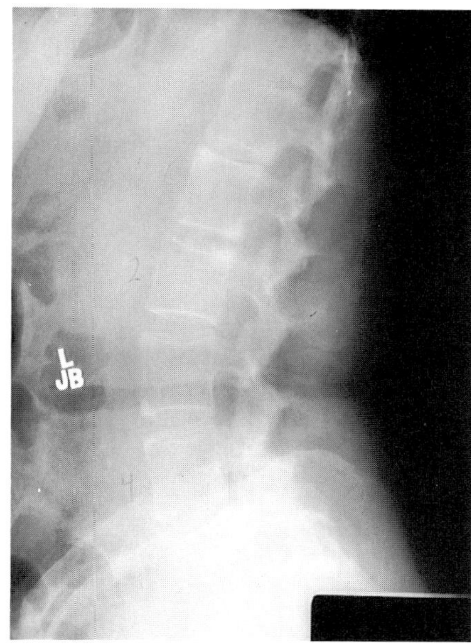

Fig 8.10 Erosions at the implants of the vertebral bodies corresponding to the joints of Luschka, which results in the rare "squaring" of the vertebral bodies in a patient with psoriatic arthritis.

The reviews by McEwen and colleagues in which radiographic findings of four diseases are compared has stood the test of time and is useful in the radiologic differential diagnosis of these diseases (Table 8.2) [42,48]. They demonstrated similarities in the axial arthritis associated with ankylosing spondylitis and ulcerative colitis and contrasted these to similarities seen in PSA and Reiter's syndrome. In addition, they call attention to the higher frequency of peripheral joint destruction in ankylosing spondylitis and Reiter's syndrome.

Most recently, the use of panoramic tomography has demonstrated involvement of the temporomandibular joints in 41% of 64 patients [69]. These changes correlated with peripheral involvement in the hands and wrists. Another series used radiolabeled granulocyte scintigraphy as a more sensitive method to quantitate inflammation in peripheral joints, which were involved but not swollen [70,71].

Cervical spine involvement

Cervical spine involvement deserves special attention. Wright noted that 25% of 118 patients with inflammatory arthritis complained of neck symptoms and showed radiographic evidence of involvement [23]. In another series of 52 patients with psoriasis, a subset of 18 patients with peripheral arthritis showed a high frequency of apophyseal sclerosis on radiographs of the cervical spine compared to age-matched controls without psoriasis [72]. Another series called attention to a high incidence of apophyseal sclerosis and anterior ligamentous calcification of the cervical spine [40]. In another radiographic evaluation of 20 patients with PSA, syndesmophytes typical of thoracic or lumbosacral involvement were seen but a high incidence of atlantoaxial subluxation was also reported. Nine patients (45%) showed this abnormality, usually not seen in ankylosing spondylitis but often

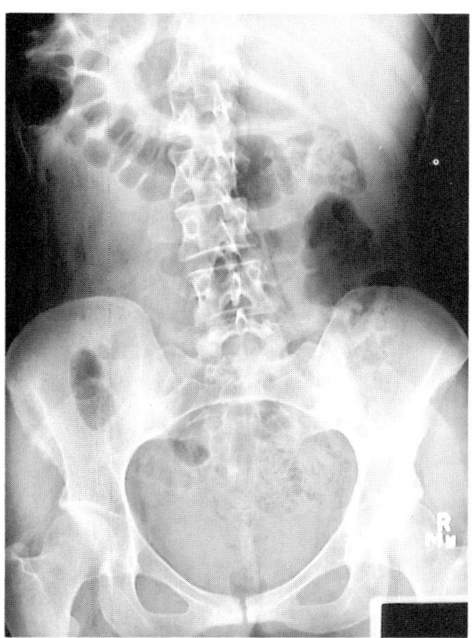

Fig 8.11 Bilateral sacroiliac involvement with sclerosis and obliteration of those joints. Note the sparing of the lumbosacral spine.

Table 8.2 Radiographic differences of the spondyloarthropathies. Adapted from Killebrew *et al.* [42]

	Ankylosing spondylitis ($n = 28$)	Ulcerative colitis ($n = 37$)	Psoriatic arthritis ($n = 38$)	Reiter's syndrome ($n = 33$)
Age at onset (years)	26	27	31	34
Only axial involvement (%)	34	39	10	9
Small joint involvement (%)	41	42	90	88
Extensive peripheral joint damage	(−)	(−)	(++)	(+)
Squaring (%)	78	46	23	37
Symmetric syndesmophytes (%)	73	52	36	36
Asymmetric syndesmophytes (%)	8	35	28	15
Unilateral syndesmophytes (%)	19	13	36	49
Bilateral sacroiliac involvement (%)	100	82	24	24

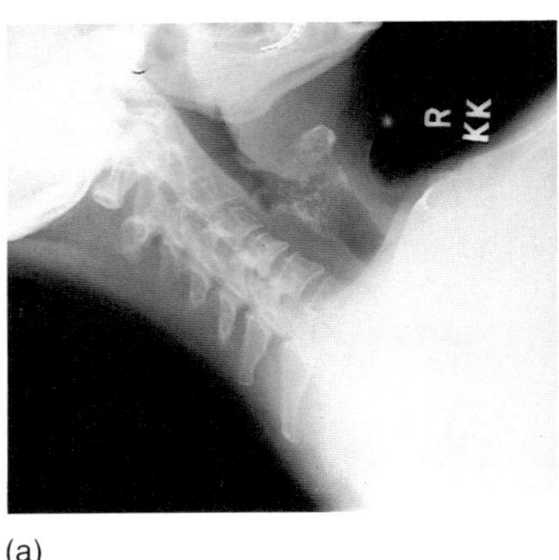

(a)

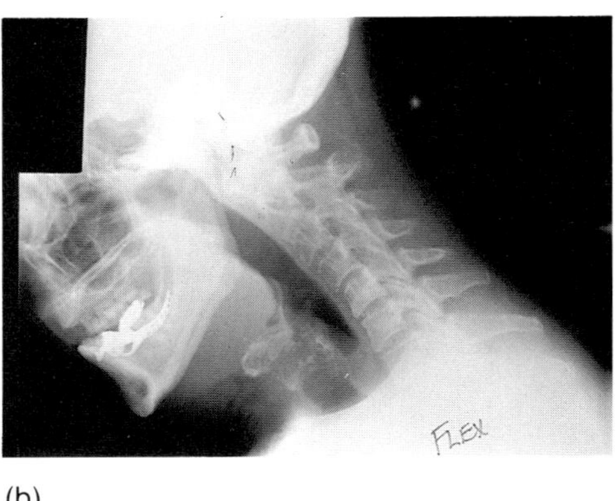

(b)

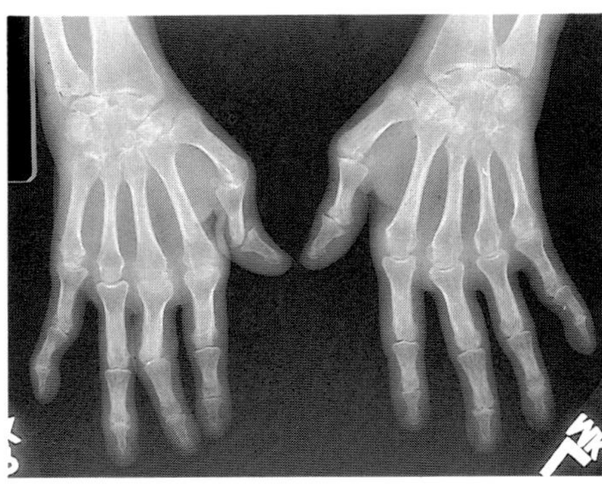

(c)

Fig 8.12 Atlantoaxial subluxation in a 41-year-old female with psoriasis and rheumatoid factor negative arthritis. In the neutral position (a), the distance between the odontoid and the anterior portion of C1 is 5 mm. This opens to 7 mm with extension (b). In both lateral cervical spine X-rays note the anterior ligamentous calcifications. (c) Shows hand films in this same patient, which demonstrates metacarpophalangeal involvement with narrowing and periarticular osteopenia more typical of rheumatoid arthritis. However, the "pencil-in-cup" appearance of the distal interphalangeal joint of the right thumb establishes the correct diagnosis.

encountered in RA, although no PSA patients showed evidence of cord compression [42]. Apophyseal sclerosis and anterior ligamentous calcification was rare. A comparison of radiographic cervical spine involvement is given in Table 8.3.

Neurologic symptoms are rare; none were described in the patients reported by Salvarani *et al.* [73] and they were reported only in three of 21 (14%) patients by Blau and Kaufman [74]. Inflammation of the cervical spine presents as the only axial involvement in up to 36% of patients [75]. In this same series of 57 patients, the best predictors of inflammatory cervical spine disease were the presence of the HLA-B39 and HLA-DR4 antigens, radial–carpal erosions and the absence of the HLA-DR5 antigen. Atlantoaxial subluxation has been reported in PSA and is associated with peripheral disease [76].

LABORATORY FINDINGS

Laboratory findings in PSA are nonspecific. Classically, rheumatoid factor is negative and the antinuclear factor is positive in approximately 10% of cases; it is not significantly higher than that seen in the general population [22]. Anemia, leukocytosis, and thrombocytosis may parallel disease activity. Acute phase reactants such as the Westergren sedimentation rate and C-reactive protein correlate well with the severity and activity of arthritis [16,33,54,77]. Recently, a battery of acute phase indicators was tested in

Table 8.3 Radiographic cervical spine involvement in three series of psoriatic arthritis patients

Author/year*	No. of patients	% Involvement	RA-like	AS-like	Atlantoaxial subluxation	Odontoid erosions	Subaxial subluxation
Salvarani (1992)	57	70	26	44	23	12	16
Blau (1987)	28	75	28	47	18	43	28
Lassoued (1989)	56	42	—	28	5	10	—

RA, rheumatoid arthritis; AS, ankylosing spondylitis.
* Data from Salvarani *et al.* [73], Blau and Kaufman [74], and Lassoued *et al.* [75].

36 patients with PSA [78]. The erythrocyte sedimentation rate (ESR) correlated best with disease activity defined as the number of tender or swollen joints, and the C-reactive protein with severity of radiographic grade. In an efficacy study of cyclosporine A, soluble interleukin-2 receptor paralleled the fall in joint count in a subset of patients [79]. This finding suggests significant participation of the T-cell immune system in the pathogenesis of PSA.

Hyperuricemia is reported by most authors and occurs in 10–20% of patients [30]. Hyperuricemia, as a measure of purine metabolism and epidermal cell turnover, reflects the severity and distribution of cutaneous involvement. Acute gout occurring in the context of hyperuricemia can present a diagnostic challenge. Although some series report normal mean uric acid values [31,32], a Swedish group has demonstrated concentrations of uric acid that were higher in synovial fluid than in serum in patients with inflammatory arthritis including PSA [80] setting the stage for acute gouty arthritis.

ETIOLOGY AND PATHOGENESIS

A primary cause of PSA has not been demonstrated. The interaction of the environment, genetic inheritance, immunologic mechanisms, and the inflammatory cascade all play a role.

The environment

The least-studied primary event resulting in PSA is trauma. For years trauma has been a suspected cause of both psoriasis and PSA [81]. Although a 1 : 1 relationship has not been shown, compelling temporal relationships have been described in case reports [82,83]. The hypothesis that trauma may be an important early event in the etiopathogenesis of cutaneous and joint manifestations comes from two venues. Espinoza and colleagues [84] propose that trauma results in a "deep Koebner phenomenon which initiates the inflammatory cascade". On the other hand, trauma is generally stressfull and information linking stress to the elaboration of neuropeptides which produce neurogenic inflammation in psoriasis allow other possible interactive mechanisms [85,86]. Add to these facts that one controlled study has proven that stress reduction in the form of meditation is efficacious in psoriasis, and the relationship of these nebulous factors to disease exacerbation seems certain in some cases [87].

A reactive etiopathogenesis much like that of acute rheumatic fever or Reiter's syndrome has also been proposed. Levels of antibodies to certain bacterial antigens including streptococci and staphylococci are elevated [88,89]. In addition, the rate of transformation of synovial fluid lymphocytes to streptococcal antigens is increased in patients with PSA [90], and the new onset or exacerbation of psoriasis is more often associated with recent streptococcal infection than in patients without exacerbation [91]. The study of heat shock proteins implicates other bacterial species. Activation of synovial fluid T lymphocytes by degradation fragments of the 65-kDa protein of *Mycobacterium tuberculosis* [92] and high serum levels of IgG and IgM antibodies to heat shock proteins which derive from *Escherichia coli* and mycobacteria [93] expand the field of possible etiologic organisms. Other proteins have been indicted including bacterial cell wall peptidoglycans produced by Gram-positive bacteria. Antibodies to soluble peptidoglycans in 22 patients with PSA were found to be higher than in patients with psoriasis alone and slightly higher than in seven patients with Reiter's syndrome [94]. Peptidoglycans or other bacterial proteins can produce arthritis by inducing macrophage-like dendritic cells to produce interleukin-1, which can directly activate T lymphocytes, plasminogen, collagenase, and lysosomal enzymes [94,95].

Genetics

Inheritance plays a role. Both psoriasis and PSA are more common in first-degree relatives of patients with PSA [17,96]. HLA antigens DR-7, B13, B17, B37, and Cw6 are seen in increased frequency in populations of patients with psoriasis [97]. The association with Cw6 seems the strongest [98,99]. Other associations which include those with DR7 and B57 may be due to linkage dysequilibrium to Cw6 [100].

Axial and peripheral joint involvement is also influenced by heredity. HLAB-27 appears to be dependent on the presence of sacroiliitis and is not overrepresented in peripheral arthritis [101–103]. HLA-DR4, while seen in increased frequency in patients with peripheral arthritis, appears to be a marker of disease severity rather than of presence or absence of arthritis [104,105]. HLAB38 shows the strongest correlation with presence of peripheral disease [99,106,107] and is most specific, being absent in patients with RA or Reiter's syndrome [106]. The presence of HLAB38 does not predict disease expression [107]. Other markers include B7 [99] and A3 [104] which are encountered more frequently in mild disease, and A26 which is a weak marker of arthritis susceptibility [99].

Different HLA frequencies are encountered in different populations. In northern Italian patients, B38 is a strong marker of the presence of peripheral arthritis [108] but is not found in a higher frequency than in normals among 104 Spanish patients with peripheral arthritis [109]. The recognition of these differences serves to emphasize the role of HLA testing in this disease as a way to establish inheritance as a factor but not as a clinical diagnostic tool. Further studies such as analysis of immunoglobulin heavy chain genes by restriction fragment length polymorphism might also provide clues about the role of inheritance in the immunopathophysiology of PSA [110].

Pathogenic mechanisms

The pathogenesis of psoriasis is not entirely understood, but much is known. Over the years, as new research tools became available and new mediators of inflammation and cellular interaction were described, these pieces were fitted into the puzzle. In the 1970s and 1980s, the chemical mediators of skin and joint inflammation were carefully scrutinized. These compounds, especially prostaglandins, leukotrienes and platelet-derived factors are clearly important in the synovial pathology of similar appearing diseases such as RA (111).

These chemical mediators of inflammation have also been shown to be important in the cutaneous manifestations of psoriasis. Leukotriene B_4 and related lipoxygenase products have been found in moderate concentration in lesional skin but not in the unaffected skin of patients with psoriasis [112]. Intradermal injection of as little as 0.15–1.5 μg produces a dermal infiltrate [113] and with higher doses (5 μg) the lesions begin to resemble the polymorphonuclear infiltrates and microabscesses of psoriasis [114]. In contrast, local application of leukotriene B_4 or 12-hydroxy-5,8,10, 14-eicosatetraenoic acid fails to reproduce skin lesions in unaffected skin of psoriatic patients [115]. These compounds appear to play an important role in cutaneous and joint disease, but Greaves and Camp [116] have published a strong argument which indicts their effects on interleukin-1 and platelet-activation factor as the key to their actions. Alternatively, leukotriene B_4 may act as a keratinocyte growth factor [117]. Whatever the effects of these chemical mediators of inflammation, their actions lie distal to the more important etiopathogenic cellular activities within the inflammatory cascade and probably tell us about primary causes.

The humoral immune system has also been studied. Autoantibodies to the stratum corneum and basal keratinocyte nuclei have been shown in psoriasis [118,119]. Further information from Hall and colleagues characterizes the nature of immune complexes in PSA [120]. Using the Raji cell method, to analyze 35 PSA patients, 28 of 35 (80%) showed significant levels of IgA-containing complexes. Thirty-seven percent and 31% of patients, respectively, showed IgG or C1q binding complexes. In addition, the levels of IgA-containing complexes correlated with disease activity. This confirmed earlier work, which showed higher than normal serum levels of immune complexes in at least 50% of PSA patients [121,122]. This also strengthened the argument that mucosal immunity played some part in the pathogenesis of PSA as exemplified by high levels of IgA in afflicted patients [123].

Autoantibodies linking PSA to RA have been described in a minority of patients. Nonspecific antiglobulin levels to cross-linked IgG were found to be elevated in PSA in the same concentration as in ankylosing spondylitis [124]. More specific testing for rheumatoid factor is generally negative in patients with typical PSA. Thirteen of 60 patients with psoriasis and arthritis were positive for rheumatoid factor by latex fixation in an analysis done in 1961 [125]. Three of 37 patients with asymmetric and/or axial disease tested positive while 10 of 36 patients with symmetric disease were positive. This pattern fits the previous findings of Wright and suggests that, at times, RA and psoriasis are present in the same patient [126].

Antinuclear factors have been reported both positive [127] and negative

[128–131] in PSA. When 48 patients with PSA were analyzed using the highly specific indirect immunofluorescent assay on HEP-2 cells eight (16.6%) were positive vs two (4.1%) healthy controls [132]. Neither anti-DNA nor anti-ENA activities were found in the antinuclear factor positive individuals.

The role of the T-cell immune system has long been appreciated. Cell-mediated responses to standard mitogens have alternatively been found depressed compared to normal and RA patients and inversely related to disease activity [133] or to be normal [123]. Decreased *in vivo* delayed hypersensitivity [134] and decreased natural killer cell function [135] have also been shown.

Recently, interest in subsets of T cells dominates the literature. One-hundred and four patients with "complicated" (10 with PSA) and "uncomplicated" psoriasis were studied using specific murine monoclonal antisera [136]. The T helper/suppressor ratio was lower in patients with more complicated disease (erythrodermic and joint manifestations) and tended to normalize with treatment using a thymus-derived extract. Lower numbers of circulating helper cells (CD4) have also been shown by Jajic *et al.* [137].

Whether psoriasis and PSA are associated with a general decrease in the number of helper lymphocytes as occurs in HIV-related disease [138] or are associated with deficient subsets of helper cells, such as the suppressor/inducer subsets CD4+ 2H4+ cells demonstrated in RA by Emery and coworkers [139] and confirmed by our group [140], was addressed by Crockard and colleagues [141]. This subset was analyzed in 12 RA patients vs 12 patients with other inflammatory arthritis including two with PSA. Although the percentage of suppressor/inducer helper T cells was called "within the reference range" in peripheral blood specimens for both patient groups, the numbers of these cells were reduced in synovial fluid in both groups. The possibility that these cells may simply be the "naive" or immature forms of memory CD4 cells designated CD4+ 4 B4+, and that their appearance represents an epiphenomenon simply associated with inflammation, has been advanced by these authors as well as others [142].

Although patients with RA and PSA do share this cellular abnormality, another T-cell subtype bearing the γ/δ receptor [143] is seen in high concentration in the synovial fluid of patients with RA but does not occur in increased numbers in the synovial fluid of patients with PSA [144]. On the other hand, when dendritic macrophage cells have been studied in the same two diseases, both RA and PSA are characterized by fewer circulating cells, but a higher than normal number of these antigen-presenting cells in synovial fluid [145], suggesting a major role for antigen presentation in the pathogenesis of both PSA and RA.

Cytokines and intercellular adhesion molecules are also important in the pathogenesis of psoriasis. Interferon-γ, which is not seen in normal skin has been demonstrated in four of five psoriatic dermal specimens [146]. Interferon-α therapy has also been associated with the *de novo* appearance of psoriasis [147]. Skin and synovial fibroblasts have an increased capacity to produce interleukin-1β and platelet-derived growth factor-β [148]. Finally, specific intercellular adhesion molecules which are important endothelial gatekeepers for the synovial circulation in patients with RA [149], have been shown to be present both on keratinocytes and endothelial cells of the skin and endothelial cells of the synovium in patients with PSA [150]. This finding of identical staining endothelial surface markers in both the arterioles of skin and synovium suggests similar cellular pathogenesis for both psoriasis and PSA.

Another "immunologic" finding clearly establishes the relationships between pathogenesis of skin disease and synovial disease as well as the "autoimmune" nature of PSA. The c-*myc* gene and c-*myc* RNA are expressed during the initial phase of DNA synthesis within the cell cycle. c-*myc* RNA then migrates to the cell nucleus [151–154] where it can be identified by monoclonal antibody and counter-staining methods. Peripheral blood lymphocytes in patients with many autoimmune diseases including RA, systemic lupus erythematosus, and Sjögren's syndrome contain significantly more c-*myc* RNA than do lymphocytes from control patients [155–157], and the percentage of positive cells correlates directly with disease activity [156]. Epithelial cells and synovial lining cells from two patients with PSA showed a much higher percentage of positive cells than did epithelial cells from uninvolved skin [158].

Histopathology

The corresponding histopathology has been reviewed and described by Laurent [16]. Although hyperplasia and hypertrophy of synovial lining cells occurs in PSA, it is not as prominent as that seen in RA. Fibrosis occurs and is more striking in erosive and chronic disease. Immunofluorescence shows the presence of IgG, IgA, and only minimal IgM. Complement components are generally not found nor are the prominent aggregations of lymphocytes often seen in RA. The synovial blood vessels show the most striking changes, with capillary wall thickening, endothelial swelling and hypertrophy, and a polymorphonuclear infiltration of the wall. Vessel wall necrosis rarely occurs.

In early disease, T lymphocytes infiltrate the synovium [159,160]. In established disease, despite clear evidence of autoimmunity, the vast majority of cells infiltrating the synovium have been identified (using monoclonal antibody technology) as type I (phagocytic) synoviocytes [161]. Synovia available from eight patients with long-standing PSA, four of whom had active disease as seen by a rise in the ESR rate above 30 mm/hour, gave negative results for the vast majority of monoclonal antibodies usually seen on B, T, and natural killer (NK) lymphocytes. Alternatively, monoclonal antibodies directed at a variety of surface proteins shared by mononuclear phagocytic-derived cells (type I synoviocytes) were consistently positive. The few scattered cells which did show staining consistent with lymphocyte derivation were identified immunohistologically as suppressor lymphocytes.

These findings suggested to the authors that in late disease, immunologically committed cells which perpetuate inflammation are mostly macrophage-derived synoviocytes.

Again, the role of the antigen-presenting cell in psoriasis appears prominent. When this information is considered in the context of the findings of Gottleib *et al.* [162], that immunochemical studies with monoclonal anti-HLA-DR antibody directed at the keratinocytes obtained from active psoriatic skin plaques identified patients who were at increased risk for the development of associated arthritis, the role for the macrophage seems pivotal.

TREATMENT

Introduction

A variety of agents meant to modify the inflammatory cascade and/or to interrupt cellular processes leading to inflammation have been studied in patients with PSA. Most of these series have been prospective or retrospective open trials of short duration (weeks to months). Very few controlled, blinded trials exist, which makes authoritative pronouncement about the best therapy difficult if not impossible. We have attempted to critically but briefly review this literature.

Nonsteroidal antiinflammatory drugs

Together with patient education, joint protection, occupational therapy, and physical therapy, nonsteroidal antiinflammatory drugs (NSAIDs) are often considered the cornerstone of therapy for osteoarthritis and RA. A review of the English language rheumatologic literature shows an absence of therapeutic trials testing NSAIDs against placebo in PSA. In fact, only one comparative trial has been done [163]. Despite this state of affairs, all textbooks of rheumatology and all review articles about PSA suggest that (by analogy with other inflammatory arthritides?) NSAIDs are useful as first-line treatment.

Clinical use and efficacy

Most controlled clinical trials involving a single NSAID in osteoarthritis and RA, demonstrate significant efficacy when compared to placebo [164]. NSAID efficacy equals aspirin in terms of controlling swelling, pain, morning stiffness, range of motion, and improving activities of daily living. Few direct comparisons of NSAIDs have been published which makes it difficult to rank them in order of efficacy. Clearly, individual patients, and to some degree, individual diseases, may show a wide spectrum of response to any single drug. In general, therapeutic trials of several drugs for 3–6 weeks each must be undertaken before an optimal NSAID is discovered [165].

NSAIDs can be considered rapid acting, first-line therapy which provides symptomatic relief by virtue of their analgesic and antiinflammatory properties. Because of their inability to reduce acute phase reactants, lower rheumatoid factor, or alter the clinical or radiologic progression of an inflammatory arthropathy, they are usually not considered to be disease modifying drugs. It is of interest, however, that at least one therapeutic trial identified a subset of RA patients who responded to NSAID therapy with significant reduction in laboratory and clinical correlates of disease activity [166]. These same investigators later identified a similar subset of patients who experienced a reduction in the number of circulating active T and B lymphocytes, ESR, C-reactive protein, and rheumatoid factor in response to NSAID therapy [167]. They speculated that this "disease modifying property" of NSAIDs may be due to significant reduction of the serum concentration of prostaglandin E_2. If this is the case, it may be reasonable to propose that NSAIDs are effective for symptomatic treatment of inflammatory arthritis and may have a limited role as disease modifying agents.

Toxicity

Although considered relatively safe drugs, NSAIDs are not without adverse effects. Twenty-one percent of patients using these medications in the USA report side effects [168]. The most serious adverse effect occurs in the gastrointestinal tract. At least 60% of patients taking these medicines for 6 months or longer report some gastrointestinal symptoms, particularly dyspepsia. Endoscopic findings, however, are often negative despite symptoms [168,169]. The converse is also true, that is, 20–30% of patients with endoscopically-proven gastric or duodenal ulcerations may be asymptomatic [170,171].

NSAIDs damage the gastric mucosa by directly breaking the mucosal barrier and increasing basal gastric acid secretion, which allows ion trapping in the mucosal cell. This latter effect permits back-diffusion of hydrogen ions. Prostaglandins play a vital role in protecting the gastric mucosa, partially through the production of gastric mucus. Inhibition of prostaglandin synthesis therefore allows for further weakening of the gastric mucosal barrier. Collectively, these factors allow for mucosal damage which manifests clinically as erosions, bleeding, and ulcerations [172]. Most patients with NSAID-induced mucosal ulceration will not suffer major morbidity in the form of upper gastrointestinal bleeding or perforated viscus. The frequency of such morbid events is estimated to be 1.5–4% of the entire population receiving NSAIDs [170–173]. Virtually all NSAIDs can inflict this injury. Furthermore, sulindac, indomethacin, and meclophenamate have extensive enterohepatic recirculation which increases the potential for gastrointestinal toxicity [174]. Patients at greatest risk for gastrointestinal toxicity include the elderly, smokers, alcohol abusers, and patients with previous peptic ulcer disease [174]. These patients may be candidates for prophylaxis against ulceration or gastric erosion which can be accomplished with H_2 blocking agents such as cimetidine, ranitidine, and famotidine or cytoprotective agents such as sucralfate or the prostaglandin analog misoprostol (Cytotec) [164,168]. Cytoprotection seems attractive, but clinical trials have not proved superiority of that strategy over standard H_2 blocker therapy.

Increasingly evident is renal dysfunction resulting from or worsened by NSAID use. Certain clinical factors may be identified that put patients at greater risk for renal toxicity. These factors include advanced age, evidence of renal–vascular disease (as manifested by hypertension), diabetes mellitus or atherosclerotic cardiovascular disease, diuretic use, preexisting renal disease, systemic lupus erythematosus, congestive heart failure, and hepatic insufficiency [175–177]. At least four pathophysiologic types of renal dysfunction can be encountered with these agents:

1 papillary necrosis;
2 interstitial nephritis;
3 acute oliguric renal failure;
4 interstitial nephritis resulting in proteinuria.

The conditions frequently overlap [176]. Associated renal insufficiency improves with discontinuation of the offending agent. Much of the apparent toxicity stems from inhibition of renal prostaglandin E_2 and I_2 synthesis. Resting renal blood flow and glomerular filtration in euvolemic, unstressed humans is only minimally, if at all, dependent on renal prostaglandin synthesis. In the presence of hypovolemia (diuretic use or sodium restriction), patients are more dependent upon renal prostaglandins and are at greater risk for decremental renal function [178]. Likewise, in patients with advanced liver disease, renal production of vasodilating prostaglandins is critical in order to maintain renal perfusion [179]. Animal studies document significant reduction in glomerular filtration rate and renal blood flow in the presence of congestive heart failure [180]. Because NSAID-induced renal insufficiency is preventable and reversible, it seems prudent to monitor carefully those patients at greatest risk.

Cutaneous reactions reported with the use of NSAIDs include erythema multiforme, toxic epidermal necrolysis, exfoliative erythroderma, purpura, petechiae, photosensitivity, fixed drug eruption, exanthem, and nail disorders. Flaring of psoriasis which reportedly occurs in some patients taking NSAIDs has curtailed the use of certain NSAIDs including indomethacin [181,182], meclophenamate [183–185], and phenylbutazone [186,187] for PSA.

Investigators describe an increase in the number of new lesions as well as increased size in preexisting lesions which develop within 1–2 weeks of initiating NSAID therapy [181]. A more serious reaction, generalized pustular psoriasis, may occasionally be precipitated in susceptible individuals [181]. Arachidonic acid metabolism, specifically leukotriene generation may play a key role in the pathogenesis of psoriasis [188,189]. These arachidonic acid products do not cause the disease, but may affect epidermal cell growth, polymorphonuclear leukocyte chemotaxis, and vascular tone. It follows logically that exacerbation of psoriasis may occur when compounds are used that inhibit the cyclooxygenase pathway (such as indomethacin) thereby allowing arachidonic acid to accumulate and subsequently shift the reaction to the lipoxygenase pathway. The formation of leukotrienes then follows. Of interest, benoxaprofen, which is no longer available, inhibited the 5-lipoxygenase pathway and was shown to be effective in the treatment of psoriasis [189] lending credence to this hypothesis.

Despite these data, our experience suggests that clinically significant flares of psoriasis rarely result from the use of medications such as indomethacin. Twenty-seven of our 103 consecutive patients seen between November 1988 and November 1989 were receiving indomethacin. A review of the charts showed that the drug was discontinued in four patients due to "possible flare" of poorly controlled psoriasis. A fifth patient developed a significant generalized flare of skin disease necessitating discontinuation of meclophenamate. However, upon rechallenge at a later date, the generalized cutaneous reaction did not recur.

Pharmacology and mechanisms of action

NSAIDs can be differentiated by chemical structure and pharmacokinetics. Table 8.4 lists the NSAIDs currently available in the USA.

When an NSAID is selected for clinical use, many factors enter the

Table 8.4 Chemical classes of available nonsteroidal antiinflammatory drugs (Trade names in parentheses)

I Oxicams
- Piroxicam (Feldene)

II Pyrazoles
- Phenylbutazone (Butazolidin)
- Oxyphenbutazone (Oxalid, Tandearil)

III Carboxylic acids
- A Salicylates
  - Aspirin
  - Choline magnesium trisalicylate (Trilisate)
  - Diflunisal (Dolobid)
  - Magnesium salicylate
  - Salsalate (Disalcid)
- B Indole acetic acids
  - Indomethacin (Indocin)
  - Sulindac (Clinoril)
  - Tolmetin (Tolectin)
- C Propionic acids
  - Fenoprofen (Nalfon)
  - Ibuprofen (Motrin, Rufin)
  - Naproxen (Naprosyn, Anaprox)
  - Ketoprofen (Orudis)
  - Etodolac (Lodine)
  - Oxaprozin (Daypro)
- D Fenemates
  - Meclofenamate (Meclomen)
  - Mefenamic acid (Ponstel)

formula, e.g., drug half-life, enteric coating, titratability, and method of administration. In the final analysis, the choice is largely empiric. There is little to suggest that one agent is superior to another or that combinations of NSAIDs are more beneficial than any one agent alone [164]. Individual responses to various nonsteroidal agents are unpredictable and may vary markedly between agents [164].

Despite apparent diversity, these agents share many similarities, and it is therefore convenient to view them as a single drug class, focusing on their common properties rather than their metabolic differences [190]. All currently available NSAIDs have analgesic, antipyretic, and antiinflammatory properties. Most are organic acids with a pK_a of 3.5–5.0 [191]. This property allows for rapid absorption and enhanced uptake into inflamed tissue where the pH may be low. Most NSAIDs are 90% bound to plasma albumin; therefore, increasing total drug concentration may disproportionately increase free drug as all available albumin sites are saturated. Because of the avidity of binding and high proportion of drug bound, the potential for displacement of other protein-bound drugs which can result in toxicity is of clinical relevance. For instance, coumarin may be displaced resulting in abnormal bleeding times.

Hepatic metabolism and renal excretion are the principal means of NSAID clearance [164]. NSAID accumulation and toxicity may result from primary liver disease and should therefore be a matter of concern in such patients [192].

At appropriate doses, NSAIDs clearly serve as effective antiinflammatory agents. Several mechanisms have been postulated to explain this action. The leading hypothesis pertains to the property of NSAIDs to inhibit prostaglandin synthesis. In response to certain inflammatory stimuli, phospholipase cleaves arachidonic acid from membrane phospholipids [164]. Arachidonic acid is then converted to cyclic endoperoxide PGG_2 by the enzyme cyclooxygenase [164]. Nonsteroidal agents perturb this enzymatic step. Figure 8.13 outlines the metabolism of arachidonic acid. Aspirin has been studied extensively and found to have analgesic and antipruritic properties only at low dose. Antiinflammatory activity requires higher doses of aspirin (4–6 g/day). Interestingly, the salicylate levels achieved with analgesic doses are inadequate to impair prostaglandin synthesis, employing a mode of action distinct from or in addition to its capacity to inhibit prostaglandin biosynthesis [193]. Further complicating the picture, prostaglandins PGE_2 and PGI_2 have both proinflammatory and antiinflammatory effects. Similarly, prostaglandins of the E-type inhibit activation of neutrophils, platelets, and mononuclear cells, without which an inflammatory effect does not occur [193–195]. Clearly then, inhibition of prostaglandin synthesis is only one of the actions by which NSAIDs act to produce antiinflammatory benefit.

The enzyme 5-lipoxygenase mediates another pathway of arachidonic acid metabolism (Fig. 8.13). In the presence of adenosine triphosphate (ATP) and calcium, this enzyme converts arachidonic acid to 5-hydroperoxyeicosatetraenoic acid (5-HPETE) [196]. This product is acted upon

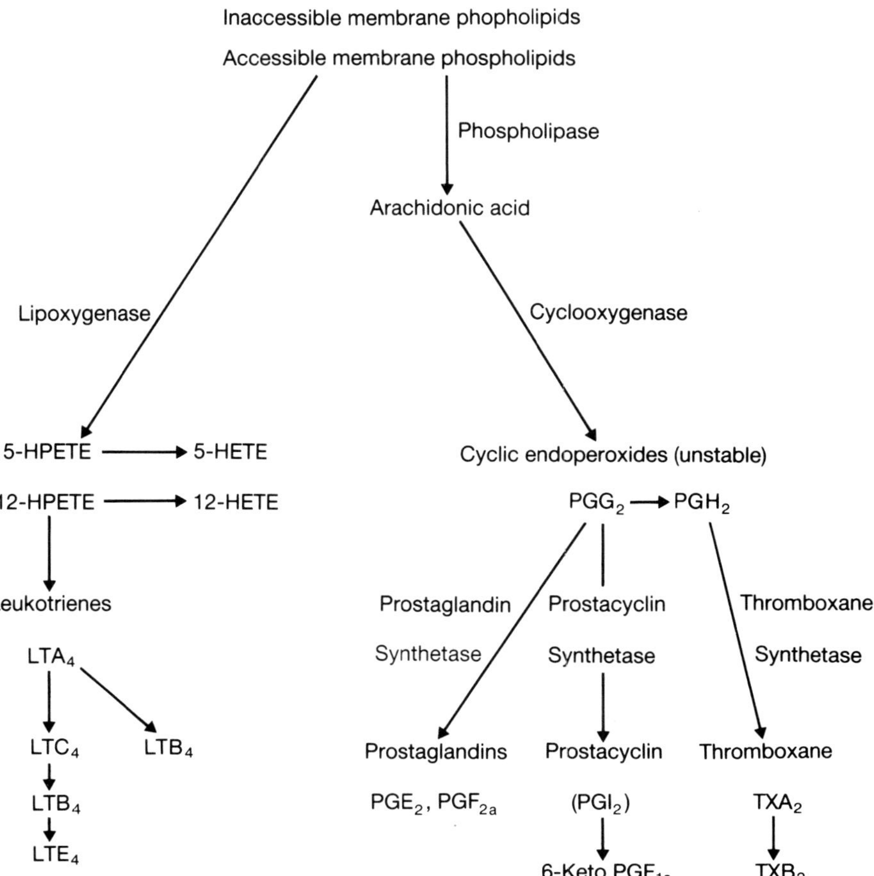

Fig 8.13 Metabolism of arachidonic acid. HPETE, hydroperoxyeicosatetraenoic acid; LT, leukotriene; PG, prostaglandin; TX, thromboxane.

enzymatically to form the unstable epoxide leukotriene A_4. Leukotrienes generated in this way are responsible for enhanced cellular chemotaxis, vasoconstriction, bronchospasm, and increased vascular permeability [196]. *In vitro* studies have shown marked inhibition of lipoxygenase by benoxaprofen [197]. Modest inhibition can be demonstrated with diclofenac and ketoprofen. No inhibition of this pathway is encountered with indomethacin, naproxen, flurbiprofen, or piroxicam [197]. Additional antiinflammatory effects of NSAIDs include: (i) inhibition of neutrophil activation [198]; (ii) inhibition of neutrophil aggregation [199]; and (iii) inhibition of the superoxide anion production [164].

No single mechanism entirely explains the beneficial effects of NSAIDs. In fact, considerable evidence suggests that the mechanism(s) of action of these agents is multifaceted, poorly understood and deserves further investigation.

Antimalarial drugs

Quinine, one of approximately 25 alkaloids derived from the bark of the Chinchona tree native to the mountains of Peru has been used for centuries to treat pneumonia, circulatory problems, thyroid disease, hemorrhoids, and dermatologic disorders [200]. Quinacrine hydrochloride, a synthetic

4-aminoquinolone was first manufactured in the late 1920s [201]. The outbreak of World War II resulted in a scarcity of Chinchona bark available to the Allies, necessitating the synthesis of chloroquine, an antimalarial less toxic than quinacrine [202]. Current 4-aminoquinolone derivatives include quinacrine, chloroquine phosphate (CHL), and hydroxy-chloroquine (HCQ).

Page was the first to publish an optimistic report of antimalarial therapy for lupus erythematosus and inflammatory arthritis [203], followed by reports of its usefulness in RA [204,205]. Two double-blind controlled studies showed favorable trends in most efficacy measures vs placebo in RA, but failed to show overall statistically significant improvement [206,207]. Because CHL and HCQ are considerably less toxic than other so-called "disease-modifying drugs," usage of these compounds and interest in them has remained. A prospective, open trial in 108 RA patients of 6–24 months' duration [208], and a controlled, blinded dosage study of HCQ in 54 patients [209], have established antimalarials as safe, moderately effective drugs for the treatment of RA.

Clinical use and efficacy

By analogy, because antimalarials are effective in RA they might be thought useful in PSA. Data, however, about efficacy are surprisingly lacking, partially due to fear of sometimes severe cutaneous toxicity in patients with psoriasis. In two case reports, a patient with PSA resistant to NSAIDs and/or parenteral gold was treated with HCQ which was discontinued at approximately 2 weeks because of the appearance of a bullous, pruritic, desquamating rash [210,211]. In another report, seven patients with inflammatory arthritis and psoriasis were treated with either HCQ or CHL [212]. Only two patients experienced worsening of psoriasis, but the authors did not describe the response of joint symptoms.

Only two series report the response of arthritis to these drugs. Unfortunately, details are lacking. The first report is part of a review of PSA published in 1979 [17]. Thirty-two patients were treated with HCQ 200–400 mg/day combined with high dose aspirin; 18 additional patients were treated with HCQ 200–400 mg alone. Sixty-eight percent achieved remission, improvement, or stabilization. Adverse effects which were generally cutaneous, occurred in 10 patients (20%) leading to drug discontinuation in six (12%). In the second less complete report, 20 patients with PSA were treated with CHL (dose not given) [213]. All patients had discontinued therapy within 3 months due to cutaneous toxicity. Favorable response to treatment was not observed; ". . no changes in arthritis nor in the value of the erythrocyte sedimentation rate was seen" [213].

We reviewed the medical records of 103 patients with PSA referred to the Department of Rheumatic and Immunologic Diseases from November 1988 through November 1989. Thirty patients with PSA were treated with HCQ 200–400 mg/day and two with CHL 250 mg/day. Treatment duration ranged from 4 to 6 years in all patients. Unfortunately, because of frequent changes of NSAIDs, efficacy was difficult to evaluate. Because all patients continued antimalarial therapy for at least 4 years, and because therapy was not escalated to include drugs such as methotrexate (MTX), circumstantial evidence exists to conclude that therapy with antimalarials was judged successful by the patients and treating physicians.

Toxicity

In RA patients, the most common adverse effect is gastrointestinal disturbance including nausea, vomiting, abdominal cramping, and bloating, possibly due to depressed contractibility of smooth muscle [214]. Pigmentary abnormalities and neuromyopathy may occur with high dose therapy, and are probably dose-dependent adverse effects [214,215]. Exacerbation or precipitation of porphyria has been reported [216].

The main deterrent to the rheumatologic use of antimalarial drugs is the occurrence of associated ocular toxicity due to deposition of the CHL or HCQ in the melanin-containing tissues of the iris, choroid, and retinal epithelium. Reports in the late 1950s and early 1960s described a high frequency of retinal toxicity associated with the use of antimalarials [217–220]. Since that time, Mackenzie and others have reported a much lower incidence of all ocular toxicity [221–224]. Ninety-nine patients with a variety of rheumatic diseases (RA, 58; systemic lupus erythematosus, 31; juvenile chronic arthritis, four; other, six) were evaluated after treatment with HCQ 400 mg/day for a mean duration of 33 months [222]. No patient was found to have visual constriction to white light. Ocular toxicity occurred in three patients including complaints of paracentral scotomata in two, and increased retinal granularity in one. Further ophthalmologic examination showed minor constriction of red vision in all three patients. Discontinuation (one patient) or reduction of the dose (two patients) resulted in complete resolution of the complaints and abnormal testing. Another report compared patients with systemic lupus erythematosus or RA who were age and disease matched and treated with either CHL or HCQ [223]. Patients treated with CHL showed a higher frequency of retinal toxicity.

Mackenzie reviewed the literature and emphasized the direct relationship of high daily dose antimalarial therapy to serious ocular toxicity [225]. He suggested guidelines, e.g., safe daily doses of CHL should not exceed 2 mg/pound (4 mg/kg), and the dose of HCQ should not exceed 3.5 mg/pound (6 mg/kg). At least yearly ophthalmologic evaluation is also indicated. In addition, from a review of the literature there is little evidence to support a role for the cumulative dose of antimalarials as an independent factor in ocular toxicity [226].

Cutaneous toxicity

The reported frequency of cutaneous toxicity associated with antimalarial therapy in psoriasis ranges from 100% with CHL in 3 months [213] to 20% over years with HCQ [17]. Of interest, the generalized erythematous, sometimes bullous, and often exfoliative reaction seen within a few weeks after initiation of therapy with quinacrine was initially considered as a treatment alternative for resistant psoriasis, because as the cutaneous adverse effect cleared, so too did preexisting psoriatic plaques (Table 8.5) [227–230].

One open study reported clearing of light-sensitive psoriasis in the majority of patients treated with short-term, high dose CHL without the appearance of erythema or need for desquamation [231]. The trial of short-term, high dose CHL by O'Quinn and colleagues is of interest because it suggested that treatment with antimalarials increases sensitivity to UV light [232]. After treatment with moderately high dose CHL, the mean erythema dose of UV light was reduced by 50%. Of further interest, none of the 14 treated patients experienced worsening of psoriasis during 13 weeks of therapy. In fact, eight patients volunteered opinions of subjective improvement.

Studies demonstrating the cutaneous toxicity of antimalarial therapies in psoriasis are listed in Table 8.6. Only one open trial was designed specifically to determine the frequency of skin toxicity in patients with psoriasis treated with 4-aminoquinolone derivatives for malaria [234]. Forty-eight patients with psoriasis stationed in Vietnam were given CHL 200 mg and primaquine 15 mg/day for 2 weeks. Twenty patients (42%) experienced some degree of worsening of psoriasis. No patient experienced erythroderma or other more severe cutaneous reactions. Short-term exposure to these antimalarials may have biased this relatively favorable report.

Table 8.5 Cutaneous toxicity in psoriatic arthritis with antimalarials

First author [reference]	No. of patients	Antimalarial used	Efficacy	Toxicity
Baker [212]	6	HCQ (1)* CHL (5)*	Not stated	Psoriasis worsened in one CHL-treated patient
Kammer [17]	50	HCQ	Improvement in 61% HCQ alone and 72% HCQ + ASA	20%, mostly cutaneous manifestations
Luzar [210]	1	HCQ	Not stated	Exacerbation of psoriasis at approximately 10 days' treatment
Trnovsky [213]	20	CHL	No favorable effect	Cutaneous reactions within 3 months in 100%

CHL, chloroquine phosphate; HCQ, hydroxychloroquine; ASA, aspirin.
* Number of patients treated.

Table 8.6 Cutaneous toxicity with antimalarials in psoriasis

First author [reference]	No. of patients	Agent	Disease	Response	Toxicity
Cormia [227]	5	Quinacrine 100 mg, t.i.d.	Psoriasis + pustular psoriasis	Erythroderma within 3 weeks. Clearing psoriasis at 6–9 weeks	100%
Ziprowski [228]	9	Quinacrine 100 mg, t.i.d.	Psoriasis	Erythroderma 1–3 weeks. Clearing psoriasis six of nine	67%
Witten [229]	1	Quinacrine	Psoriasis	Erythroderma at 2–3 weeks. Psoriasis cleared	100%
Cornbleet [230]	6	Quinacrine 100 mg/day, CHL 250 mg/day, HCQ 200 mg/day simultaneously	Psoriasis	Five of six patients experienced erythroderma and improved	100%
Bielicky [231]	24	CHL 250 mg, t.i.d., 3–6 weeks	Light sensitive psoriasis vs nonlight sensitive psoriasis	Light sensitive disease improved 10 of 14, nonlight sensitive psoriasis worsened eight of 10	80% nonlight sensitive psoriasis
O'Quinn [232]	14	CHL 250 mg, t.i.d., tapered to 250 mg/day 13 weeks	Psoriasis	Eight of 14 subjectively improved	Minimal erythema dose of UV light fell by 50%
Olson [233]	1	CHL 500 mg/ week	Psoriasis	"Worse"	100%
Kuflik [234]	48	200 mg/day + Quinacrine 15 mg/ day × 2 weeks	Malaria prophylaxis in psoriasis patients	20 patients worsened	42%

CHL, chloroquine phosphate; HCQ, hydroxychloroquine.

Of the 32 patients with PSA treated at the Cleveland Clinic for 4–6 years, only three were judged by examining dermatologists to have experienced a "possible flare." These adverse effects consisted of increased cutaneous photosensitivity in one patient, poorly controlled generalized psoriasis in a second and new palmar pustular psoriasis in a third. All three of these patients were receiving HCQ. Neither of the two patients receiving CHL experienced a deleterious change in skin disease.

Based on our experience and this review, quinacrine and CHL should probably be avoided in patients with PSA because of the likelihood of worsening psoriasis and more severe adverse cutaneous reactions. A recent report that the manufacture and distribution of quinacrine has been discontinued [235] makes the point moot for that agent. From the perspective of safety, the cautious use of HCQ is appropriate, but further efficacy studies are necessary before any strong recommendation for its use can be made.

Mechanism of action

The definitive mechanism(s) of action of antimalarials in rheumatic diseases and dermatologic conditions is not known. Initial hypotheses included a sun-screening effect [203] or alteration of glucose metabolism [236]. Most recent hypotheses suggest both antiinflammatory and immunosuppressive effects. Lysosomal stabilization [237], suppression of monocyte chemotaxis [238], enzyme inhibition [239], and inhibition of polymorphonuclear leukocyte activity [240,241] support antiinflammatory activity. Interactions with DNA [242], inhibition of RNA and DNA polymerase [243], and potentiation of cancer chemotherapeutic agents [244,245] support a role for immunosuppression.

Gold compounds

Ragan and Tyson were the first to report the use of parenteral gold in PSA [246]. They reported their experience while treating 142 patients with inflammatory arthritis; 11 of these had PSA. Overall, 50% of patients showed clinically important improvement and 33% experienced limiting toxicity. Of the psoriasis patients, four (36%) dropped out due to adverse effects and two (18%) showed marked improvement. This similar frequency of toxicity comparing PSA patients to RA patients was confirmed by Moll and Wright in a comparative study of 48 PSA patients and 42 RA cases [15].

A restrospective review of 27 PSA patients given 30 mg of gold sodium thiomalate each week, documented a response rate of 52% and toxicity of 33% [247]. All patients who responded had polyarticular disease with an RA-like pattern. Rheumatoid factor status was not given in this report. Of interest, five (19%) suffered exacerbation of psoriasis with treatment.

Dorwart and colleagues [248] compared the response to chrysotherapy of 42 patients with RA to 14 patients with PSA. Clinically, significant improvement was seen in 59% of the RA patients and 71% of the PSA patients. Although adverse reactions were more common in the PSA patients (73% vs 57%), cessation of therapy was only necessary in two of 10 PSA patients due to toxicity. Exacerbation of psoriasis was not seen.

Dequeker *et al.* [249] were the first to report the use of oral gold in PSA. They compared 20 RA patients to 11 PSA patients in an open, prospective, 2-year study. Both groups showed significant improvement in ESR and articular index at 1 and 2 years compared to baseline. Although gastrointestinal and mucocutaneous adverse effects occurred in approximately 50% of patients, no PSA patient was withdrawn from treatment. Exacerbation of psoriasis was not seen.

Barbieri *et al.* [250] reported similar findings in a 2-year open study of 22 patients given 6 mg of auranofin daily. Radiographic worsening was seen in only three of 10 patients in whom comparative X-rays were available. Both of these uncontrolled reports suggest that oral gold was useful therapy.

Carette and colleagues [251] performed the only prospective, blinded, placebo-controlled study of auranofin in PSA. At the conclusion of this 6-month trial of 6–9 mg/day oral gold in 238 patients, only the physician's global assessment and daily activity functional scores showed statistically significant improvement. In fact, efficacy was very modest. Although duration of morning stiffness was reduced by approximately 40% in treated patients, the number of tender joints only fell from a mean of 18.2 at time zero to 14.2 at 6 months in treated patients compared to 18.8 at time zero to 15.1 at 6 months in placebo patients. As in past open studies, mild side effects were common (67%) but withdrawals due to toxicity were few (10%).

Palit and colleagues [252] conducted the most recent trial of gold in PSA, in which they compared 26 placebo-treated patients, 29 patients receiving auranofin 6 mg/day and 27 patients given parenteral gold sodium thiomalate during a 24-week study. Neither agent was highly effective. Although minor trends in the direction of improvement occurred in the auranofin-treated patients, no change in disease variables reached statistical significance. In the parenteral gold-treated patients, pain score, Ritchie index, and ESR were statistically significantly improved; however, the changes were barely clinically significant (Ritchie index improvement of 14 at time zero to nine at 24 weeks). Adverse effects were rare (13%) in the auranofin patients, and although rash occurred in six (19%) parenteral gold patients, worsening of psoriasis was not seen.

It appears that auranofin is relatively safe for the treatment of PSA but not very effective. Parenteral gold seems to be tolerated no worse than in RA but is less efficacious in PSA.

D-Penicillamine

The French literature documents response in 12 of 18 patients with PSA treated with long-term maintenance D-penicillamine (dPN) [253]. An 11-patient, double-blind, 4-month crossover study using 750 mg of dPN per day has been reported [254]. Significant decreases were noted in the visual analog pain scale and the ESR. Three of five patients with polyarticular disease showed the best response. The paucity of patients and heterogeneity of disease did not allow any definitive recommendation about the use of dPN in PSA. Adverse effects, if they occurred, were not reported.

Corticosteroids

High dose (0.5–1 mg/kg prednisone equivalent) corticosteroids can worsen psoriasis when they are discontinued, and their use is usually contraindicated [255,256]. However, these drugs are probably indicated in low dose when they are used as "bridge therapy" while the clinician and patient await the onset of action of maintenance drugs such as antimalarials or MTX [257]. Despite its dangers, this agent is used in the "real" world. Disease was severe enough in 180 Spanish patients that 32 (17.7%) required chronic corticosteroid treatment [258]. In addition, intravenous methylprednisolone pulse has been used successfully in a French population of PSA patients without causing exacerbation of skin disease [259].

Sulfasalazine

An uncontrolled, open 1-year trial of sulfasalazine (SSZ) in which 34 patients were given 2 g daily showed a response in 67% of patients and documented limiting toxicity in only eight patients (24%) [260]. In another uncontrolled prospective trial, 10 patients experienced a mean fall in the number of tender joints from 30 at time zero to 10 at 16 weeks [261]. This study also demonstrated a fall in immunoglobulin levels and total B cells with treatments, suggesting an immunologic effect of SSZ.

The efficacy of SSZ was confirmed in a 30-patient placebo-controlled, blinded 6-month study by Farr and colleagues [262]. Early morning stiffness, articular index, the number of painful joints, and the pain score showed statistical improvement after only 1 month. At 6 months, grip strength had also statistically increased in treated patients. These changes were clinically significant. For instance, the number of painful joints fell from 11 at time zero to five at 6 months and the ESR from 31 to 14 mm/hour, respectively. Only three patients (20%) in the SSZ limb discontinued treatment due to adverse effects. Psoriasis was neither improved nor worsened.

Sulfasalazine appears to be a relatively effective safe therapy for patients with PSA who have not optimally responded to NSAIDs.

Colchicine

An open study of eight patients with psoriasis treated with colchicine suggested improvement in joint pain [263]. On the basis of that report, a controlled study was undertaken and reported [264]. Fifteen patients were entered into a 16-week, placebo-controlled, double-blind crossover study. Patients were treated with colchicine 0.5 mg three times daily. Although psoriatic skin lesions did not improve, statistically significant improvement was noted in the grip strength, Ritchie's index, joint size, joint pain, and overall therapeutic assessment. The raw data are not given but 10 of 12 patients felt that placebo was less effective than colchicine. Three patients did not complete the study, two due to gastrointestinal disturbances and one due to unrelated surgery. Five additional patients noted some diarrhea, which responded to reduction of the daily dose of colchicine.

Because of the relative benignity of this drug, it might even be considered in lieu of possibly more dangerous NSAIDs.

Methotrexate

Clinical efficacy

The most extensive use of MTX for nonmalignant disease was as treatment for psoriasis [265–269]. Fairly rapid, significant benefit for cutaneous involvement was demonstrated in a blinded study in 1962 [270]. The same authors also reported their experience with arthritis associated with psoriasis [271]. MTX was continued in an open phase in which 6-day courses of 2.5–5.0 mg/day were given. Nineteen of 22 patients experienced clinically significant joint improvement without experiencing limiting toxicity.

At this writing, 11 case reports or series that describe the use of MTX in PSA in a total of 230 patients have been published (Table 8.7). In two reports daily doses of 2.5–5.0 mg were given [271,272]. Three series describe results using 0.1–0.2 mg/kg per week [273–275]. Three series and one case report describe treatment with doses generally exceeding 0.2 mg/week up to 40 mg/m^2 [276–279]. Cumulative review of the literature shows that the 100 patients receiving less than 0.2 mg/kg per week showed the best response to therapy (76% good to excellent) and had the lowest percentage of patients who discontinued the drug due to toxicity (10%).

Patient populations in all studies may not have been comparable. For instance, the case report of a 34-year-old woman with explosive onset of pustular psoriasis, fever, weight loss, and multiple joint involvement showed an initial Westergren sedimentation rate (WSR) of 110 mm/hour, had failed several NSAIDs and topical corticosteroids, and clearly was sicker than most [279]. PUVA and parenteral MTX 40 mg/m^2 was initiated. At 8 weeks, rash and arthralgias remitted. Oral MTX was continued at 15 mg/week for one more month and then discontinued. At 8 months' followup, no recurrence was noted. This favorable response of uncharacteristically severe PSA resistant to nonstandard treatment is impressive and suggests that under certain clinical circumstances, careful high-dose MTX therapy may be appropriate.

Two double-blind controlled studies have been performed. The first trial was a crossover study of 21 patients published in 1964 [280]. Very high doses of parenteral MTX were given at 10-day intervals; 1 mg/kg, 2 mg/kg, and finally 3 mg/kg, which proved very effective but remarkably toxic. Numbers of swollen, tender joints fell from a mean of 24.2 to 11.8 and the WSR fell 29% during the 30 days of treatment. Unfortunately, 27 adverse effects were experienced by these 21 patients and laboratory abnormalities included leukopenia or thrombocytopenia in eight (38%). Further, during the study period and/or immediately after, two mortalities occurred, probably not directly as a result of MTX therapy. Because of the high frequency and frightening severity of adverse effects, the authors caution against the use of MTX for inflammatory arthritis. Of interest, however, in the discussion they presented eight patients who continued MTX at 40–60 mg/week and maintained benefit for weeks to months.

The second report, a parallel, controlled 12-week trial, employed a more conservative weekly oral dose of MTX, 7.5–15 mg [281]. Although

Table 8.7 Methotrexate for psoriatic arthritis

First author [Reference]	No. of patients	Dose	Period of followup	Efficacy	Toxicity
Hunter [271]	22 (18 MTX alone)	6 day courses of 2.5–5 mg/day	1 week–2 months	11 improved or symptom free (50%), 7 unchanged (32%)	4 (19%)
Kragballe [273]	59	Initial 15 mg 1 week — then lower	1–11 years; median 3 years	21 modest (40%), 22 signs of inflammation disappeared (42%), 9 no response (18%)	7 (12%), 2 GI, 1 vertigo, 2 cirrhosis, 1 ↑ HE
Feldges [275]	10 AZA 2.5 mg/kg per day 5 MTX 10–25 mg/week	Mean 15 mg/week	17 months	1 fair (20%), 2 good (40%), 2 excellent (40%)	4 GI (80%)
Kersley [272]	11 (1 RA, 1 SLE)	Mean 3 mg/day; given 2 week courses	ND	7 "arthritis benefited greatly" (64%), 1 "some response" (9%), 3 "no response" (27%)	4 (36%) stomatitis, 1 (9%) stomatitis and alopecia
Chaouat [276]	26	25–50 mg, i.m. q 2 weeks	ND	4 excellent (15%), 11 good (42%), 5 doubtful (19%), 6 no response (23%)	16 GI (62%), 4 WBC (15%), 3 other (12%)
Black [280]	21	1 mg/kg 3 mg/kg q 10 days (3 days)	30 days	Statistically significant improvement in joint index and ESR	16 GI (72%), 7 WBC (33%)
Willkens [281]	16 MTX 21 Placebo	2.5–5 mg q 12 hours × 3 1 week	12 weeks	Statistically significant improvement in physician's global assessment only	3 (19%) GI or stomatitis
Dunky [277]	31	5 mg/week start; as high as 50 mg q 4 weeks	2 years	17 improved (55%)	5 (16%)
Nyfors [278]	41	7.5–50 mg/week	ND	30 improved	ND

Continued

Table 8.7 *Continued*

First author [reference]	No. of patients	Dose	Period of followup	Efficacy	Toxicity
Eeckhout [279]	1	40 mg/m^2 per week × 8 weeks, then 15 mg/ week × 4 weeks then 0	8 months	Joint disease rash in remission 8 months later	None
Espinoza [274]	36	9.8 mg/week	22 months	34 (95%) "Excellent or good response"	1 HE (3%), 1 GI (3%)
Total*	232	100 patients < 0.2 mg/kg per week	76 (76%)	10 (10%)	
		99 patients > 0.3 mg/kg per week	55 (55%)	46 (48%)	
		33 daily	19 (58%)	9 (27%)	

AZA, azathioprine; ESR, erythrocyte sedimentation rate; GI, gastrointestinal; HE, hepatic enzymes; MTX, methotrexate; ND, not described; RA, rheumatoid arthritis; SLE, systemic lupus erythematosus; WBC, white blood cell count.
* Only 47 patients with toxicity data.

at this dose, none of the 16 treated patients discontinued MTX due to adverse effects, the efficacy data were not very impressive. Only the physician's assessment improved significantly. Trends towards improvement were seen in reduction of early morning stiffness, the patient's assessment, and the WSR. The small number of patients and short duration of this trial may have allowed a type II error. Most rheumatologists interpret this report as a positive study.

Toxicity

From the perspective of practical therapeutics, only agents which are well tolerated by the majority of patients for years can be useful treatments. The frequency and severity of adverse effects with MTX as treatment for RA has been carefully studied and compared to other effective drugs. It has proven to be among the safest [282,283]. Nevertheless, minor toxicity occurs including gastrointestinal problems (nausea, vomiting, and diarrhea in 10–20%, stomatitis in 10%), alopecia in 5%, and headaches in 4% [284–293]. More worrisome, pulmonary toxicity may occur in up to 6% of patients at any time after initiation of therapy [294–300]. Clinically, pulmonary toxicity resembles acute viral pneumonitis and can be life threatening. Treatment includes discontinuation of MTX, supportive care, and short-term prednisone equivalent of 1 mg/kg per day. Cytopenia is rare except in the presence of renal insufficiency [284]. Although hepatic enzymes may be elevated in up to 20% of treated patients [294–301], serious liver histopathology is rare [290,302–307]. At present, in the absence of previous liver disease, alcohol abuse, renal insufficiency, chronic elevation of liver enzymes, or unexplained gastrointestinal symptoms, liver biopsy is not recommended [308,309]. In RA, while teratogenesis may be a concern [310], oncogenesis has not been proven [311–315].

If patients are carefully chosen and those with liver or renal disease, cytopenia, and alcohol abuse are excluded, low dose treatment with 0.1–0.2 mg/kg per week MTX should be quite safe, as it is in RA. Although not studied in PSA, folate supplementation (equivalent of 1–2 mg folic acid per day) has been shown to reduce the frequency of toxicity without reducing effectiveness and should be considered [316,317].

Mechanism of action

MTX inhibits the enzyme dihydrofolate reductase and in high dose cancer chemotherapy, exerts an antiproliferative effect [318]. Its mechanisms(s) of action in low dose pulse therapy for RA is not as clear. The swift onset of action, within 2–4 weeks, suggests antiinflammatory effects [319]. Its properties to decrease the synthesis of leukotriene B_4, to slow the generation of superoxide anion, and to inhibit mononuclear chemotaxis, all support an antiinflammatory mechanism [320,321]. Alternatively, decreased antibody production, inhibition of mononuclear cell IgM rheumatoid factor production and modulation of T-cell subsets all favor immunomodulatory effects [322–326]. The observation that the effectiveness of MTX is abolished if folinic acid is given shortly after MTX to patients with RA, suggests that antifolate, antiproliferative effects are important [327].

Other immunosuppressive agents

Azathioprine (AZA) was first reported as a useful treatment of PSA in a letter by Menkes *et al.* [328]. Five patients were treated with variable doses and followed for 6 months to 4 years. All patients tolerated treatment and showed improvement. A 12-month, double-blind, placebo-controlled crossover study of six PSA patients given 3 mg/kg per day showed 50% reduction in mean active joint count with marked improvement in four of six treated patients [329]. In an open study, 10 patients who received 2.5 mg/kg of AZA per day with a followup of 4.5–67 months also suggested that the drug was effective [275]. Nine of 10 treated patients showed an excellent or good response. At that dose leukopenia was encountered in two patients.

6-Mercaptopurine was reported as useful in a 13-patient open experience [330]. Eleven of the patients showed improvement within 3 weeks, and although the authors described this improvement as "complete," residual joint tenderness was documented in some patients. Continued benefit after discontinuation of the drug was seen for a mean of 4.3 months. Leukopenia, nausea and vomiting [329] and elevation of hepatic transaminase complicated therapy in five patients.

Azaribine, an antipyrimidine drug (6-azauridine triacetate) in daily doses of approximately 200 mg/kg was shown to be effective for skin manifestations of psoriasis in a double-blind, controlled trial [331]. An open trial of five patients treated with 125–270 mg/kg per day demonstrated some improvement in all patients (W.H. Kammerer and M. Rivelis, personal communication, 1972). A prospective trial in 32 patients with polyarthritis in 27 (84%) documented remission or marked improvement in 20 patients (63%) using a daily dose of 2–10 grams [332]. The mean joint count fell from 13.9 to 6.8 and mean duration of morning stiffness from 136 to 46 min at 6 months' followup. Ten patients (32%) discontinued the drug due to leukopenia [329] mental confusion [275] and gastrointestinal intolerance [331]. The drug is provided as 500 mg pills. Unfortunately, the daily dose of 2–10 grams requires patients to take large numbers of pills each day and may be a drawback to its use.

Razoxane, a derivative of ethylenediamine tetraacetic acid was given in doses ranging from 375–750 mg/day, 2 days each week to 36 patients [333]. The drug was principally given for recalcitrant cutaneous disease. However, six patients had severe, polyarticular arthritis. These patients were treated for 6–24 months and generally showed 50% improvement in ESR, active joint count, and morning stiffness at 6 months. Unfortunately, neutropenia is a very common side effect which was seen in 35 to 36 patients at 6 months. The mean neutrophil count at the start of treatment was 6.0×10^9 cells/l which fell to 2.1×10^9 cells/l at 6 months.

Nitrogen mustard, either alone or in combination has been reported in two separate cases [334,335]. In the first case, reported in 1966, a 53-year-old male patient with erythrodermic psoriasis and arthritis was treated first with oral cyclophosphamide 50 mg/day followed by nitrogen mustard given in a single 20 mg intravenous dose, which produced remission of skin disease but had little effect on the arthritis. A repeat 20 mg parenteral dose later in the patient's course again cleared cutaneous manifestations but did not improve joint symptoms. Later, 6-mercaptopurine 100 mg/day was initiated, which resulted in improvement of joint symptoms.

We reported some response of pauciarticular arthritis to nitrogen mustard in a 40-year-old male who had not responded to parenteral MTX 25–50 mg/week [335]. Intravenous nitrogen mustard was given in divided doses over 5 days to a total dose of 0.3 mg/kg. At 14 days, active joint count fell from 24 to 19 and duration of morning stiffness from 4 hours to 1 hour. Followup treatment initiated on day 14 included the reintroduction of MTX 12.5 mg/week and AZA 50 mg/day. One month later, the active joint count had fallen to six and the WSR from an initial value of 123 to 45 mm/hour.

The mechanism(s) of action of these drugs in PSA has not been well investigated. All of these agents have antiproliferative potential, and this is thought to be important to their activity in psoriatic disease.

Cyclosporine

Open studies which suggested that cyclosporine was effective as therapy for recalcitrant psoriasis [336,337] were confirmed in a 21-patient, 4-week, double-blind trial employing high-dose oral therapy (14 mg/kg per day) [338]. Seventeen patients (81%) experienced moderate improvement to total clearing which began after approximately 7 days of therapy. Although adverse effects, including hypertension, headaches, and paresthesias were common, no patient exited the study due to toxicity. Elevation of serum creatinine, although universal, was not significant and reversed when cyclosporine was discontinued.

Controlled studies in PSA have not yet been performed. However, three open studies suggest effectiveness in relatively resistant disease. In an open study of six patients treated for 8 weeks with 6 mg/kg per day cyclosporine, the mean number of tender joints was reduced by greater than 50% at 8 weeks [339]. Although skin manifestations improved quickly, within 2–4 weeks, joint symptoms responded later at 6–8 weeks. Eight episodes of toxicity occurred in six patients, but none prompted discontinuation of cyclosporine.

Two 6-month, open studies using 3 mg/kg per day in 12 patients [79] and 3.5 mg/kg per day in eight patients [340] are very hopeful. Seventeen of 20 patients had failed either MTX or etretinate. Still, 14 of 20 (70%) experienced 50% reduction of disease activity measured as joint count, global assessment and/or morning stiffness at the study conclusion. With lower dose therapy, adverse effects (eight episodes in 20 patients) were less common. Serum levels of soluble interleukin-2-receptor fell in parallel with joint symptom improvement in one study [79] suggesting an immunologic mechanism of action.

Oral retinoids

Etretinate, a synthetic derivative of vitamin A, has been shown to be effective in the control of skin disease in which epidermal cell proliferation and keratinization play important roles including psoriasis [341]. Numerous open studies suggest that it is effective in PSA [342–348]. In one study of 20 patients first given etretinate 1 mg/kg per day and then followed for 2 years on maintenance therapy 10–25 mg per day, positive therapeutic effects were described in all patients, sometimes occurring as early as 4–6 weeks [347]. Acute phase reactants normalized within 2–5 months after starting treatment. "Many" patients complained of dose-related mucocutaneous toxicity.

In another two-center open experience, 40 patients who received a mean of 50 mg of etretinate per day, were followed for a mean of 22 weeks [348]. Response in this study was generally seen at 12 weeks. The active joint count fell from 22 at entry to 11 at the completion of evaluation and the ESR from 39 to 23 mm/hour. Thirty-nine of 40 patients complained of some mucocutaneous reactions including dry cracked lips, dry cracked skin, alopecia, pruritus, and increased nose bleeds. In addition, mild elevation of liver enzymes was encountered in eight patients, and in two cases the elevation was graded "severe." Adverse effects led to discontinuation of therapy in nine patients before the end of 24 weeks.

The very high incidence of mucocutaneous adverse effects has made controlled trials difficult. Nevertheless, 20 patients were entered into a comparative, blinded 24-week study in which etretinate 0.5 mg/kg per day was compared to ibuprofen 1600 mg/day [349]. Eleven patients continued etretinate for 24 weeks, seven discontinuing therapy due to cutaneous toxicity and two due to lack of efficacy. Only one of 20 patients continued ibuprofen for 24 weeks with dropouts largely due to inefficacy. In most patients who completed the study, favorable trends were seen with etretinate, but statistical significance was not achieved. The ESR fell from 42 mm/hour at entry to 30 mm/hour at 24 weeks and the articular index decreased from 16.5 to 11. This study and others demonstrated initial worsening of disease during the first few weeks followed by gradual improvement.

The concurrent use of MTX and etretinate for the treatment of skin manifestations has been reported in two patients [350,351]. In one of these cases, arthritis was prominent [350]. This 51-year-old man with severe exfoliative, erythrodermic skin disease failed to respond to MTX 30 mg/week. The addition of etretinate 80 mg/day controlled skin disease but did not control arthritis. Neither synergistic nor severe additive toxicity was encountered in these two cases.

PUVA therapy: as monotherapy

Twenty-seven PSA patients with either axial involvement [6] or peripheral arthritis [20] were treated using photochemotherapy with 8-methoxypsoralen [352], which has been useful in the treatment of psoriasis [353,354]. Patients were treated two to three times each week until less than 5% of the skin was still involved with psoriatic plaques. Eight patients with peripheral arthritis experienced 60% improvement and six patients 30–60% improvement. In contrast, 16% deterioration in articular index was experienced by the group with spondylitis. Because photochemotherapy has no known antiarthritic properties, the authors speculated that skin activity influences articular response and control of skin activity improves arthritis.

Psoralen UVA combined with other modalities

In order to obtain a faster result with retinoid therapy, psoralen UVA (PUVA) was combined with retinoid therapy in nine patients [355,356]. Five of these nine patients responded favorably to combined therapy.

In another report, five patients were treated with extracorporeal photochemotherapy (photopheresis) [357]. Two hours prior to treatment, each patient received 0.6–0.8 mg per kg of 8-methoxypsoralen. Approximately 2.5×10^9 lymphocytes were collected in conventional apheresis centrifuges and exposed to UVA irradiation for 4.5 hours. These damaged lymphocytes were then reinfused. Treatment was performed for the first two days of each month over a followup period of 20–60 weeks. Modest improvement including increased grip strength and decreased joint swelling was seen in three of five patients.

Interferon-γ

The newer biologic agents including monoclonal antibodies, cytokines, and agents which block the action of cytokines have not enjoyed the popularity which they have achieved in the treatment of RA. In fact the only full length report which describes any of these agents suggests that recombinant human interferon-γ may exacerbate PSA.

Three patients who were participating in a larger study to document the role of interferon-γ in the treatment of psoriasis unexpectedly developed arthritis during treatment [358]. Two of the patients experienced a generalized flare of polyarticular arthritis involving the small joints of the hands, the neck, and the shoulders; and one patient experienced new shoulder and heel pain. These symptoms remitted within days after discontinuation of interferon-γ. The authors suggested that the mechanism of arthritic symptoms may be due to the potential for interferon-γ to increase expression of class II antigens on keratinocytes. This phenomenon marks patients with psoriasis who develop arthritis [162].

Somatostatin

Growth hormone may play some part in the pathogenesis of psoriasis [359]. Somatostatin (SOM), an effective inhibitor of growth hormone release, was given to 18 PSA patients, 12 with polyarthritis. The protocol of treatment is problematic. SOM is given intravenously for 48 hours at 250 μg/hour. Patients in this study were assessed immediately before treatment, at the end of the infusion, and 15 days later. Measures of joint tenderness and pain were statistically significantly different immediately after therapy and at 15 days. Improvement was more marked at the 15-day visit. Adverse effects included leukocytosis in all patients, nausea in eight (45%), erythroderma in one patient and severe abdominal pain in another which necessitated withdrawal of the two latter patients from the study. This series is in agreement with previously reported series of patients with psoriasis and PSA [360–364].

1,25-Dihydroxyvitamin-D_3

1,25-Dihydroxyvitamin-D_3 (vitamin D_3) has been shown to be useful as therapy for psoriasis resulting in significant clearing in up to 70% of patients [365]. Based on this experience, a 6-month, open-label trial of oral vitamin D_3, 2 μg/day given to 10 patients with active PSA was undertaken [366]. Four of 10 patients experienced 50% improvement. Six patients completed the study, two exiting due to hypercalcemia. Of those completing the study, the mean tender joint count fell from 17.9 to 11.8, ESR from 24 to 14 mm/hour and grip strength rose from 145.5 to 167.3 mmHg. The authors speculate that the beneficial effects seen may be due to an inhibitory effect on T-helper cells [367].

Miscellaneous treatments

Bromocriptine inhibits the action of growth hormone which may have a role in the pathogenesis of psoriasis [96]. In one study, using up to 30 mg/day, 77% of 35 patients were said to have experienced significant improvement of arthritic symptoms [368]. The authors, however, only present four patients, one of whom had failed oral MTX, who received 20 mg/day of bromocriptine and showed some response at 3 months.

Total lymphoid irradiation to a total of 2000 rads was reported in one 31-year-old male patient whose arthritis was worsening on 20 mg of prednisone per day [369]. At 14 months' followup, the patient was doing well.

Peptide-T, a synthetic octapeptide mimicking a portion of the glycoprotein envelope of the human immunodeficiency virus, was reported useful in one patient with severe psoriasis and monoarthritis [370]. In an open trial, polyunsaturated ethyl esters, given orally as dietary supplements improved the subjective symptoms of joint pain during a 4-week study [371]. In a prospective study of eight PSA patients, cimetidine ranging from 600 mg to 1 g/day, given for 14–28 days did not provide improvement in either skin or joint involvement [372].

A 6-week, double-blind, placebo-controlled trial of zinc sulfate 220 mg three times daily showed statistically significant improvement in only pain assessment [373]. Eleven patients continued for 24 additional weeks and experienced further significant reduction in the duration of morning stiffness and global assessment.

PROGNOSIS

Prognosis in PSA is generally better than in RA [30], and depends on the clinical subset. Oligoarticular and axial disease is clearly less disabling than ankylosing spondylitis. In one series of 52 patients [44] at 57 months' followup, most patients were less disabled than at entry despite increasing numbers of syndesmophytes and increasing sacroiliac erosions. The presence of HLA-B27 influenced the number of new syndesmophytes and sacroiliac progression, but did not influence symptoms or disability.

Most authors [17,28] consider severe disability a rare occurrence in patients with peripheral arthritis except those with arthritis mutilans. In one large series, 71% of patients were judged adequate for normal activities [28]. However, some disability does occur. Fifty percent of patients in another large series were found to be at least marginally disabled, a much higher frequency than seen in patients with psoriasis alone [31]. In this series, as in others, poor prognosis was associated with early onset (especially before age 20), the severity of cutaneous involvement and a family history of arthritis. The presence of HLA-DR4 has also been shown to be associated with more severe peripheral erosive disease and a more guarded prognosis [104,105,374].

Two recent publications suggest that polyarticular disease, either symmetric or asymmetric, is the most common subset, but disagree about prognosis. In the first series, of 220 patients, only 28% had mild, pauciarticular, asymmetric disease [22]. In this series, 67% of all patients had erosive disease which would seem to predict a poor outcome.

The second series, however, gives a dissenting opinion about prognosis. In this prospective longitudinal study, 40 hospitalized psoriasis patients with associated polyarthritis were followed for a mean of 8 years [375]. During that time, only seven patients (18%) became more disabled and 28 (58%) became less disabled. The authors segregated patients on the basis of disease duration and found that 73% of patients treated within the first 5 years of disease showed improvement in functional class. Only 43% of patients treated after 10 years of PSA showed improvement in functional class. The authors emphasize that all patients were treated aggressively. Ninety percent received at least one disease-modifying agent and 26 (65%) received two such agents simultaneously, usually consisting of parenteral gold and hydroxychloroquine. They further compared the PSA patients to 112 similarly treated RA patients and demonstrated that PSA patients fared better. This is the only long-term longitudinal study that emphasizes therapy and suggests that when disease is treated soon after onset, prognosis may improve.

In summary, patients with axial disease and pauciarticular disease have an excellent long-term prognosis. Patients with polyarticular onset, before age 20, with extensive skin involvement, and a family history of arthritis have a more guarded prognosis and should be treated early and aggressively. In the last few years, rheumatologists have reconsidered their approach to therapy in RA. Long-term followup has demonstrated progression of both joint destruction and disability despite appropriate therapy based on the paradigm of the therapeutic pyramid [376–378]. Now, many advocate very early use of effective therapy which might include HCQ and MTX given in an attempt to normalize acute phase reactants and limit the number of swollen tender joints in the first year of therapy [378–380]. No prospective series have yet been reported although some are in progress [379,380].

We have also learned recently that PSA patients with symmetric polyarthritis predominate and that these patients may progress much as do patients with RA [23,32]. Clinical assessment of joint activity as in RA has been shown to be reliable in PSA [381]. The ESR has proven to be an accurate measure of disease activity in PSA [78]. The time may come soon when NSAIDs will not be considered the mainstay of therapy for erosive PSA, and more aggressive therapy, especially for this subset, will be the rule.

REFERENCES

1 Colombo FF. El job de la Ley de Gracia retratado en la admirable Madrid, Imprenta Real, 1674.
2 Van Romunde LK, Valkenburg HA, Swart-Bruinsma W, Cats A, Hermans J. Psoriasis and arthritis. I. A population study. *Rheumatol Int* 1984;4:55–60.
3 Van Romunde LKJ, Cats A, Hemans J, Valkenburg HA. Psoriasis and arthritis. II. A cross-sectional comparative study of patients with "psoriatic arthritis" and sero-negative and sero-positive polyarthritis: clinical aspects. *Rheumatol Int* 1984; 4:61–5.
4 Van Romunde LKJ, Cats A, Hermans J, Valkenburg HA, De Vries E. Psoriasis and arthritis. III. A cross-sectional comparative study of patients with "psoriatic arthritis" and sero-negative and sero-positive polyarthritis: radiologic and HLA aspects. *Rheumatol Int* 1984;4:67–73.
5 Wright V. Psoriasis and arthritis. *Ann Rheum Dis* 1956;15:348–56.
6 Wright V. Psoriatic arthritis: a comparative radiographic study of rheumatoid arthritis and arthritis associated with psoriasis. *Ann Rheum Dis* 1961;20:123–32.
7 Murray C, Mann DL, Gerber LN, *et al.* Histocompatibility alloantigens in psoriasis and psoriatic arthritis: evidence for the influence of multiple genes in the major histocompatibility complex. *J Clin Invest* 1980;66:670–5.
8 Lambert JR, Wright V, Rajah SM, Moll JM. Histocompatibility antigens in psoriatic arthritis. *Ann Rheum Dis* 1976;35:526–30.
9 Metzger AL, Morris RI, Bluestone R, Terasaki PI. HL-A W27 in psoriatic arthritis. *Arthritis Rheum* 1975;18:111–5.
10 Seingnalet J, Sany J, Serre H. HL-A antigens and arthropathies in psoriasis. *Lancet* 1974;i:1350.
11 Espinoza LR, Vasey FB, Olt JH, Wilkinson R, Osterland CK. Association between HLA-BW38 and peripheral psoriatic arthritis. *Arthritis Rheum* 1978;21:72–5.
12 Kellgren L. Association between rheumatoid arthritis and psoriasis in total populations. *Acta Rheumatol Scand* 1969;15:316–26.
13 Lawrence JS. *Rheumatism in Populations.* London: Heinemann, 1977.
14 Leczinsky CG. The incidence of arthropathy in a 10 year series of psoriasis cases. *Acta Derm Venereol* 1948;28:483–7.
15 Moll JM, Wright V. Psoriatic arthritis. *Semin Arthritis Rheum* 1973;3:55–78.
16 Laurent MR. Psoriatic arthritis. *Clin Rheum Dis* 1985;11:61–85.
17 Kammer GM, Soter NA, Gibson DJ, Shur PH. Psoriatic arthritis: a clinical, immunologic and HLA study of 100 patients. *Semin Arthritis Rheum* 1979;9: 75–97.
18 Baker H. Epidemiological aspects of psoriasis and arthritis. *Br J Dermatol* 1966; 78:249–61.
19 McEwen C, DiTata D, Lingg C, Porini A, Good A, Rankin T. Ankylosing spondylitis and spondylitis accompanying ulcerative colitis, regional enteritis, psoriasis and Reiter's syndrome. A comparative study. *Arthritis Rheum* 1971;14: 291–318.
20 Bywaters EG, Dixon AS. Paravertebral ossification in psoriatic arthritis. *Ann Rheum Dis* 1965;24:313–31.
21 Biondi Oriente CB, Scarpa R, Pucino A, Oriente P. Psoriasis and psoriatic arthritis. Dermatological and rheumatological cooperative clinical report. *Acta Derm Venereol* 1989;146(Suppl.):69–71.
22 Gladman DD, Shuckett R, Russell ML, Thorne JC, Schachter JK. Psoriatic arthritis — an analysis of 220 patients. *Q J Med* 1987;62:127–41.
23 Wright V. Rheumatism and psoriasis: a re-evaluation. *Am J Med* 1959;27: 454–62.
24 Roberts ME, Wright V, Hill AG, Mehra AC. Psoriatic arthritis. Follow-up study.

Ann Rheum Dis 1976;35:206–12.
25 Gladman DD. Psoriatic arthritis: recent advances in pathogenesis and treatment. *Rheum Dis Clin North Am* 1992;18:247–56.
26 Helliwell P, Marchesoni A, Peters M, Barker M, Wright V. A reevaluation of the osteoarticular manifestations of psoriasis. *Br J Rheumatol* 1991;30:339–45.
27 Scarpa R, Oriente P, Pucino A, *et al.* Psoriatic arthritis and psoriatic patients. *Br J Rheumatol* 1984;23:246–50.
28 Molin L. Joint involvement in psoriasis. *Acta Derm Venereol* 1973;53(Suppl. 72):37–68.
29 Reed WB. Psoriatic arthritis. A complete clinical study of 86 patients. *Acta Derm Venereol* 1961;41:396–402.
30 Aguilar JL, Espinoza LR. Psoriatic arthritis: a current perspective. *J Musculoskeletal Med* 1989:11–28.
31 Stern RS. The epidemiology of joint complaints in patients with psoriasis. *J Rheumatol* 1985;12:315–20.
32 Little H, Harvie JN, Lester RS. Psoriatic arthritis in severe psoriasis. *Can Med Assoc J* 1975;112:317–9.
33 Leonard DG, O'Duffy JD, Rogers RS. Prospective analysis of psoriatic arthritis in patients hospitalized for psoriasis. *Mayo Clin Proc* 1978;53:511–8.
34 Hammerschlag WA, Rice JR, Caldwell DS, Goldner JL. Psoriatic arthritis of the foot and ankle: analysis of joint involvement and diagnostic errors. *Foot Ankle* 1991;12:35–9.
35 Miles DA, Kaugars GA. Psoriatic involvement of the temporomandibular joint. A literature review and report of two cases. *Oral Surg Oral Med Oral Pathol* 1991;71:770–4.
36 Cecire AA, Austin BW, Ng PK. Polyp of the external ear canal arising from the temporomandibular joint: a case report. *J Otolaryngol* 1991;20:168–70.
37 Buskila D, Langevitz P, Gladman DD, Urowitz S, Smythe HA. Patients with rheumatoid arthritis are more tender than those with psoriatic arthritis. *J Rheumatol* 1992;19:1115–9.
38 Denko CW, Aponte J, Gabriel P, Petricevic M. Serum beta endorphin in rheumatic disorders. *J Rheumatol* 1982;9:827–33.
39 Green L, Meyers OL, Gordon W, Briggs B. Arthritis in psoriasis. *Ann Rheum Dis* 1981;40:366–9.
40 Lambert JR, Wright V. Psoriatic spondylitis: a clinical and radiological description of the spine in psoriatic arthritis. *Q J Med* 1977;184:411–25.
41 Jajic I. Radiological changes in the sacrociliac joints and spine of patients with psoriatic arthritis and psoriasis. *Ann Rheum Dis* 1968;27:1–6.
42 Killebrew K, Gold RH, Sholkoff SD. Psoriatic spondylitis. *Radiology* 1973;108:916.
43 Dixon AS, Lience E. Sacroiliac joint in adult rheumatoid arthritis and psoriatic arthropathy. *Ann Rheum Dis* 1961;20:247–57.
44 Hanly JG, Russell ML, Gladman DD. Psoriatic spondyloarthropathy: a long-term prospective study. *Ann Rheum Dis* 1988;47:386–93.
45 Moller P, Vinge O. Arthropathy and sacro-iliitis in severe psoriasis. *Scand J Rheumatol* 1980;9:113–7.
46 Shore A, Ansell BM. Juvenile psoriatic arthritis: an analysis of 60 cases. *J Pediatr* 1982;100:529–35.
47 Sills EM. Psoriatic arthritis in childhood. *Johns Hopkins Med J* 1980;146:49–53.
48 Ansell BM. Juvenile chronic polyarthritis, series 3. *Arthritis Rheum* 1977;20: 176–8.
49 Calabro JJ. Psoriatic arthritis in children. *Arthritis Rheum* 1977;20:415–6.
50 Southwood TR, Petty RE, Malleson PN, *et al.* Psoriatic arthritis in children. *Arthritis Rheum* 1989;32:1007–13.
51 Lambert JR, Ansell BM, Stephenson E, Wright V. Psoriatic arthritis in children.

Clin Rheum Dis 1976;2:339–52.

52 Wesolowska H. Clinical course of psoriatic arthropathy in children. *Mater Med Pol* 1985;55:185–7.

53 Eastmond CJ, Wright V. The nail dystrophy of psoriatic arthritis. *Ann Rheum Dis* 1979;38:226–8.

54 Wright V, Moll JMH. *Seronegative Polyarthritis*. Amsterdam: Elsevier/North Holland, 1976.

55 Kvedar JC, Baden HP. Nail changes in cutaneous disease. *Semin Dermatol* 1991; 10:65–70.

56 Kahn MF, Bouvier M, Palazzo E, Tebib JG, Colson F. Sternoclavicular pustulotic osteitis (SAPHO): 20-year interval between skin and bone lesions. *J Rheumatol* 1991;18:1104–8.

57 Szanto E, Linse V. Arthropathy associated with palmoplantar pustulosis. *Clin Rheumatol* 1991;10:130–5.

58 Hein G, Abendroth K, Muller A, Wessel G. Studies on psoriatic osteopathy. *Clin Rheumatol* 1991;10:13–17.

59 Bruneau C, Villiaumey J, Avouac B, *et al.* Seronegative spondyloarthropathies and IgA glomerulo nephritis: a report of four cases and a review of the literature. *Semin Arthritis Rheum* 1986;15:179–84.

60 Jennette JC, Ferguson AL, Moore MA, Freeman DG. IgA nephropathy associated with seronegative spondyloarthropathies. *Arthritis Rheum* 1982;25:144–9.

61 Krothapalli R, Neeland B, Small S, *et al.* IgA nephropathy in a patient with ankylosing spondylitis and solitary kidney. *Clin Nephrol* 1984;21:134–7.

62 Muna WF, Roller DH, Craft J, Shaw RK, Ross AM. Psoriatic arthritis and aortic regurgitation. *JAMA* 1980;244:363–5.

63 Rowe IF, Gibson DG, Keat AC, Brewerton DA. Echocardiographic diastolic abnormalities of the left ventricle in inflammatory joint disease. *Ann Rheum Dis* 1991;50:227–30.

64 Guzman LR, Gall EP, Pitt M, Lull G. Psoriatic spondylitis. Association with advanced nongranulomatous upper lobe pulmonary fibrosis. *JAMA* 1978;239: 1416–7.

65 Avila R, Pugh DG, Slocumb CH, Winkelmann RK. Psoriatic arthritis: a roentgenologic study. *Radiology* 1960;75:691–701.

66 Resnick D, Broderick TW. Bony proliferation of terminal toe phalanges in psoriasis. The “ivory” phalanx. *J Can Assoc Radiol* 1977;28:187–91.

67 McEwen C, Ziff M, Carmel P, DiTata D, Tanner M. The relationship to rheumatoid arthritis of its so-called variants. *Arthritis Rheum* 1958;1:481–96.

68 Yeadon C, Dumas JM, Karsh J. Lateral subluxation of the cervical spine in psoriatic arthritis: a proposed mechanism. *Arthritis Rheum* 1983;26:109–12.

69 Kononen M, Wolf J, Kilpinen E, Melartin E. Radiographic signs in the temporomandibular and hand joints in patients with psoriatic arthritis. *Acta Odontol Scand* 1991;49:191–6.

70 Rydgren L, Wollmer P, Hultquist R, Gustafon T. 111-Indium-labelled leukocytes for measurement of inflammatory activity in arthritis. *Scand J Rheumatol* 1991; 20:319–25.

71 Holzmann H, Werner RJ, Hor G, Maul FD. The significance of hot spots in psoriatic skeletal involvement. *Hautarzt* 1991;42:564–9.

72 Kaplan D, Plotz CM, Nathanson L, Frank L. Cervical spine in psoriasis and in psoriatic arthritis. *Ann Rheum Dis* 1964;23:50–6.

73 Salvarani C, Macchioni P, Cremonesi T, *et al.* The cervical spine in patients with psoriatic arthritis: a clinical, radiological, and immunogenic study. *Ann Rheum Dis* 1992;51:73–7.

74 Blau RH, Kaufman RL. Erosive and subluxing cervical spine disease in patients

with psoriatic arthritis. *J Rheumatol* 1987;14:111–7.

75 Lassoued S, Hamidou M, Fournie B, Fournie A. Cervical spine involvement in psoriatic arthritis. *J Rheumatol* 1989;16:251–2.

76 Suarez-Almazor ME, Russell AS. Anterior atlantoaxial subluxation in patients with spondyloarthropathies: association with peripheral disease. *J Rheumatol* 1988;15:973–7.

77 Lodin A, Gentele H, Langerholm B, Karltorp N. Psoriatic arthritis and an elevated ESR. *Acta Derm Venereol* 1957;37:459–64.

78 Helliwell PS, Marchesoni A, Peters M, Platt R, Wright V. Cytidine deaminase activity, C-reactive protein, histidine, and erythrocyte sedimentation rate as measures of disease activity in psoriatic arthritis. *Ann Rheum Dis* 1991;50: 362–5.

79 Salvarani C, Macchioni P, Boiardi L, *et al.* Low dose cyclosporine A in psoriatic arthritis: relation between soluble interleukin 2 receptors and response to therapy. *J Rheumatol* 1992;19:74–9.

80 Gudbjornsson B, Zak A, Niklasson F, Hallgren R. Hypoxanthine, xanthine, and urate in synovial fluid from patients with inflammatory arthritides. *Ann Rheum Dis* 1991;50:669–72.

81 Vasey FB. Etiology and pathogenesis of psoriatic arthritis: In Gerber LH, Espinoza LR, eds. *Psoriatic Arthritis.* Orlando: Grune and Stratton, 1985:45.

82 Langevitz P, Buskila D, Gladman D. Psoriatic arthritis precipitated by physical trauma. *J Rheumatol* 1990;17:695–7.

83 Goupille P, Soutif D, Valat JP. Psoriatic arthritis precipitated by physical trauma (Letter). *J Rheumatol* 1991;18:633.

84 Espinoza LR, Cuellar ML, Silveira LH. Psoriatic arthritis. *Curr Opin Rheumatol* 1992;4:470–8.

85 Ryan GM. Psoriatic arthritis and Koebner phenomenon. *J Hand Surg* 1991;16: 180–1.

86 Farber EM, Rein G, Lanigan SW. Stress and psoriasis. Psychoneuroimmunologic mechanisms. *Int J Dermatol* 1991;30:8–12.

87 Gaston L, Crombez C, Lassonde M, Bernier-Buzzanga J, Hodgins S. Psychological stress and psoriasis: experimental and prospective correlational studies. *Acta Derm Venereol* 1991;156(Suppl.):37–43.

88 Whyte J, Baughman RD. Acute guttate psoriasis and streptococcal infection. *Arch Dermatol* 1964;89:350–6.

89 Vasey FB, Deitz CB, Frenske NA, Germain BF, Espinoza LR. Possible involvement of group A streptococci in the pathogenesis of psoriatic arthritis. *J Rheumatol* 1982;9:719–22.

90 Sheldon P. Specific cell-mediated responses to bacterial antigens and clinical correlations in reactive arthritis. Reiter's syndrome and ankylosing spondylitis. *Immunol Rev* 1985;86:5–25.

91 Telfer NR, Chalmers RJ, Whale K, Colman G. The role of streptococcal infection in the initiation of guttate psoriasis. *Arch Dermatol* 1992;128:39–42.

92 Pope RM, Wallis RS, Sailer D, Buchanan TM, Pahlavani MA. T-cell activation by mycobacterial antigens in inflammatory synovitis. *Cell Immunol* 1991;133: 95–108.

93 Jarjour WN, Jeffries BD, Davis JS IV, Welch WJ, Mimura T, Winfield JB. Autoantibodies to human stress proteins: a survey of various rheumatic and other inflammatory diseases. *Arthritis Rheum* 1991;34:1133–8.

94 Rahman MU, Ahmed S, Schumacher HR, Zeiger AR. High levels of antipeptidoglycin antibodies in psoriatic and other seronegative arthritides. *J Rheumatol* 1990;17:621–5.

95 Vasey FB, Seleznick MJ, Fenske NA, Espinoza LR. New signposts on the road to understanding psoriatic arthritis (Editorial). *J Rheumatol* 1989;16:1405–7.

96 Moll JM, Wright V. Familial occurrence of psoriatic arthritis. *Ann Rheum Dis* 1973;32:181–201.

97 Espinoza LR. Psoriatic arthritis: further epidimiologic and genetic considerations. In Gerber LH, Espinoza LR, eds. *Psoriatic Arthritis*. Orlando: Grune and Stratton, 1985:9.

98 Tiilikainen A, Lassus A, Karnoven J, *et al*. Psoriasis and HLA-CW6. *Br J Dermatol* 1980;102:179–84.

99 Murray C, Mann DL, Gerber LN, *et al*. Histocompatibility alloantigens in psoriasis and psoriatic arthritis. Evidence for the influence of multiple genes in the major histocompatibility complex. *J Clin Invest* 1980;66:670–5.

100 Hawkins BR, Tiwari JL, Lowe N, *et al*. HLA and psoriasis. In Terasaki PI, ed. *Histocompatibility Testing*. Los Angeles, CA: UCLA Tissue Typing Laboratory, 1980:711–4.

101 Arnett FC. Psoriatic arthritis: relationship to other spondyloarthropathies. In Gerber LH, Espinoza LR, eds. *Psoriatic Arthritis*. Orlando: Grune and Stratton, 1985:95–108.

102 Kantor SM, Hsu SH, Bias WB, Arnett FC. Clinical and immunogenic subsets of psoriatic arthritis. *Clin Exp Rheumatol* 1984;2:105–9.

103 Lambert JR, Wright V, Rajah SM, Moll JM. Histocompatibility antigens in psoriatic arthritis. *Ann Rheum Dis* 1976;35:526–30.

104 Gerber LH, Murray CL, Perlman SG, *et al*. Human lymphocyte antigens characterizing psoriatic arthritis and its subtypes. *J Rheumatol* 1982;9:703–7.

105 McHugh NJ, Laurent MR, Treadwell BL, Tweed JM, Dagger J. Psoriatic arthritis: clinical subgroups and histocompatibility antigens. *Ann Rheum Dis* 1987;46:184–8.

106 Espinoza LR, Vasey FB, Gaylord SW, *et al*. Histocompatibility typing in the seronegative spondyloarthropathies: a survey. *Semin Arthritis Rheum* 1982;11: 375–81.

107 Espinoza LR, Vasey FB, Oh JH, Wilkinson R, Osterland CK. Association between HLA-BW38 and peripheral psoriatic arthritis. *Arthritis Rheum* 1978;21:72–5.

108 Salvarani C, Macchioni PL, Zizzi F, *et al*. Clinical subgroups and HLA antigens in Italian patients with psoriatic arthritis. *Clin Exp Rheumatol* 1989;7:391–6.

109 Lopez-Larrea C, Torre Alonso JC, Rodriguez Perez AR, Coto E. HLA antigens in psoriatic arthritis subtypes of a Spanish population. *Ann Rheum Dis* 1990;49: 318–9.

110 Sakkas LI, Marchesoni A, Kerr L-A, *et al*. Immunoglobulin heavy chain gene polymorphisms in Italian patients with psoriasis and psoriatic arthritis. *Br J Rheumatol* 1991;30:449–50.

111 Hunder GG, Bunch TW. Treatment of rheumatoid arthritis. *Bull Rheum Dis* 1982;32:1–7.

112 Brain S, Camp R, Dowd P, Black AK, Greaves M. The release of leukotriene B4-like material in biologically active amounts from the lesional skin of patients with psoriasis. *J Invest Dermatol* 1984;83:70–3.

113 Camp RDR, Coutts AA, Greaves MW, Kay AB, Walport MJ. Responses of human skin to intradermal injection of leukotrienes C4, D4 and B4. *Br J Pharmacol* 1983;80:497–502.

114 Camp R, Jones RR, Brain S, Wollard P, Greaves M. Production of intraepidermal microabscesses by topical application of leukotriene B4. *J Invest Dermatol* 1984; 82:202–4.

115 Wong E, Camp RD, Greaves MW. The responses of normal and psoriatic skin to single and multiple topical applications of leukotriene B4. *J Invest Dermatol* 1985;84:421–3.

116 Greaves MW, Camp RDR. Prostaglandins, leukotrienes, phospholipase, platelet activating factor and cytokines: an integrated approach to inflammation of human

skin. *Arch Dermatol Res* 1988;280(Suppl.):S33–41.
117 Kragballe K, Herlin T. Benoxaprofen improves psoriasis. A double-blind study. *Arch Dermatol* 1983;119:548–52.
118 Krogh HK. Antibodies to stratum corneum in man. In Beutner EH, Chorzelski TP, Bean SF, Jordan RE, eds. *Immunopathology of the Skin.* Stroudsburg: Dowden, Hutchinson, and Ross, 1973:402–14.
119 Cormane RH. Immunopathology of psoriasis. *Arch Dermatol Res* 1981;270: 201–15.
120 Hall RP, Gerber LH, Lawley TJ. IgA-containing immune complexes in patients with psoriatic arthritis. *Clin Exp Rheumatol* 1984;2:221–5.
121 Karsh J, Espinoza LR, Dorval G, Vasey F, Wilkinson R, Osterland CK. Immune complexes in psoriasis with and without arthritis. *J Rheumatol* 1978;5:314–9.
122 Laurent MR, Panayi GS, Shepherd P. Circulating immune complexes, serum immunoglobulins and acute phase proteins in psoriasis and psoriatic arthritis. *Ann Rheum Dis* 1981;40:66–9.
123 Sany J, Clot J. Immunological abnormalities in psoriatic arthropathy. *J Rheumatol* 1980;7:438–44.
124 Howell FA, Chamberlain MA, Perry RA, Torrigiani G, Roitt IM. IgG antiglobulin levels in patients with psoriatic arthropathy, ankylosing spondylitis and gout. *Ann Rheum Dis* 1972;31:129–31.
125 Reed WB, Heiskell CL, Becker SW. Negative latex-fixation test in psoriatic arthritis. *Arch Dermatol* 1961;83:653–6.
126 Wright V. Psoriatic arthritis. *Arch Dermatol* 1959;80:65–73.
127 Sonnichsen N, Apostologg G. On the evidence of antinuclear factors in various forms of psoriasis. *Arch Klin Exp Dermatol* 1966;227:247–9.
128 Sonnichsen N. Immunologic studies on the nosology of psoriasis arthropathica. *Allerg Asthma* 1969;15:124.
129 Sonnichsen N, Kluge K, Miemic E. The clinical picture and nosology of psoriasis arthropathica. *Z Gesamte Inn Med* 1971;26:742.
130 Zachariae H, Zachariae E. Antinuclear factors, the antihuman globulin consumption test and Wassermann reaction in psoriatic arthritis. *Acta Rheumatol Scand* 1969;15:62.
131 Lambert JR, Scott G, Wright V. Psoriatic arthritis and anti-nuclear factor. *Br J Dermatol* 1977;96:11–4.
132 Calzavara PG, Cattaneo R, Franceschini F, Tosoni C, Martinelli M, Carlino A. Antinuclear antibodies in psoriatic arthritis and its subgroups. *Acta Derm Venereol* 1989;146(Suppl.):31–2.
133 Espinoza LR, Gaylord SW, Vasey FB, Osterland CK. Cell-mediated immunity in psoriatic arthritis. *J Rheumatol* 1980;7:218–24.
134 Krueger GG, Hill HR, Jederberg WW. Inflammatory and immune cell function in psoriasis — a subtle disorder. I. *In vivo* and *in vitro* survey. *J Invest Dermatol* 1978;71:189–94.
135 Kaminski M, Szmurlo A, Pawinska M, Jablonska S. Decreased natural killer cell activity in generalized pustular psoriasis (von Zumbusch type). *Br J Dermatol* 1984;110:565–8.
136 Rubins AY, Merson AG. Subpopulations of T-lymphocytes in psoriasis patients and their changes during immunotherapy. *J Am Acad Dermatol* 1987;17:972–7.
137 Jajic Z, Jajic I, Jajic I, Lukac J, Dekaris D. Immunological reactivity in psoriatic arthritis. *Acta Med Iugosl* 1991;45:141–50.
138 Fuchs D, Hausen A, Reibnegger G, *et al.* Interferon-gamma concentrations are increased in sera from individuals infected with human immunodeficiency virus type I. *J AIDS* 1989;2:158–62.
139 Emery P, Gentry KC, Mackay IR, Muriden KD, Rowley M. Deficiency of the suppressor inducer subset of T-lymphocytes in rheumatoid arthritis. *Arthritis*

Rheum 1987;30:849–56.
140 Calabrese LH, Taylor JV, Wilke WS, Segal AM, Valenzuela R, Clough JD. Response of immunoregulatory lymphocyte subsets to methotrexate in rheumatoid arthritis. *Cleve Clin J Med* 1990;57:232–41.
141 Crockard AD, Finch MB, Fay AC, McNeill TA, Bell AL, Roberts SD. Comparative analysis of CD4 subsets in peripheral blood and synovial fluid of patients with inflammatory joint disease. *Scand J Rheumatol* 1990;19:157–61.
142 Pitzalis C, Kingsley G, Murphy J, Panayi G. Abnormal distribution of the helper inducer and the suppressor inducer T-lymphocyte subsets in the rheumatoid joint. *Clin Immunol Immunopathol* 1987;45:252–8.
143 Reme T, Portier M, Frayssinoux F, *et al.* T-cell receptor expression and activation of synovial lymphocyte subsets in patients with rheumatoid arthritis. Phenotyping of multiple synovial sites. *Arthritis Rheum* 1990;33:485–92.
144 Meliconi R, Pitzalis C, Kingsley GH, Panayi GS. (gamma/delta) T-cells and their subpopulations in blood and synovial fluid from rheumatoid arthritis and spondyloarthritis. *Clin Immunol Immunopathol* 1991;59:165–72.
145 Stagg AJ, Harding B, Hughes RA, Keat A, Knight SC. The distribution and functional properties of dendritic cells in patients with seronegative arthritis. *Clin Exp Immunol* 1991;84:66–71.
146 Barker JN, Karabin GD, Stoof TJ, Sarma BJ, Dixit VM, Nickoloff BJ. Detection of interferon-gamma mRNA in psoriatic epidermis by polymerase chain reaction. *J Dermatol Sci* 1991;2:106–11.
147 Jucgla A, Marcoval J, Curco N, Servitje O. Psoriasis with articular involvement induced by interferon alpha. *Arch Dermatol* 1991;127:910–11.
148 Agular JL, Berman A, Silveiria LH, Martinez-Osuna P, Jara L, Espinoza LR. Psoriatic fibroblasts: participation in the pathogenesis of the proliferative and inflammatory responses seen in psoriasis and psoriatic arthritis. *Arthritis Rheum* 1991;34(Suppl.): S194(abstract).
149 Ziff M. Role of the endothelium in chronic inflammatory synovitis. *Arthritis Rheum* 1991;34:1345–52.
150 Horrocks C, Duncan JI, Oliver AM, Tomson AW. Adhesion molecule expression in psoriatic skin lesions and the influence of cyclosporin-A. *Clin Exp Immunol* 1991;84:157–62.
151 Rabbitts TH, Forster A, Hamlyn P, Baer R. Effective somatic mutation within translocated c-*myc* genes in Burkitt's lymphoma. *Nature* 1984;309:592–7.
152 Watt RA, Shatzman AR, Rosenberg M. Expression and characterization of the human c-*myc* DNA-binding protein. *Mol Cell Biol* 1985;5:448–56.
153 Kaczmarek L, Hyland JK, Watt R, Rosenberg M, Baserga R. Microinjected c-*myc* as a competence factor. *Science* 1985;228:1313–5.
154 Studzinski GP, Brelvi ZS, Feldman SC, Watt RA. Participation of c-*myc* protein in DNA synthesis of human cells. *Science* 1986;234:467–70.
155 Klinman DM, Mushinski JF, Steinberg AD. Oncogene expression in systemic lupus erythematosus. *Clin Res* 1985;33(Suppl.):558a.
156 Boumpas DT, Tsokos GC, Mann DL, *et al.* Increased proto-oncogene expression in peripheral blood lymphocytes from patients with systemic lupus erythematosus and other autoimmune diseases. *Arthritis Rheum* 1986;29:755–60.
157 Gay S, Tanaka A, Tarkowski A, Gay RE, Fassbender H. Expression of oncogenes *ras* and c-*myc* in proliferating synovial lining cells in rheumatoid arthritis. *Arthritis Rheum* 1988;31(Suppl.):R40 (abstract).
158 Osterland CK, Wilkinson RD, St Louis EA. Expression of c-*myc* protein in skin and synovium in psoriasis and psoriatic arthritis. *Clin Exp Rheumatol* 1990;8: 145–50.
159 Gladman DD. The role of immunological factors in the pathogenesis of psoriatic arthritis. In Gerber LH, Espinosa LR, eds. *Psoriatic Arthritis*. Orlando: Grune and

Stratton, 1985:3–44.
160 Braathen LR, Fyrand O, Mellbye OJ. Predominance of cells with T-markers in the lymphocytic infiltrates of synovial tissue in psoriatic arthritis. *Scand J Rheumatol* 1979;8:75.
161 Taccari E, Fattorossi A, Moretti S, Riccieri V, Fasani M, Zoppini A. Phenotypic profile of major synovial cell populations in long standing psoriatic arthritis. *J Rheumatol* 1987;14:525–30.
162 Gottlieb AB, Fu SM, Carter DM, Fotino M. Marked increase in the frequency of psoriatic arthritis and psoriasis patients with HLA-DR + keratinocytes. *Arthritis Rheum* 1987;30:901–7.
163 Lassus A. A comparative pilot-study of azapropazone and indomethacin in the treatment of psoriatic arthritis and Reiter's disease. *Curr Med Res Opin* 1976; 4:65–9.
164 Schlegel SI, Paulus HE. Update on NSAID use in rheumatic diseases. *Bull Rheum Dis* 1986;36:1–8.
165 Wasner C, Britton MC, Kraines RG, *et al.* Nonsteroidal anti-inflammatory agents in rheumatoid arthritis and ankylosing spondylitis. *JAMA* 1981;246:2168–72.
166 Cush JJ, Lipsky PE, Postlethwaite AE, Schrohenloher RE, Saway A, Koopman WJ. Correlation of serologic indicators of inflammation with effectiveness of NSAID therapy in rheumatoid arthritis. *Arthritis Rheum* 1990;33:19–28.
167 Cush JJ, Jasin HE, Johnson F, Lipsky PE. Relationship between clinical efficacy and laboratory correlates of inflammatory and immunologic activity in rheumatoid arthritis patients treated with nonsteroidal anti-inflammatory drugs. *Arthritis Rheum* 1990;33:623–33.
168 Ehsanullah RSB, Page ME, Tildestey G, Wood JR. Prevention of gastroduodenal damage by NSAID, controlled trial of ranitidine. *Br Med J* 1988;297:1017–21.
169 Graham DY, Smith JL. Aspirin and the stomach. *Ann Intern Med* 1986;104: 390–8.
170 Barrier CH, Hirschowitz BI. Controversies in the detection of nonsteroidal anti-inflammatory drug-induced side effects of the upper gastrointestinal system. *Arthritis Rheum* 1989;32:926–32.
171 Skander MP, Ryan FP. Nonsteroidal anti-inflammatory drugs and pain free peptic ulceration in the elderly. *Br Med J* 1988;297:833–4.
172 Schoen RT, Vender RJ. Mechanisms of nonsteroidal anti-inflammatory drug-induced gastric damage. *Am J Med* 1989;86:449–58.
173 Faulkner G, Prichard P, Somerville K, Langman MJ. Aspirin and bleeding peptic ulcers in the elderly. *Br Med J* 1988;297:1311–3.
174 Roth SH, Bennett RE. Nonsteroidal anti-inflammatory drug gastropathy. *Arch Int Med* 1987;147:2093–100.
175 Blackshear JL, Davidman M, Stillman T. Identification of risk for renal insufficiency from nonsteroidal anti-inflammatory drugs. *Arch Intern Med* 1983;143: 1130–4.
176 Bender WL, Whelton A, Beschorner WE, Darwish MO, Hall-Craggs M, Solez K. Interstitial nephritis, proteinuria and renal failure caused by nonsteroidal anti-inflammatory drugs. Immunologic characterization of the inflammatory infiltrate. *Am J Med* 1984;76:1006–12.
177 Zipser RD, Henrich WL. Implications of nonsteroidal antiinflammatory drug therapy. *Am J Med* 1986;81(Suppl. 1A):78–84.
178 Sedor JR, Davidson EW, Dunn MJ. Effects of nonsteroidal antiinflammatory drugs in healthy individuals. *Am J Med* 1986;81(Suppl. 2B):58–70.
179 Zipser RD. Role of renal prostaglandins and the effects of nonsteroidal anti-inflammatory drugs in patients with liver disease. *Am J Med* 1986;81(Suppl. 2B):95–103.
180 Cannon PJ. Prostaglandins in congestive heart failure and the effects of non-

steroidal anti-inflammatory drugs. *Am J Med* 1986;91(Suppl. 2B):123–32.

181 Katayama H, Kawada A. Exacerbation of psoriasis induced by indomethacin. *J Dermatol* 1981;8:323–7.

182 Ellis CN, Fallon JD, Heezen JL, Voorhees JJ. Topical indomethacin exacerbates lesion of psoriasis. *J Invest Dermatol* 1983;80:362 (abstract).

183 Paller AS, Wishner A, Roenigk HH. Meclophenamate for psoriasis. *Arch Dermatol* 1984;120:438.

184 Meyerhoff JO. Exacerbation of psoriasis with meclofenamate. *N Engl J Med* 1983;309:496.

185 Ellis CN, Goldfarb MT, Roenigk HH Jr, Rosenbaum M, Wheeler S, Voorhees JJ. Effects of oral meclophenamate therapy in psoriasis. *J Am Acad Dermatol* 1986; 14:49–52.

186 Reshad H, Hargreaves GK, Vickers CF. Generalized pustular psoriasis precipitated by phenylbutazone and oxyphenbutazone. *J Dermatol* 1983;108:111–3.

187 Voorhees JJ. Leukotrienes and other lipoxygenase products in the pathogenesis and therapy of psoriasis and other dermatoses. *Arch Dermatol* 1983;119:541–7.

188 Albe A, DiCicco LM, Orenberg EK, Fraki E, Farber EM. Drugs in exacerbation of psoriasis. *J Am Acad Dermatol* 1986;15:1007–22.

189 Kragballe K, Herlin T. Benoxaprofen improves psoriasis. A double-blind study. *Arch Dermatol* 1983;119:548–52.

190 Mazanec DJ. Nonsteroidal anti-inflammatory drug-therapy. Clinical use in a high-risk group — the elderly. *Cleve Clin J Med* 1988;55:419–24.

191 O'Brien WM. Pharmacology of non-steroidal anti-inflammatory drugs. Practical review for clinicians. *Am J Med* 1983;75(Suppl. 4B):32–9.

192 Juhl RP, Van Thiel DH, Dittert LW, Albert KS, Smith RB. Ibuprofen and sulindac kinetics in alcoholic liver disease. *Clin Pharmacol Ther* 1983;34:104–9.

193 Abramson SB, Weissmann G. The mechanisms of actions of nonsteroidal anti-inflammatory drugs. *Arthritis Rheum* 1989;132:1–9.

194 Tateson JE, Mocada S, Vane JR. Effects of prostacyclin (PGX) on cyclic AMP concentrations in human platelets. *Prostaglandins* 1977;13:389–92.

195 Weksker BB, Knapp JM, Jaffe EA. Prostacyclin (PG12) synthesized by cultured endothelial cells modulates PMN function. *Blood* 1977;50:287(abstract).

196 Samuelsson B. Leukotrienes: mediators of immediate hypersensitivity reactions and inflammation. *Science* 1983;220:568–75.

197 Dawson W, Boot JR, Harvey J, Walker JR. The pharmacology of benoxaprofen with particular reference to effects on lipoxygenase product formation. *Eur J Rheumatol Inflamm* 1982;5:61–8.

198 Abramson S, Edelson H, Kaplan H, Ludewig R, Weissmann G. Inhibition of neutrophil activation by nonsteroidal anti-inflammatory drugs. *Am J Med* 1984; 77(Suppl. 4B):3–6.

199 Weissmann G. Pathogenesis of inflammation: effects of pharmacologic manipulation of arachidonic acid metabolism on the cytotoxical response to inflammatory stimuli. *Drugs* 1987;33(Suppl. 1):28–37.

200 Leden I. Anti-malarial drugs — 350 years. *Scand J Rheumatol* 1981;10:307–12.

201 Goodman L, Gillman A. Drugs used in chemotherapy of malaria. In *The Pharmacologic Basis of Therapeutics*, 5th edn. New York: MacMillan, 1975:1062–5.

202 Wyler DJ. Landmark perspective: The ascent and decline of chloroquine. *JAMA* 1984;251:2420–2.

203 Page F. Treatment of lupus erythematosus with mepacrine. *Lancet* 1951;ii:755–8.

204 Kersley GD, Palin AG. Amodiaquine and hydroxychloroquine in rheumatoid arthritis. *Lancet* 1959;ii:886–8.

205 Haydu GG. Rheumatoid arthritis therapy: rationale and use of chloroquine diphosphate. *Am J Med Sci* 1953;225:71–5.

206 Mainland D, Sutcliffe MI. Hydroxychloroquine sulfate in rheumatoid arthritis. A

six month, double-blind trial. *Bull Rheum Dis* 1962;13:287–90.
207 Hamilton EB, Scott JT. Hydroxychloroquine sulfate (Plaquenil) in treatment of rheumatoid arthritis. *Arthritis Rheum* 1962;5:502–11.
208 Adams EM, Yocum DE, Bell CL. Hydroxychloroquine in the treatment of rheumatoid arthritis. *Am J Med* 1983;75:321–6.
209 Pavelka K Jr, Sen KP, Peliskova Z, Vacha J, Trnavsky K. Hydroxychloroquine sulphate in the treatment of rheumatoid arthritis: a double-blind comparison of two dose regimens. *Ann Rheum Dis* 1989;48:542–6.
210 Luzar MJ. Hydroxychloroquine in psoriatic arthropathy: exacerbations of psoriatic skin lesions. *J Rheumatol* 1982;9:462–4.
211 Slagel GA, James WD. Plaquenil-induced erythroderma. *J Am Acad Dermatol* 1985;12:857–62.
212 Baker H. The influence of chloroquine and related drugs on psoriasis and keratoderma blenorrhagicum. *Br J Dermatol* 1966;78:161–6.
213 Trnavsky K, Zbojanova M, Vlcek F. Anti-malarials and psoriatic arthritis. *J Rheumatol* 1983;10:833–4.
214 Scherbel AL, Schuchter SL. Comparison of the effects of 2 antimalarial agents, hydroxychloroquine sulfate and chloroquine phosphate in patients with rheumatoid arthritis. *Cleve Clin Q* 1957;24:98–104.
215 Tuffanelli D, Abraham RK, Dubois EL. Pigmentation from anti-malarial therapy. Its possible relationship to ocular lesions. *Arch Dermatol* 1963;88:419–26.
216 Baler GR. Porphyria precipitated by hydroxychloroquine treatment of systemic lupus erythematosus. *Cutis* 1976;17:96–8.
217 Cambiaggi A. Unusual ocular lesions in the case of systemic lupus erythematosus. *Arch Ophthalmol* 1957;57:451–3.
218 Hobbs HE, Sorsby A, Freedman A. Retinopathy following chloroquine therapy. *Lancet* 1959;ii:478–80.
219 Dubois EL. *Lupus Erythematosus*. New York: McGraw-Hill, 1966:222.
220 Henkind P, Rothfield NF. Ocular abnormalities in patients treated with synthetic anti-malarial drugs. *N Engl J Med* 1963;269:433–9.
221 Mackenzie AH, Scherbel AL. Chloroquine and hydroxychloroquine in rheumatological therapy. *Clin Rheum Dis* 1980;6:545–66.
222 Rynes RI, Krohel G, Falbo A, Rienecke D, Wolfe B, Bartholomew LE. Ophthalmologic safety of long-term hydroxychloroquine treatment. *Arthritis Rheum* 1979;22:832–6.
223 Finbloom DS, Silver K, Newsome DA, Gunkel R. Comparison of hydroxychloroquine and chloroquine use and the development of retinal toxicity. *J Rheumatol* 1985;12:692–4.
224 Johnson MW, Vine AK. Hydroxychloroquine therapy in massive total doses without retinal toxicity. *Am J Ophthalmol* 1987;104:139–44.
225 Mackenzie AH. An appraisal of chloroquine. *Arthritis Rheum* 1970;13:280–91.
226 Maksymowych W, Russell AS. Antimalarials in rheumatology: efficacy and safety. *Semin Arthritis Rheum* 1987;16:206–21.
227 Cormia FE, Noun MH. Treatment of pustular psoriasis and pustular bacteria with quinacrine (Atabrine). *Arch Dermatol Syphilol* 1953;68:337–8.
228 Ziprkowski L, Haim S, Bank H. Atabrine in psoriasis. *Acta Med Orient* 1954;13: 45–52.
229 Witten VH, Sulzberger MB. Psoriasis — an unusual response following Atabrine. *Arch Dermatol* 1956;74:210–11.
230 Cornbleet T. Action of synthetic anti-malarial drugs on psoriasis. *J Invest Dermatol* 1956;26:435–6.
231 Bielicky T. Light-sensitive psoriasis and antimalarial drugs. *J Invest Dermatol* 1963;41:1–2.
232 O'Quinn SE, Kennedy CB, Naylor LZ. Psoriasis, ultraviolet light and chloroquine.

Arch Dermatol 1964;90:211–6.

233 Olsen TG. Chloroquine and psoriasis. *Ann Intern Med* 1981;94:546–9.

234 Kuflik EG. Effect of antimalarial drugs on psoriasis. *Cutis* 1980;26:153–5.

235 Anonymous. Manufacturer says raw materials for drug not available. *Dermatol World* 1992;2:1.

236 Bielicky T, Malina L, Sonka J. Glucose metabolism and clinical alterations in psoriasis under chloroquine therapy. *Acta Derm Venereol* 1966;46:72–7.

237 Weissmann G. Labilisation and stabilization of lysosomes. *Fed Proc* 1964;23: 1038–44.

238 Ward PA. The chemosuppression of chemotaxis. *J Exp Med* 1966;124:209–25.

239 Wibo M, Poole B. Protein degradation in cultured cells. II. The uptake of chloroquine by rat fibroblasts and the inhibition of cellular protein degradation and cathepsin B_1. *J Cell Biol* 1974;63:430–40.

240 Chang YH. Studies on phagocytosis. II. Effect of nonsteroidal anti-inflammatory drugs on phagocytosis and urate crystal-induced canine joint inflammation. *J Pharmacol Exp Ther* 1972;183:235–44.

241 Jones CJP, Jayson MI. Chloroquine: its effect on leucocyte auto- and heterophogacytosis. *Ann Rheum Dis* 1984;43:205–12.

242 Cohen SN, Yielding KL. Spectrophotometric studies on the interaction of chloroquine and deoxyribonucleic acid. *J Biol Chem* 1965;240:3123–31.

243 Cohen SN, Yielding KL. Inhibition of DNA and RNA polymerase reactions by chloroquine. *Proc Natl Acad Sci USA* 1965;54:521–7.

244 Gaudin D, Yielding KL. Response of a "resistant" plasmacytoma to alkylating agents and X-ray in combination of the "excision" repair inhibitors caffeine and chloroquine. *Proc Soc Exp Biol Med* 1969;131:1413–6.

245 Ramakrishnan S, Houston LL. Inhibition of human acute lymphoblastic leukemia cells by immunotoxins: potentiation by chloroquine. *Science* 1984;223:58–61.

246 Ragan C, Tyson TL. Chrysotherapy in rheumatoid arthritis. A 3-year study of 142 cases. *Am J Med* 1946;1:252–6.

247 Richter MB, Kinsella P, Corbett M. Gold in psoriatic arthropathy. *Ann Rheum Dis* 1980;39:279–80.

248 Dorwart BB, Gall EP, Schumacher HR, Krauser RE. Chrysotherapy in psoriatic arthritis. Efficacy and toxicity compared to rheumatoid arthritis. *Arthritis Rheum* 1978;21:513–5.

249 Dequecker J, Verdickt W, Gevers G, Vanschoubroek M. Long term experience with oral gold in rheumatoid arthritis and psoriatic arthritis. *Clin Rheumatol* 1984;3(Suppl.):67–74.

250 Barbieri P, Ciompi ML, Bini C, Pasero G. Long term experience with oral gold in psoriatic arthritis. *Clin Rheumatol* 1986;5:274–5.

251 Carette S, Calin A, McCafferty JP, Wallin BA. A double-blind placebo-controlled study of auranofin in patients with psoriatic arthritis. *Arthritis Rheum* 1989;32: 158–65.

252 Palit J, Hill J, Capell HA, *et al.* A multicentre double-blind comparison of auranofin, intramuscular gold thiomalate and placebo in patients with psoriatic arthritis. *Br J Rheumatol* 1990;29:280–3.

253 Roux H, Schiano A, Maestracci D, *et al.* Our experience in the treatment of psoriatic rheumatism with D-penicillamine. *Rev Rhum Mal Osteoartic* 1979; 46:631–3.

254 Price R, Gibson T. D-penicillamine and psoriatic arthropathy. *Br J Rheumatol* 1986;25:228.

255 Rivet JP, Richard A. Volatarene, an antiinflammatory agent in rheumatology. *Gaz Med Fr* 1977;84:3547–54.

256 Zboganova M, Trnavsky K, Vicek F. Indomethacin in the treatment of psoriatic arthritis. *Czech Dermatol* 1974;49:129–32.

257 Rondier J. Comment je traite un rhumatisme psoriasique. *Gaz Med Fr* 1972;85: 419–20.

258 Torre Alonso JC, Rodriguez Perez A, Arribas Castrillo JM, Ballina Garcia J, Riestra Noriega JL, Lopez Larrea C. Psoriatic arthritis (PA): a clinical, immunological and radiological study of 180 patients. *Br J Rheumatol* 1991;30:245–50.

259 Hilliquin P, Gregoir C, Menkes CJ. Efficacité des bolus de corticoides dans le rhumatisme psoriasique. *Rev Rhum Mal Osteoartic* 1990;10:715(abstract E15).

260 Farr M, Kitas GD, Waterhouse L, Jubb R, Felix-Davies DD, Bacon PA. Treatment of psoriatic arthritis with sulphasalazine. A one year open study. *Clin Rheumatol* 1988;7:372–7.

261 Newman ED, Perruquet JL, Harrington TM. Sulfasalazine therapy in psoriatic arthritis: clinical and immunologic response. *J Rheumatol* 1991;18:1379–82.

262 Farr M, Kitas GD, Waterhouse L, Jubb R, Felix-Davies D, Bacon PA. Sulfasalazine in psoriatic arthritis: a double-blind placebo-controlled study. *Br J Rheumatol* 1990;29:46–9.

263 Wahba A, Cohen HS. Therapeutic trials with oral colchicine in psoriasis. *Acta Derm Venereol* 1980;60:515–20.

264 Seideman P, Fjellner B, Johannesson A. Psoriatic arthritis treated with oral colchicine. *J Rheumatol* 1987;14:777–9.

265 Gubner R. Effect of aminopterin on epithelial tissues. *Arch Dermatol* 1951;64: 688–99.

266 Rees RB, Bennett JH, Bostick WL. Aminopterin for psoriasis. *Arch Dermatol* 1955;72:133–43.

267 Edmundson WF, Guy WB. Treatment of psoriasis with folic acid antagonists. *Arch Dermatol* 1958;78:200–3.

268 Rees RB, Bennett JH. Further observations on aminopterin for psoriasis. *J Invest Dermatol* 1959;32:61–6.

269 Rees RB, Bennett JH. Methotrexate versus aminopterin for psoriasis. *Arch Dermatol* 1961;83:970–2.

270 Hunter GA, Turner AN. Methotrexate in the treatment of psoriasis: a controlled clinical trial. *Australas J Dermatol* 1962;6:248–53.

271 Hunter GA, Millazzo SC. Response of psoriatic arthropathy to methotrexate. *Australas J Dermatol* 1965;8:137–41.

272 Kersley GD. Amethopterin (methotrexate) in connective tissue disease — psoriasis and polyarthritis. *Ann Rheum Dis* 1968;27:64–6.

273 Kragballe K, Zachariae E, Zachariae H. Methotrexate in psoriatic arthritis: a retrospective study. *Acta Derm Venereol* 1983;63:165–7.

274 Espinoza LR, Gutierrez F, Vasey F, Germain B. Clinical experience with methotrexate in psoriatic arthritis (PSA). *Arthritis Rheum* 1990;33(Suppl.):S160.

275 Feldges DH, Barnes CG. Treatment of psoriatic arthropathy with either azathioprine or methotrexate. *Rheumatol Rehab* 1974;13:120–4.

276 Chaouat Y, Kanovitch B, Faures B, Grupper CH, Bourgeois-Spinasse J. Psoriatic rheumatism. Treatment with methotrexate. *Rev Rhum Mal Osteoartic* 1971;38: 453–60.

277 Dunky A. Low dose methotrexate therapy in psoriatic arthritis. In Rau R, Lasch H-G (eds). *Low-dose Methotrexate Therapy in Rheumatic Diseases (Rheumatology, No. 9)*. Basel/New York: Karger, 1986:88–95.

278 Nyfors A. Methotrexate therapy in psoriasis and psoriatic arthritis. In Rau R, Lasch H-G (eds). *Low-dose Methotrexate Therapy in Rheumatic Diseases (Rheumatology, No. 9)*. Basel/New York: Karger, 1986:69–87.

279 Eeckhout E, Suys E, Buydens P, Van Belle S, Berbruggen LA. Short-term, high-dose methotrexate therapy in a case of severe psoriatic arthritis. *Br J Rheumatol* 1988;27:160–2.

280 Black RL, O'Brien WM, Van Scott EJ, Auerbach R, Eisen AZ, Bunim JJ. Meth-

otrexate therapy in psoriatic arthritis. Double-blind study on 21 patients. *JAMA* 1964;189:743–7.

281 Willkens RF, Williams HJ, Ward JR, *et al.* Randomized, double-blind, placebo controlled trial of low-dose pulse methotrexate in psoriatic arthritis. *Arthritis Rheum* 1984;27:376–81.

282 Willkens RF. Resolve: methotrexate is the drug of choice after NSAIDs in rheumatoid arthritis. *Semin Arthritis Rheum* 1990;20:76–80.

283 Zatarain E, Williams CA, Fries JF. Comparison of adverse reactions of methotrexate and other disease-modifying drugs. *Arthritis Rheum* 1988;31(Suppl.):S116.

284 Gispen JG, Alarcon GS, Johnson JJ, Acton RT, Barger BO, Koopman WJ. Toxicity of methotrexate in rheumatoid arthritis. *J Rheumatol* 1987;14:74–9.

285 Groff GD, Shenberger KN, Wilke WS, Taylor TH. Low dose oral methotrexate in rheumatoid arthritis: an uncontrolled trial and review of the literature. *Semin Arthritis Rheum* 1983;12:333–47.

286 Boh LE, Schuna AA, Pitterle ME, Abrams EM, Sundstrom WR. Low dose weekly oral methotrexate therapy for inflammatory arthritis. *Clin Pharm* 1986;5:503–8.

287 Szanto E. Low-dose methotrexate in rheumatoid arthritis: effect and tolerance. An open trial and a double-blind randomized study. *Scand J Rheumatol* 1986; 15:97–102.

288 Andersen PA, West SG, Nordstrom DM. Toxicity of chronic therapy with pulse methotrexate (MTX) in rheumatoid arthritis: potential increased risk of infection. *Arthritis Rheum* 1987;30(Suppl.):S60.

289 Kremer JM, Lee JK. The safety and efficacy of the use of methotrexate in long-term therapy for rheumatoid arthritis. *Arthritis Rheum* 1986;29:822–31.

290 Weinstein A, Marlowe S, Korn J, Farouhar F. Low-dose methotrexate treatment of rheumatoid arthritis: long-term observations. *Am J Med* 1985;79:331–7.

291 Wilke WS, Calabrese LH, Krall PL, Segal AM. Incidence of toxicity in patients with rheumatoid arthritis treated with methotrexate. In Rau R, Lasch H (eds). *Low-dose Methotrexate Therapy in Rheumatic Disease (Rheumatology, No. 9)*. Basel/New York: Karger, 1986:134–44.

292 Hoffmeister RT. Methotrexate therapy in rheumatoid arthritis: 15 years experience. *Am J Med* 1983;75:69–73.

293 Segal AM, Koo AP, Calabrese LH, *et al.* 20 year experience of methotrexate (MTX) toxicity in rheumatoid arthritis (RA). *Arthritis Rheum* 1987;30(Suppl.): S59.

294 From E. Methotrexate pneumonitis in a psoriatic. *Br J Dermatol* 1975;93: 107–10.

295 Sostman HD, Matthay RA, Putman CE, Walker-Smith GJ. Methotrexate-induced pneumonitis. *Medicine* 1976;55:371–88.

296 Louie S, Lillington GA. Low-dose methotrexate pneumonitis in rheumatoid arthritis. *Thorax* 1986;41:703–4.

297 Engelbrecht JA, Calhoon SL, Scherrer JJ. Methotrexate pneumonitis after low-dose therapy for rheumatoid arthritis. *Arthritis Rheum* 1983;26:1275–8.

298 Maier WP, Leon-Perez R, Miller SB. Pneumonitis during low-dose methotrexate therapy. *Arch Intern Med* 1986;146:602–3.

299 Cannon GW, Ward JR, Clegg DO, Samuelson CO Jr, Abbott TM. Acute lung disease associated with low-dose pulse methotrexate therapy in patients with rheumatoid arthritis. *Arthritis Rheum* 1983;26:1269–74.

300 Carson CW, Cannon GW, Egger MJ, Ward JR, Clegg DO. Pulmonary disease during the treatment of rheumatoid arthritis with low-dose pulse methotrexate. *Semin Arthritis Rheum* 1987;16:186–95.

301 Segal AM, Wilke WS. Toxicity of low-dose methotrexate in rheumatoid arthritis. In Wilke WS, ed. *Methotrexate Therapy in Rheumatic Disease*. New York: Marcel Dekker, Inc., 1989:147–8.

302 DiBartolomeo AG, Mayes MD, Bathon JM. Methotrexate in rheumatoid arthritis: a longitudinal study of liver biopsy. *Arthritis Rheum* 1984;27(Suppl.):S61.
303 Mackenzie AH. Hepatotoxicity of prolonged methotrexate therapy for rheumatoid arthritis. *Cleveland Clin Q* 1985;52:129–35.
304 Aponte J, Petrelli M. Hepatic histology following prolonged treatment of rheumatoid arthritis with bolus methotrexate. *Arthritis Rheum* 1985;28(Suppl.):S37.
305 Kremer JM. A long-term prospective study of methotrexate (MTX) in rheumatoid arthritis (RA). *Arthritis Rheum* 1985;28(Suppl.):S68.
306 Koo AP, Mackenzie AH, Tuthill RJ, Leatherman JR. Liver histology in rheumatoid arthritis. *Arthritis Rheum* 1985;28(Suppl.):S14.
307 Rau R, Karger T. Liver biopsy findings in patients with rheumatoid arthritis (RA) psoriatic arthritis (PSA) on long-term treatment with methotrexate. *Arthritis Rheum* 1986; 29(Suppl.):S76.
308 Wilke WS. Practical considerations: dose, route, and monitoring. In Wilke WS, ed. *Methotrexate Therapy in Rheumatic Disease*. New York: Marcel Dekker, Inc., 1989:261–83.
309 Grisanti JM, Wilke WS. Proper use of disease-modifying agents. *Consultant* 1992; 32:23–6.
310 Kozlowski RD, Steinbrunner JV, MacKenzie AH, Clough JD, Wilke WS, Segal AM. Outcome of first-trimester exposure to low-dose methotrexate in eight patients with rheumatic disease. *Am J Med* 1990;88:589–92.
311 Rustin GJ, Rustin F, Dent J, *et al*. No increase in second tumors after cytotoxic chemotherapy for gestational trophoblastic tumors. *N Engl J Med* 1983;308: 473–6.
312 Stern RS, Zierler S, Parrish JA. Methotrexate used for psoriasis and the risk of noncutaneous malignancy. *Cancer* 1982;50:869–72.
313 Bailin PL, Tindall JP, Roenigk HH, Hogan MD. Is methotrexate therapy for psoriasis carcinogenic? A modified retrospective analysis. *JAMA* 1975;232: 359–62.
314 Nyfors A, Jensen H. Frequency of malignant neoplasms in 248 long-term methotrexate-treated psoriatics. A preliminary study. *Dermatologica* 1983;167:260–1.
315 Grunwald HW, Rosner F. Acute leukemia in immunosuppressive drug use. A review of patients undergoing immunosuppressive therapy for non-neoplastic diseases. *Arch Intern Med* 1979;139:461–6.
316 Morgan SL, Baggott JE, Vaughn WH, *et al*. Effect of folic acid supplementation on the toxicity of low-dose methotrexate in patients with rheumatoid arthritis. *Arthritis Rheum* 1990;33:9–18.
317 Stewart KA, Mackenzie AH, Clough JD, Wilke WS. Folate supplementation in methotrexate-treated rheumatoid arthritis patients. *Semin Arthritis Rheum* 1991; 20:332–8.
318 Jolivet J, Cowan KH, Curt GA, *et al*. The pharmacology and clinical use of methotrexate. *N Engl J Med* 1983;309:1094–104.
319 Wilke WS, Calabrese LH, Scherbel AL. Methotrexate in the treatment of rheumatoid arthritis: pilot study. *Cleveland Clin Q* 1980;47:305–9.
320 Sperling R, Larkin J, Coblyn J, Austen KF, Weinblatt M. Methotrexate decreases leukotriene B4 (LTB4) production in rheumatoid arthritis. *Arthritis Rheum* 1989; 32(Suppl.):S43.
321 Nesher G, Moore TL. Effect of methotrexate on chemotaxis and superoxide production of normal monocytes. *Arthritis Rheum* 1989;32(Suppl.):S60.
322 Suarez CR, Pickett WC, Bell DH, McClintock DK, Oronsky AL, Kerwar SS. Effect of low-dose methotrexate on neutrophil chemotaxis induced by leukotriene B4 and complement C5A. *J Rheumatol* 1987;14:9–11.
323 Andersen PA, West SG, O'Dell JR, Via CS, Claypool RG, Kotzin BL. Weekly pulse methotrexate in rheumatoid arthritis: clinical and immunologic effects in a random-

ized double-blind study. *Ann Intern Med* 1985;103:489–96.
324 Olsen NJ, Callahan LF, Pincus T. Immunologic studies of rheumatoid arthritis patients treated with methotrexate. *Arthritis Rheum* 1987;30:481–8.
325 Olsen NJ, Murray LM. Antiproliferative effects of methotrexate on peripheral blood mononuclear cells. *Arthritis Rheum* 1989;32:378–85.
326 Calabrese LH, Taylor JV, Wilke WS, Segal AM, Valenzuela R, Clough JD. Response of immunoregulatory lymphocyte subsets to methotrexate in rheumatoid arthritis. *Cleveland Clin J Med* 1990;57:232–41.
327 Joyce DA, Will RK, Hoffman DM, Laing B, Blackbourn SJ. Exacerbation of rheumatoid arthritis in patients treated with methotrexate after administration of folinic acid. *Ann Rheum Dis* 1991;50:913–4.
328 Menkes CJ, Simon F, Delbarre F. Letter: Treatment of psoriatic polyarthritis by azathioprine. *Nouv Presse Med* 1975;4:585.
329 Levy J, Paulus HE, Barnett EV, Sokoloff M, Bangert R, Pearson CM. A double-blind controlled evaluation of Azathioprine treatment in rheumatoid arthritis and psoriatic arthritis. *Arthritis Rheum* 1972;15:116–17.
330 Baum J, Hurd E, Lewis D, Ferguson JL, Ziff M. Treatment of psoriatic arthritis with 6-mercaptopurine. *Arthritis Rheum* 1973;16:139–47.
331 Vogler WR, Olansky S. A double-blind study of Azaribine in the treatment of psoriasis. *Ann Intern Med* 1970;73:951–6.
332 Levine S, Paulus HE. Treatment of psoriatic arthritis with azaribine. *Arthritis Rheum* 1976;19:21–8.
333 Atherton DJ, Wells RS, Laurent MR, Williams YF. Razoxane (ICRF 159) in the treatment of psoriasis. *Br J Dermatol* 1980;102:307–17.
334 Higgins LC Jr, Thompson JG. Psoriasis with arthritis: chemotherapy with cyclophosphamide, nitrogen mustard, and six-mercaptopurine. *South Med J* 1966;59: 1191–3.
335 Wilke WS, Sexton C, Steck W. Parenteral nitrogen mustard for inflammatory arthritis. *Cleve Clin J Med* 1990;57:643–6.
336 Griffiths CE, Powles AV, Leonard JN, *et al.* Clearance of psoriasis with low dose cyclosporin. *Br Med J* 1986;293:731–2.
337 Wentzel JM, Baughman RD, O'Connor GT, Bernier GM Jr. Cyclosporine in the treatment of psoriasis. *Arch Dermatol* 1987;123:163–5.
338 Ellis CN, Gorsulowsky DC, Hamilton TA, *et al.* Cyclosporin improves psoriasis in a double-blind study. *JAMA* 1986;256:3110–16.
339 Gupta AK, Matteson EL, Ellis CN, *et al.* Cyclosporin in the treatment of psoriatic arthritis. *Arch Dermatol* 1989;125:507–10.
340 Steinsson K, Jonsdottir I, Valdimarsson H. Cyclosporin-A in psoriatic arthritis: an open study. *Ann Rheum Dis* 1990;49:603–6.
341 Grekin RC, Ellis CN, Voorhees JJ. Retinoids in the treatment of psoriasis. Monotherapy in combinations. *Dermatol Clin* 1984;2:439–54.
342 Stollenwerk R, Fischer-Hoinkes H, Komenada K, Schilling F. Clinical observations on oral retinoid therapy of psoriatic arthropathy. In Orfanos CE, ed. *Retinoids. Advances in Basic Research and Therapy*. Berlin: Springer-Verlag, 1981:205–9.
343 Bitter T, Bahaus I, Rosenthal M. All-*trans* retinoic acid: a remission aim in the treatment of psoriatic arthritis. *Ann Rheum Dis* 1981;40:209.
344 Woo J, Yip SY, Wang SWS. The use of etretinate in psoriatic arthropathy. *Postgrad Med J* 1985;61:843.
345 Seppala J, Laulainen M, Reunala T. Comparison of etretinate (Tigason) and parenteral gold in the treatment of psoriatic arthropathy. *Clin Rheumatol* 1988;7: 498–503.
346 Klinkhoff AV, Gertner E, Chalmers A, *et al.* Pilot study of etretinate in psoriatic arthritis. *J Rheumatol* 1989;16:789–91.
347 Chieregato GC, Leoni A. Treatment of psoriatic arthropathy with etretinate: a

two-year follow-up. *Acta Derm Venereol* 1986;66:321–4.

348 Fritsch P, Ranschmeier W, Neuhofer J. Response of psoriatic arthropathy to a retinoid: a pilot study. In Cunliffe WJ, Miller AJ, eds. *Retinoid Therapy*. Lancaster: MTP Press, 1984:329–33.

349 Hopkins R, Bird HA, Jones H, *et al.* A double-blind controlled trial of etretinate (Tigason) and ibuprofen in psoriatic arthritis. *Ann Rheum Dis* 1985;44:189–93.

350 VanDerveen EE, Ellis CN, Campbell JP, Case PC, Voorhees JJ. Methotrexate and etretinate as concurrent therapies in severe psoriasis. *Arch Dermatol* 1982;118: 660–2.

351 Rosenbaum MM, Roenigk HH Jr. Treatment of generalized pustular psoriasis with etretinate (Ro 10–9359) and methotrexate. *J Am Acad Dermatol* 1984;10: 357–61.

352 Perlman SG, Gerber LH, Roberts RM, Nigra TP, Barth WF. Photochemotherapy and psoriatic arthritis. A prospective study. *Ann Intern Med* 1979;91:717–22.

353 Parrish JA, Fitzpatrick TB, Tanenbaum L, Pathak MA. Photochemotherapy of psoriasis with oral methoxsalen and long wave ultraviolet light. *N Engl J Med* 1974;291:1207–11.

354 Melski JW, Tanenbaum L, Parrish JA, Fitzpatrick TB, Bleich HL. Oral methoxsalen photochemotherapy for the treatment of psoriasis: a cooperative clinical trial. *J Invest Dermatol* 1975;68:328–35.

355 Thivolet J, Robart S, Vignon E. Combination aromatic retinoid-PUVA therapy in the treatment of psoriatic arthritis. Preliminary study. *Ann Dermatol Venereol* 1979;106:1037–8.

356 Thivolet J, Robart S, Vignon E. Combined oral retinoid and PUVA therapy in the treatment of psoriasis and psoriatic arthropathy. *Ann Dermatol Venereol* 1981; 108:131–7.

357 Wilfert H, Honigsmann H, Stiener G, Smolen J, Wolff K. Treatment of psoriatic arthritis by extracorporeal photochemotherapy. *Br J Dermatol* 1990;122:225–32.

358 O'Conell PG, Gerber LH, Digiovanna JJ, Peck GL. Arthritis in patients with psoriasis treated with gamma-interferon. *J Rheumatol* 1992;19:80–2.

359 Weber G, Klughardt G, Neidhardt M. Psoriasis and human growth hormone: aetiology and therapy. *Arch Dermatol Res* 1981;270:361–5.

360 Matucci-Cerinic M, Lotti T, Cappugi P, Boddi V, Fattorini L, Panconesi E. Somatostatin treatment of psoriatic arthritis. *Int J Dermatol* 1988;27:56–8.

361 Weber G, Klughardt G, Neidhardt M, *et al.* Treatment of psoriasis with somatostatin. *Arch Dermatol Res* 1982;272:31–6.

362 Ghirlanda G, Uccioli L, Perri F, *et al.* Epidermal growth factor, somatostatin and psoriasis. *Lancet* 1983;i:65.

363 Venier A, Desimone C, Forni L, *et al.* Treatment of severe psoriasis with somatostatin. Four years of experience. *Arch Dermatol Res* 1988;280(Suppl.):551–4

364 Dinter L, Muler W. Somatostatin in active psoriatic arthritis. *Z Rheumatol* 1984; 43:291–3.

365 Smith EL, Pincus SH, Donovan L, Holick MF. A novel approach for the evaluation and treatment of psoriasis. *J Am Acad Dermatol* 1988;19:516–28.

366 Huckins D, Felson DT, Holick M. Treatment of psoriatic arthritis with oral 1,25-Dihydroxyvitamin-D_3: a pilot study. *Arthritis Rheum* 1990;33:1723–7.

367 Gepner P, Amor B, Fournier C. 1,25-Dihydroxyvitamin-D_3 potentiates the *in vitro* inhibitory effects of cyclosporin-A on T-cells from rheumatoid arthritis patients. *Arthritis Rheum* 1989;32:31–6.

368 Weber G, Frey H. Treatment of psoriatic arthritis with bromocriptine. *J Am Acad Dermatol* 1987;16:388–9.

369 Yazini H, Bilge N, Kinay M. Total lymphoid irradiation for psoriatic arthritis: Case report. *Arthritis Rheum* 1983;26:1052.

370 Marcusson JA, Wetterberg L. Peptide-T in the treatment of psoriasis and psoriatic

arthritis. *Acta Derm Venereol* 1989;69:86–8.

371 Lassus A, Dahlgren AL, Halpern MJ, Santalahti J, Happonen HP. Effects of dietary supplementation with polyunsaturated ethyl ester lipids (Angiosan) in patients with psoriasis and psoriatic arthritis. *J Int Med Res* 1990;18:68–73.

372 Manger BF, Stix R, Beck AL, Kalden JR. Cimetidine and psoriatic arthritis. *Arch Dermatol* 1983;119:792.

373 Clemmensen OJ, Siggaard-Andersen J, Worm AM, Stahl D, Frost F, Bloch I. Psoriatic arthritis treated with oral zinc sulphate. *Br J Dermatol* 1980;103:411–5.

374 Armstrong RD, Panayi GS, Welsh KI. Histocompatibility antigens in psoriasis, psoriatic arthritis and ankylosing spondylitis. *Ann Rheum Dis* 1983;42:142–6.

375 Coulton BL, Thomson K, Symmons DPM, Popert AJ. Outcome in patients hospitalized for psoriatic arthritis. *Clin Rheumatol* 1989;8:261–5.

376 Wolfe F, Hawley DJ, Cathey MA. Clinical and health status measures over time: prognosis and outcome assessment in rheumatoid arthritis. *J Rheumatol* 1991; 18:1290–7.

377 Pincus T. Rheumatoid arthritis: disappointing long-term outcomes despite successful short-term clinical trials. *J Clin Epidemiol* 1988;41:1037–41.

378 McCarty DJ. Treatment of rheumatoid arthritis. In McCarty DJ, Coopman WJ, eds. *Arthritis and Allied Conditions*, A *Textbook of Rheumatology* 12th edn. Philadelphia: Lea & Febiger, 1993:877–86.

379 Wilske KR, Healey LA. Remodeling the pyramid — a concept whose time has come. *J Rheumatol* 1989;16:565–7.

380 Wilke WS, Clough JD. Therapy for rheumatoid arthritis: combinations of disease modifying drugs and new paradigms of treatment. *Semin Arthritis Rheum* 1991; 21(Suppl. 1):21–34.

381 Gladman DD, Farewell V, Buskila D, *et al.* Reliability of measurements of active and damaged joints in psoriatic arthritis. *J Rheumatol* 1990;17:62–4.

nine

Psoriasis, Psoriatic Arthritis, and Reiter's Syndrome Associated with HIV Infection

Arun L. Pathy

INTRODUCTION

In recent years, there has been increasing recognition of the myriad mucocutaneous and rheumatologic complications in syndromes resulting from HIV infection. The coexistence of psoriasis and AIDS was first reported in 1985 [1]. Since then, numerous case reports and series have appeared in the medical literature describing the simultaneous occurrence of these diseases. The further association of related nonneoplastic epidermal proliferative disorders such as seborrheic dermatitis, Reiter's syndrome, and erythroderma with HIV infection has led some observers to speculate that psoriasis belongs to a continuum of papulosquamous dermatoses of varying severity, which are all triggered by HIV infection through some common underlying mechanism [2,3]. The further investigation of the association of psoriasis, psoriatic arthritis, and Reiter's syndrome with HIV infection will be of much benefit to clinicians since it may yield clues regarding the role of the immune system and infectious agents in the etiopathogenesis of these conditions in normal hosts.

EPIDEMIOLOGY

Psoriasis occurs in 1–2% of white people [4]. With as many as 40 million persons worldwide expected to be infected with HIV by the year 2000 [5], it should come as no surprise that both entities coexist in some persons. What remains unclear is whether psoriasis occurs more commonly in HIV-infected patients than in the general population. This uncertainty is due in part to the marked discordance among published studies in reported prevalence rates of psoriasis, psoriatic arthritis, and Reiter's syndrome in the setting of HIV infection.

Duvic and coworkers [3] reported 13 cases of psoriasis in a population of 1000 HIV-infected persons (a prevalence of 1.3%). Kaplan and colleagues [6] observed eight patients with psoriasis in their series of 400 patients with HIV disease (2%). These rates are comparable to those in the normal population. In a prospective study in Tampa, Florida [7], five of 101 consecutive HIV-positive patients had psoriasis (5%). Winchester *et al.* [8], in a similar prospective study found a prevalence of 13 of 65 (20%) in their cohort. The reasons for this considerable variability in reported frequencies are not clear. In the future, properly controlled cohort studies comparing HIV-infected populations with noninfected populations matched for behavioral factors (e.g., homosexuality/bisexuality, intravenous drug abuse) and HLA distribution will be required to determine unequivocally whether HIV infection is an independent risk factor for the development of psoriasis.

Psoriatic arthritis develops in approximately 5.4–7% of psoriasis patients [9]. In HIV-associated psoriasis, however, the incidence is reportedly much higher: in the range of 23–50% [7,8,10,11]. HIV-infected psoriatics who are HLA-B27 positive have a 12-fold higher risk of peripheral arthritis compared with HIV-infected psoriatics who do not express this antigen [11].

Reiter's syndrome is broadly defined as a reactive arthropathy occurring in genetically susceptible hosts (most of whom are HLA-B27 positive) in response to infections of the lower genitourinary and gastrointestinal tracts. In its classical form it comprises a triad of urethritis, conjunctivitis, and arthritis in association with the mucocutaneous lesions of keratoderma blennorrhagia and balanitis circinata. In the general population, it is typically a disease of young men with a prevalence of 0.04–0.06%. In contrast, prospective studies in HIV clinics have demonstrated frequencies as high as 1.7–10% [7,8,12]. Larger retrospective studies by Clark *et al.* [13] and Hochberg *et al.* [14] found that while homosexual/bisexual men had a 10-fold increase in the prevalence of Reiter's syndrome (0.5%), the HIV-infected men in their cohorts were no more likely to develop Reiter's syndrome than their noninfected counterparts. Therefore, it remains uncertain at this time whether HIV infection remains an independent risk factor for Reiter's syndrome after one takes into account the increased risk of infections associated with homosexual/bisexual practices and intravenous drug abuse.

CLINICAL FEATURES AND ETIOPATHOGENESIS

A number of nonneoplastic epidermal proliferative dermatoses have been described in HIV infection states. Most of these occur as helper T-cell counts fall below $150/mm^3$ [2]. Seborrheic dermatitis, which may represent the mild end of this disease continuum, occurs in 40–80% of AIDS patients [15]. While it remains controversial whether psoriasis occurs more frequently in the setting of HIV infection, there is little doubt that HIV infection modifies the clinical course of the disease: previously stable, localized psoriasis may flare severely or it may arise *de novo* and progress rapidly coincident with the onset of HIV-induced immunodeficiency [3,16]. Patients who have coexistent HIV infection and psoriasis may be otherwise asymptomatic, have symptomatic HIV infection (AIDS-related complex;

ARC), or have full blown AIDS [17]. Indeed, psoriasis may be the initial manifestation of HIV disease. The explosive onset of psoriasis or an otherwise unexplained flare of preexisting disease should prompt the physician to inquire about risk factors for HIV infection. This should be followed up by serologic testing if the clinical history indicates any likelihood of infection.

It has been suggested that psoriasis in the HIV-infected host occurs in two distinct clinical patterns [2]. Lesions may consist of discrete plaques or a more diffuse and widespread psoriasiform dermatitis with palmoplantar keratoderma, which often results in erythroderma. In Duvic's series of 13 patients [3], the most commonly observed skin lesions were large plaques (92%), guttate plaques (85%), and acral keratotic papules and pustules plus onychodystrophy (85%). Less commonly observed were sebopsoriasis of intertriginous areas (77%) and exfoliative erythroderma (46%). The histopathologic appearance of psoriasis lesions in HIV-infected patients has distinctive features which include the lack of suprapapillary epidermal thinning, a paucity of Munro microabscesses, and a moderate perivascular and diffuse lymphoid infiltrate which may contain many macrophages and plasma cells [21]. Psoriatic arthritis as discussed above, is a relatively common feature of HIV-associated psoriasis. When it occurs in this setting, it tends to be more severe and poorly responsive to antiinflammatory drugs.

Kaye [19], in a review of 51 reported cases of HIV-infected patients with Reiter's syndrome, found that most had a severe persistent oligoarticular arthritis primarily affecting the large joints of the lower extremities. Other clinical features included urethritis (57%), conjunctivitis (45%), circinate balanitis (27%), and keratoderma blennorrhagicum (18%). These findings occurred before or simultaneously with the onset of overt immunodeficiency in two-thirds of cases. The frequency of HLA-B27 expression in these patients is increased (70–80% for white people) and is similar to that seen in non-HIV-associated Reiter's syndrome. Only 20% of the general HLA-B27-positive population will progress to Reiter's syndrome after exposure to appropriate bacterial antigens [20]. To account for the high incidence of Reiter's syndrome in the HIV population observed in prospective studies [7,10,12], some have speculated that nearly all HIV-infected, HLA-B27-positive patients develop arthritis or Reiter's syndrome during the course of their illness [21]. There can be considerable clinical overlap between psoriasis with peripheral arthritis, pustular psoriasis, and Reiter's syndrome in the setting of HIV infection. The finding of increased HLA-B27 expression among HIV-infected psoriatics with peripheral arthritis has raised the possibility that psoriasis, psoriatic arthritis, and Reiter's syndrome are all variants of the same disease in the context of HIV infection [11]. The clinical overlap between HIV-associated psoriasis and Reiter's syndrome is more likely to occur in cases where the psoriasis arises *de novo* following HIV infection [17].

Theories to explain the exacerbation or onset of psoriasis with HIV infection have understandably focused on the role of the immune system and infectious agents. In the skin, HIV infects CD4+ helper T lymphocytes, epidermal Langerhans cells and dermal dendrocytes of monocytic origin causing a relative depletion of the former two populations [22]. This disrupts the intricate cytokine network regulating cutaneous immunity. An alteration of this cytokine milieu may trigger local epidermal hyperproliferation. Support for this theory comes from observations that non-HIV-infected hosts who receive pharmacologic doses of interferons and interleukin-2 experience flares of psoriasis. The efficacy of cyclosporine A, an inhibitor of T-cell cytokines, in the treatment of psoriasis underscores the importance of these molecules in the pathogenesis of psoriatic lesions. It has also been observed that patients with end-stage AIDS with markedly depressed CD4 counts experience a spontaneous clearing of their psoriasis, perhaps due to an inability to produce the cytokines necessary to drive epidermal hyperproliferation.

Bacterial, fungal, and viral agents have all been implicated as initiating factors in the onset or exacerbation of psoriasis. For example, the association between streptococcal infection and acute guttate psoriasis is well established [23]. *Staphylococcus aureus* is often cultured from the skin and nails of patients with AIDS-associated psoriasis [3]. Jaffe *et al.* [24] reported three cases of HIV-positive men with generalized psoriasis and staphylococcal sepsis whose skin disease cleared with systemic antibiotic therapy. Duvic and co-workers have demonstrated that infusion of glucan, a component of *Pityrosporum* yeast cells and Gram-positive cocci, produces psoriasiform skin lesions in patients with AIDS and ARC [25]. It is still not clear whether it is the infectious agents themselves or the host immune responses to these infections that are responsible for psoriatic flares.

Recent studies involving transgenic mice carrying the HIV TAT gene and the entire proviral genome have suggested that HIV gene products may directly promote epidermal acanthosis and hyperkeratosis [26]. This may explain why the antiretroviral agent zidovudine has a dramatic antipsoriatic effect in the HIV-infected patient. Further investigation in the areas of superimposed retroviral infections and derangements of calcium metabolism in the HIV-infected host may yield additional clues regarding the etiopathogenesis of the spectrum of psoriatic disease in this setting.

TREATMENT

The onset or exacerbation of psoriasis in HIV-infected persons is associated with worsening immunodeficiency and usually portends a poor overall prognosis [2,21]. The psoriasis itself often proves to be refractory to conventional first-line therapies such as topical corticosteroids and tar preparations. Anthralin tends to be excessively irritating in many patients with HIV-associated psoriasis [27]. Unfortunately, many standard systemic therapies utilized for severe psoriasis are associated with the potential problem of inducing further immunosuppression in an already severely immunodeficient person. This is clearly illustrated by the uniformly disappointing results reported with the use of methotrexate in this setting. Observed complications have included leukopenia, initial appearance of

Kaposi's sarcoma lesions or *Pneumocystis carinii* pneumonia, encephalopathy, and possible acceleration of the course of AIDS leading to death [1,3,8]. Limited experience with cyclosporine in severe AIDS-related psoriasis suggests that this agent may significantly improve skin lesions in some patients without shortening their survival [28]. It seems reasonable to recommend avoidance of routine use of conventional antipsoriatic immunosuppressives in the setting of HIV infection until more experience with their use is reported.

UVB and psoralen plus UVA (PUVA) phototherapy are effective treatment modalities in HIV-associated psoriasis, but their use is limited by several practical and theoretical drawbacks. The practical problems include difficulty in administering therapy to debilitated patients and the risk of contamination of phototherapy units by HIV particles in psoriatic scales [29] and bodily secretions [16]. While UVA (320–400 nm) irradiation with psoralen inactivates HIV *in vitro* [30], irradiation with shorter UV wavelengths was found to induce active production of HIV infectious particles from a low producer HIV-infected promonocytic cell line [31]. Furthermore, human studies have demonstrated that UV irradiation has inhibitory systemic effects on the immune system, including suppression of cell-mediated immune responses and cutaneous hypersensitivity reactions. These effects may be mediated through a reduction in the number and antigen presenting capacity of Langerhans cells. Thus, phototherapy also carries the theoretical risk of potentiation of HIV-induced immunosuppression. In Duvic's series [3], UVB and PUVA phototherapies were linked with the appearance or exacerbation of Kaposi's sarcoma and life-threatening infections in some patients. However, in a larger series [17], the cumulative survival at 1 year after AIDS diagnosis for psoriasis patients receiving UVB therapy was no different than that of patients receiving other modalities of treatment. A study by Ranki and colleagues [32] on the effect of PUVA on immunologic and virologic parameters in HIV-infected patients failed to demonstrate any suppression of T-lymphocyte numbers or lymphocyte proliferative capacity as a result of the phototherapy. They conclude that systemic PUVA is safe and well tolerated in early HIV infection. A lack of alteration in systemic immune functions has also been demonstrated in a group of HIV-positive patients undergoing UVB phototherapy for pruritic papular eruption [33]. Hopefully, the controversy surrounding the issue of safety of phototherapy in HIV-infected patients will be resolved as further clinical experience is accumulated with the use of this modality in psoriasis and other UV-responsive dermatoses.

The synthetic retinoid, etretinate, has been shown to be effective in the treatment of AIDS-related psoriasis and Reiter's syndrome, often producing dramatic improvement in both cutaneous and articular lesions [3,16,34,35]. Topical calcipotriol has been used as an effective adjunct to etretinate [36]. Some have pointed out that a potential disadvantage of retinoid therapy in the AIDS patient is the difficulty in distinguishing between drug adverse effects (arthralgias, headaches, hepatic dysfunction) and the onset of an occult infection [2,21]. Recently, zidovudine has become the drug of choice in the treatment of severe AIDS-related psoriasis [6,27,37,38]. Patients who receive this drug benefit from both its antiretroviral activity and antipsoriatic activity. The basis for zidovudine's antipsoriatic activity is unclear. Its effect seems to correlate better with the development of red blood cell macrocytosis than with preservation of the helper T-cell count [6]. It is not yet known whether the newer antiretroviral agent dideoxycytidine will have a place in the management of AIDS-related psoriasis.

Summary

In summary, topical corticosteroids and tar preparations should be tried first for mild localized psoriasis in the HIV-infected patient. Topical calcipotriol is also safe and beneficial in this situation. For more extensive disease in the patient who is in the very early stages of HIV infection, PUVA may be of benefit. Zidovudine is appropriate for patients with recalcitrant or widespread disease, most of whom will meet current criteria for treatment with this drug on the basis of their immune status. Etretinate may be useful in cases which are refractory to zidovudine and in patients who cannot tolerate zidovudine. Nonsteroidal antiinflammatory drugs may be added to the regimen when articular symptoms fail to respond to the antipsoriatic medications alone. Prompt recognition and treatment of concurrent infections is essential to controlling the skin disease. In some cases, complete clearing of widespread cutaneous lesions has been achieved with antistaphylococcal [24] or anti-*Pneumocystis carinii* [39] therapy alone.

CASE STUDIES

Case 1

HIV-associated exacerbation of preexisting psoriasis vulgaris.

A 48-year-old homosexual white man had limited plaque-type psoriasis since age 20 years. The eruption had been well controlled with topical corticosteroids and natural sunlight exposure. In 1987, an enzyme-linked immunosorbent assay test for HIV antibodies was noted to be positive. His helper T-cell count was 592 cells/mm^3. Cutaneous examination at that time revealed only small plaques of psoriasis over both elbows with no palmoplantar or articular involvement. These plaques cleared completely when he underwent systemic chemotherapy for an HIV-associated lymphoma in 1989. Six months later, he developed psoriasis of his scalp, axillae, and groin folds. These lesions initially responded well to topical steroids and coal tar preparations. When he presented 8 months later, there were extensive psoriatic plaques over his scalp, trunk, and extremities. Some plaques were surmounted by pustules. Treatment with zidovudine 200 mg five times daily and ketoconazole 200 mg daily resulted in rapid and significant clearing of his cutaneous plaques. When the psoriasis flared again 6 months later, he was maintained on the zidovudine and switched *from ketoconazole to fluconazole. This resulted in only slight improvement. He was subsequently lost to followup and died 1 year later of disseminated aspergillosis.*

Case 2

HIV-associated exacerbation of preexisting psoriasis vulgaris and new onset of psoriatic arthritis.

A 62-year-old homosexual white man with a 50-year history of plaque-type psoriasis was diagnosed with AIDS when he developed cerebral toxoplasmosis. Prior to that, his psoriasis (consisting of plaques on the extensor aspect of his extremities) had been well controlled with intramuscular methotrexate treatments every 4 weeks. When the methotrexate was discontinued, he rapidly developed thick psoriatic plaques of his palms, soles, and scalp. He also developed pain and swelling of several proximal interphalangeal joints on the right hand. No pustules were observed. Two additional doses of intramuscular methotrexate were administered at monthly intervals. The cutaneous and articular lesions improved transiently and then flared again when the methotrexate was withdrawn. The patient refused further treatment and had a rapid downhill clinical course culminating in death 4 months later.

Comment

These two patients presented here were initially cleared of psoriasis after the administration of zidovudine. A recent report has demonstrated that zidovudine inhibited the growth and DNA synthesis of an hyperproliferative human keratinocyte line in culture [40]. The inhibitory effects were dose-dependent in micromolar concentrations and were reversible. Most of the effects were cytostatic, but evidence of morphologic and biochemical cytotoxicity was seen at the highest concentration tested (100 μm). The concentration of zidovudine in the skin of HIV-infected patients is not known. The authors proposed that as a thymidine analog, zidovudine's antimetabolite activity is responsible for inhibiting the rapidly proliferating cells in psoriasis.

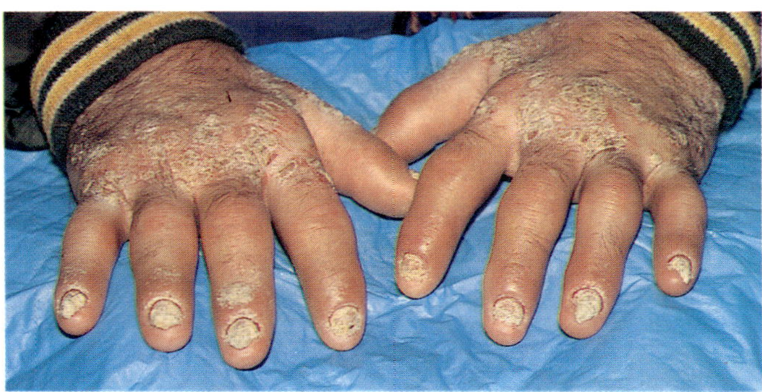

Fig 9.1 Case 2. Psoriasiform changes on dorsa of hands, synovitis of interphalangeal joints, and fingernail changes.

Case 3

Probable HIV-associated Reiter's syndrome.

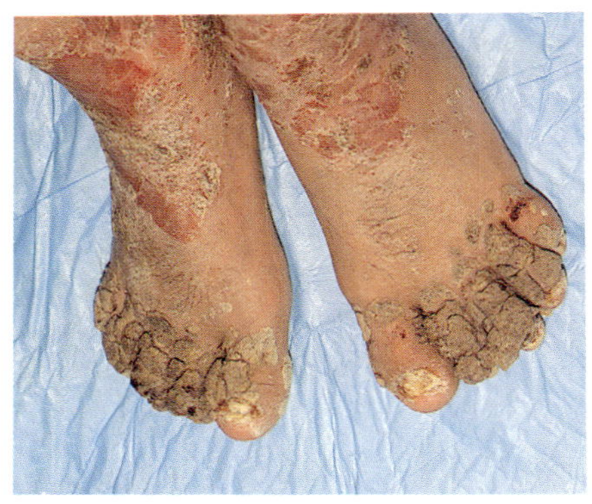

Fig 9.2 Case 3. Psoriasiform plaques on ankles and verrucous encrustation on dorsa of toes.

A 32-year-old white man, intravenous drug abuser, with no personal or family history of psoriasis was found to be HIV positive when he presented with herpes zoster ophthalmicus. Six months later, he presented with scaling and arthralgias of his hands and feet. Cutaneous examination revealed extensive palmoplantar hyperkeratosis with numerous pustules. There was marked onychodystrophy of all fingernails and toenails (Figs 9.1, 9.2). Active synovitis was noted in several proximal interphalangeal joints of both the hands (Fig. 9.1) and feet. In addition, he had psoriatic plaques on his extremities (Fig. 9.2) and circinate balanitis. Cultures of the acral pustules were negative for bacteria and fungus. His CD4 count at that time was 112 cells/mm^3. Topical tar and steroid preparations failed to improve the skin lesions. The arthritis was refractory to high doses of phenylbutazone. He was subsequently started on zidovudine 200 mg three times daily. This resulted in marked improvement of his arthritis within 1 month and near total clearing of his cutaneous lesions within 2 months. He has remained on the zidovudine and subsequent flare-ups of his cutaneous lesions have been successfully managed with topical steroids.

Comment

The patient had pustulosis with hyperkeratosis of the palms and soles. For all practical purposes these changes are indistinguishable from those seen in Reiter's syndrome called keratoderma blennorrhagicum. The patient did not have arthritis of the axial skeleton or sacroiliac involvement and was not screened for HLA-B27 which would clinch that diagnosis. It is interesting to note that improvement in the arthropathy was also temporally related to zidovudine administration.

REFERENCES

1 Johnson TM, Duvic M, Rapini RP, *et al.* Acquired immunodeficiency syndrome exacerbates psoriasis (Letter). *N Engl J Med* 1985;313:1415.

2 Sadick NS, McNutt NS, Kaplan MH. Papulosquamous dermatoses of acquired immunodeficiency syndrome. *J Am Acad Dermatol* 1990;22:1270–7.

3 Duvic M, Johnson TM, Rapini RP, *et al.* Acquired immunodeficiency syndrome-associated psoriasis and Reiter's syndrome. *Arch Dermatol* 1987;123:1622–32.

4 Baker H. Epidemiologic aspects of psoriasis and arthritis. *Br J Dermatol* 1966;78: 249–61.

5 World Health Organization. In point of fact. Geneva: World Health Organization, May 1991. (No. 74). Cited in Anonymous, the HIV/AIDS epidemic: the first 10 years. *Arch Dermatol* 1991;127:1465.

6 Kaplan MH, Sadick NS, Weider J, *et al.* Antipsoriatic effects of zidovudine in human immunodeficiency virus-associated psoriasis. *J Am Acad Dermatol* 1989; 20:76.

7 Berman A, Espinoza LR, Diaz JD, *et al.* Rheumatologic manifestations of human immunodeficiency virus infection. *Am J Med* 1988;85:59–64.

8 Winchester R, Brancato L, Itescu S, *et al.* Implications from the occurrence of Reiter's syndrome and related disorders. *Scand J Rheumatol* 1988;74(Suppl.): 89–93.
9 Finzi AF, Gibelli E. Psoriatic arthritis. *Int J Dermatol* 1991;30:1–7.
10 Solomon G, Brancato LJ, Itescu S, *et al.* Arthritis, psoriasis, and related syndromes associated with human immunodeficiency virus infection. *Arthritis Rheum* 1988; 31(Suppl. 2):S12(Abstract).
11 Reveille JD, Conant MA, Duvic M. Human immunodeficiency virus-associated psoriasis, psoriatic arthritis and Reiter's syndrome: a disease continuum? *Arthritis Rheum* 1990;33:1574–8.
12 Calabrese LH, Kelley DM, Meyers A, *et al.* Rheumatologic symptoms and human immunodeficiency virus infection: the influence of clinical and laboratory variables in a longitudinal cohort study. *Arthritis Rheum* 1991;34:257–63.
13 Clark M, Kinsolving M, Chernoff D. The prevalence of arthritis in two human immunodeficiency virus-infected cohorts. *Arthritis Rheum* 1989;32(Suppl.):S85.
14 Hochberg MC, Fox R, Nelson KE, *et al.* Human immunodeficiency virus infection is not associated with Reiter's syndrome: data from the Johns' Hopkins multicenter AIDS cohort study. *AIDS* 1990;4:1149–51.
15 Mathes BM, Douglas MC. Seborrheic dermatitis in patients with acquired immunodeficiency syndrome. *J Am Acad Dermatol* 1985;15:482–6.
16 Lazar AP, Roenigk HH Jr. Acquired immunodeficiency syndrome and psoriasis. *Cutis* 1987;39:347–51.
17 Obuch ML, Maurer TA, Becker B, *et al.* Psoriasis and human immunodeficiency virus infection. *J Am Acad Dermatol* 1992;27:667–73.
18 McNutt NS, Shu A, Sadick NS, *et al.* Psoriasiform dermatitis of acquired immunodeficiency syndrome. *J Cutan Pathol* 1989;16:317.
19 Kaye BR. Rheumatologic manifestations of infection with human immunodeficiency virus. *Ann Intern Med* 1989;111:158–67.
20 Woodrow JC. Genetics of B27-associated diseases. *Ann Rheum Dis* 1979;38(Suppl. 1):135–41.
21 Arnett FC, Reveille JD, Duvic M. Psoriasis and psoriatic arthritis associated with human immunodeficiency virus infection. *Rheumatol Dis Clin North Am* 1991;17: 59–78.
22 Mahoney SE, Duvic M, Nickoloff BJ, *et al.* Human immunodeficiency virus transcripts identified in human immunodeficiency virus-related psoriasis and Kaposi's sarcoma lesions. *J Clin Invest* 1991;88:174–85.
23 Telfer NR, Chalmers RJG, Whale K. The role of streptococcal infection in the initiation of guttate psoriasis. *Arch Dermatol* 1992;128:39–42.
24 Jaffe D, May LP, Sanchez M, *et al.* Staphylococcus sepsis in human immunodeficiency virus antibody seropositive psoriasis patients. *J Am Acad Dermatol* 1991;24: 970–2.
25 Duvic M, Reisman M, Findley V, *et al.* Glucan induced keratoderma in acquired immunodeficiency syndrome. *Arch Dermatol* 1987;123:751–6.
26 Duvic M. Immunology of acquired immunodeficiency syndrome related to psoriasis. *J Invest Dermatol* 1990;95:S38–40.
27 Ruzicka T, Froschl M, Hohenleutner U, *et al.* Treatment of human immunodeficiency virus induced retinoid-resistant psoriasis with zidovudine. *Lancet* 1987;ii:1469–70.
28 Allen BR. Use of cyclosporin for psoriasis in HIV-positive patient (Letter). *Lancet* 1992;339:686.
29 Tschachler E, Groh V, Popovick M, *et al.* Epidermal Langerhans's cells: target for HTLV-III/LAV infection. *J Invest Dermatol* 1987;88:233–7.
30 Quinnan G, Wells M, Wittek A, *et al.* Inactivation of human T-cell lymphotrophic virus type III by heat, chemicals, and irradiation. *Transfusion* 1986;26:481–3.
31 Stanley S, Folks T, Fauci A. Induction of expression of human immunodeficiency

virus in a chronically infected promonocytic cell line by ultraviolet irradiation. *AIDS Res Hum Retroviruses* 1989;5:375–84.

32 Ranki A, Puska P, Matinen S, *et al.* Effect of PUVA on immunologic and verologic findings in human immunodeficiency virus infected patients. *J Am Acad Dermatol* 1991;24:404–10.

33 Pardo RJ, Bogaert MA, Penneys NS, *et al.* UVB phototherapy of pruritic papular eruption of the acquired immunodeficiency syndrome. *J Am Acad Dermatol* 1992; 26:423–8.

34 Belz J, Breneman DL, Nordlund JJ, *et al.* Successful treatment of a patient with Reiter's syndrome and acquired immunodeficiency syndrome using etretinate. *J Am Acad Dermatol* 1989;20:898–903.

35 Williams HC, Du Vivier AWP. Etretinate and acquired immunodeficiency syndrome-related Reiter's disease. *Br J Dermatol* 1991;124:389–92.

36 Gray JD, Bottomley W, Layton AM, *et al.* The use of calcipotriol in HIV-related psoriasis. *Clin Exp Dermatol* 1992;17:342–3.

37 Duvic M, Rios A, Brewton GW. Remission of acquired immunodeficiency syndrome-associated psoriasis with zidovudine. *Lancet* 1987;ii:627.

38 Diez F, Del Hoyo M, Serrano S. Zidovudine treatment of psoriasis associated with acquired immunodeficiency syndrome. *J Am Acad Dermatol* 1990;22:146–7.

39 Rasokat H. Psoriasis and acquired immunodeficiency syndrome: complete remission with high dose trimethoprim and sulfamethoxyzole therapy. *Z Hautkr* 1986;61:991.

40 Bonnekoh B, Wevers A, Geisel J, *et al.* Antiproliferative potential of zidovudine in human keratinocyte cultures. *J Am Acad Dermatol* 1991;25:483–90.

Part three Treatment of Psoriasis

ten

Corticosteroids

INTRODUCTION

The first successful use of topical hydrocortisone for skin disease was published in 1952. Synthetic alteration of the parent compound has allowed for the proliferation of molecules which express potent glucocorticoid activity. Although their long-term efficacy is questionable topical corticosteroids have been prescribed for the majority of patients with localized psoriasis for the past three decades in the USA. A 1992 survey of 225 members of the American Academy of Dermatology revealed that the most potent agents improved less than one-third of patients with mild psoriasis [1]. Furthermore, only 40% remained relatively clear 1 month after stopping therapy. The mid- and low-potency preparations were rated considerably lower in effectiveness.

What are the reasons for this discrepancy? First, it is rational to exploit the topical corticosteroids for localized psoriasis. The drugs are small molecules which penetrate the stratum corneum and bind to steroid receptors in the cytosol of living keratinocytes; ultimately they alter DNA synthesis and gene transcription. Potency of the drug correlates with the affinity of the receptor for it. Glucocorticoids also exert both receptor-mediated and direct inhibitory effects on the inflammatory cells seen in biopsies of psoriasis. They also inhibit mediators of inflammation such as phospholipase A_2, the enzyme that liberates arachidonic acid, which is the precursor to the prostaglandins, leukotrienes, and 12-hydroxyheptadecatrienoic acid (12-HETE).

CLINICAL USE

Efficacy

The ideal topical corticosteroid would have all of the following characteristics: penetration, clinical efficacy, no tachyphylaxis, no side effects, cosmetic elegance, and low cost. Not unexpectedly, no one drug embodies all of these features. Increasing potency correlates with increasing local and systemic toxicity. The superpotent corticosteroids are generally the latest and the most expensive compounds. Penetration is enhanced in thinner skin. Thus, penetration through eyelid skin is 36–40 times that of palms or soles. Increased hydration and temperature increase penetration, factors which are exploited with application after a warm bath or occlusion of the corticosteroid with plastic wrap or tape. Increasing the concentration of drug does not necessarily result in greater penetration or potency.

Potency, that is, clinical efficacy, is increased by molecular modification of the parent compound such as halogenation, producing acetonide or valerate analogs, changing the vehicle by adding 1–2% azone [2] or high concentrations of propylene glycol (optimized vehicle).

The vasoconstrictor assay was introduced by McKenzie and Stoughton in 1962 and has been used ever since for screening new corticosteroids and as an indirect bioassay of clinical effectiveness [3]. In its current modification, the formulation is applied to the volar surface of the forearms of normal volunteers, covered with an elevated perforated guard for 16 hours, washed off, and read 2 hours later on a blind basis by an experienced investigator. Readings of vasoconstriction are quantified as follows: 0, none; 1, mild; 2, moderate; 3, intense. The results are analyzed statistically using the Wilcoxon test based on the sum of signed ranks of differences.

There is an excellent correlation between the vasoconstrictor assay and bilateral symmetric paired comparisons of psoriatic target lesions treated once to three times daily for 2–3 weeks for 30 of 32 different compounds [4]. Correlation did not exist for aclometasone ointment 0.05% (II vs VI) and hydrocortisone valerate cream 0.2% (III vs V), giving greater vasoconstriction than clinical effectiveness, respectively. The authors agree that the most precise method of evaluating the potency of a topical steroid is by well-controlled clinical studies comparing one drug with another or its vehicle. Psoriasis is particularly well-suited for study because lesions tend to be bilateral, symmetric, and of equal severity on either side.

The literature abounds with this type of study. When it has been determined in which group in the Stoughton vasoconstriction ranking classification the drug resides, the manufacturers sponsor studies comparing their drug to the others in the same group jockeying for any edge in clinical efficacy, rapidity of action, patient acceptance, side effect profile, and relapse rate. The competition is most intense among the group I or super high potency corticosteroids. For example, clobetasol propionate ointment 0.05% significantly improved the mean severity of signs of psoriasis more than betamethasone dipropionate ointment 0.05% in optimized vehicle (OV) after 14 days of treatment and 2 weeks after the 14-day treatment course [5]. Clobetasol propionate ointment 0.05% cleared 21% of lesions on day 15 of treatment and 21% at the 2-week followup visit compared to 9 and 4% for diflorasone diacetate ointment 0.05%, respectively [6].

Another study comparing diflorasone diacetate ointment 0.05% and clobetasol propionate ointment 0.05% confirmed that reductions in severity scores were greater on the clobetasol side but emphasized that "preatrophy" was also more evident [7]. Preatrophy is a term used by Katz *et al.* [8] to represent the visualization with 8× magnification of the normally covert subpapillary vascular plexus resulting from thinning of the epidermis and papillary dermis. It was twice as likely to occur in women. In another twice weekly 2-week study diflorasone ointment was as effective as betamethasone dipropionate in optimized vehicle (BDOV) [10].

Two double-blind multicenter studies compared halobetasol propionate ointment 0.05% to clobetasol ointment 0.05% or BDOV ointment 0.05% [9]. The success rate defined as "healed" or "marked improvement" after 28 days of twice-daily application, was 96% vs 91% for halobetasol vs clobetasol, but the authors emphasized that "early healing" within 24 days was more frequently seen with halobetasol than clobetasol (69% vs 56%). None of the differences were statistically significant. Similar trends for more marked and faster healing were demonstrated for halobetasol vs BDOV. In the latter study the patients judged the ointments for "cosmetic acceptability and ease of application," and the authors emphasized that the results were statistically significant in favor of halobetasol ($P = 0.02$).

In practice, none of the distinctions among the superpotent class I corticosteroids highlighted by the authors are clinically significant for short-term localized treatment.

Superpotent topical corticosteroids

Until recently clobetasol propionate was considered the most potent topical steroid available [11]. It has modifications that impart increased activity and bioavailability such as a double bond at the 1,2 position, a fluorine atom at the 9 position, esterification of the 17 position and halogenation at the 21 position which appears to inhibit deesterification at the 17 position (Fig. 10.1). A new ultrapotent steroid, halobetasol propionate, is structurally similar to clobetasol with the exception of an additional fluorine atom in the 6-α position (Fig. 10.1). Halobetasol appears to be equivalent to clobetasol in terms of pharmacodynamic and pharmacologic activity responses [9].

Potency in the vasoconstrictor assay is generally correlated with clinical

Fig 10.1 Chemical structures of some topical corticosteroids.

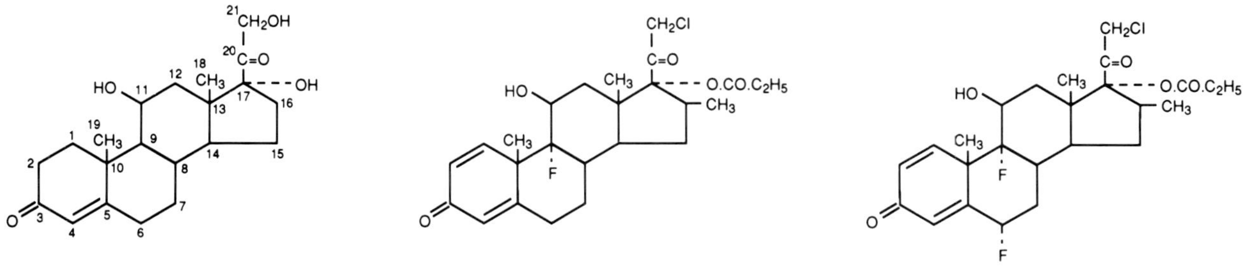

Hydrocortisone (prototype of structure of glucocorticosteroids)

Clobetasol 17-propionate

Halobetasol propionate

efficacy in psoriasis [4]. Potency is also correlated with bioavailability and adverse effects, both local and systemic. Therefore, the advent of superpotent steroids opens new vistas for dermatologists. On the one hand, plaques of psoriasis may be completely cleared after 2–4 weeks of twice-daily application, but more importantly, maintenance of remission by intermittent pulsing of topical therapy has become a reality. Unfortunately, serious unwanted effects such as striae and hypothalamic–pituitary–adrenal (HPA) axis suppression can occur, and the spectre of abuse of these agents by patients, pharmacists, and physicians exists.

In an unpublished postal survey of 174 members of a USA dermatologic society in 1990 there were 65% who "usually" or "always" prescribed superpotent steroids, presumably for acute phase management (H.I. Katz unpublished data). Only 13% preferred to use them for maintenance. Clinically significant HPA-axis suppression or iatrogenic Cushing's syndrome had been observed by 8 and 11% of respondents, respectively. Abusive usage (not otherwise defined by the questionnaire) by dermatologists (40%) and by nondermatologists (74%) was also reported. Such abusive or inappropriate use may have included more than twice-daily application (wasteful), use under occlusion and use in children under 12 years (more atrophogenic and increased systemic absorption), use on the face or intertriginous areas (more risk of steroid-induced rosacea and atrophy with telangiectasia or striae), use for more than 2 consecutive weeks or more than 50 g/week.

In a bilateral paired comparison of psoriasis, clobetasol and BDOV gave nearly identical results with twice-daily application for 2 weeks: 28 of 59 and 26 of 59 were 75–100% cleared, respectively [12]. In a separate parallel design study for 3 weeks, 15 of 18 and 17 of 19 obtained similar results [13]. Both studies showed that the majority of patients (60–74%) who were cleared or almost cleared by conventional twice-daily application of BDOV for 2–4 weeks could be maintained in remission status for up to 6 months by applying three consecutive doses of 3.5 g at 12-hour intervals each week (e.g., Saturday a.m., Saturday p.m., Sunday a.m.). Eighty percent of patients who were randomized to the placebo vehicle experienced exacerbation of their disease. No serious local or systemic adverse effects were reported. There were no "substantial" alterations in plasma cortisol, urinary cortisol or 17-ketosteroid levels in the 12-week study; in the multicenter study two of 48 (4%) patients in the BDOV-treated group had subnormal a.m. cortisol levels.

Gammon *et al.* [14] used successive courses of clobetasol ointment 0.05% (twice daily for 14 days) separated by 1 or more weeks determined by the rate of relapse. The treatment was effective, but mild local adverse effects and transient low a.m. plasma cortisol levels were found in 20% and 12% of patients, respectively.

The effects of two superpotent steroids, 3.5 g applied twice daily for 3 weeks, on the HPA-axis were studied and showed that both clobetasol and BDOV dramatically suppressed a.m. plasma cortisol ($< 5\ \mu g\%$) and urinary-free cortisol ($< 35\ \mu g\%$) in eight of 40 (20%) patients [13]. Most of the abnormal values were first recorded between treatment days 3 and 8. The group treated with clobetasol had a more sustained decrease than BDOV, 24 days vs 10 days, respectively. None of the patients manifested any classical signs of adrenal insufficiency, and none was stress-challenged. One patient's a.m. cortisol declined from 18.0 at baseline to 0.9 μg% at days 4–5 while using clobetasol and required a full week off therapy for recovery.

Clinical effectiveness with the superpotent topical steroids parallels suppression of the HPA-axis [11]. Clobetasol is the most suppressive at 7 g daily for 1 week; even one of nine patients became suppressed using 2 g daily (one sample tube of cream or ointment!). Halobetasol ointment 0.05% applied 7 g daily for 1 week to seven psoriasis patients did not decrease a.m. plasma cortisol or 24-hour urinary 17-hydroxy-corticosteroid below the lower limit of normal in any patient [15]. Ranking among the superpotent agents is probably clobetasol > halobetasol > BDOV > diflorasone diacetate.

Patients whose plasma a.m. cortisol drops below 5 μg% could conceivably develop clinically significant adverse effects if they sustained coincident serious trauma, infection, or underwent major surgery with anesthesia. Therefore, the following guidelines for the use of the superpotent agents have been suggested [3,11,16]:

1 do not use more than 50 g/week;
2 do not use under occlusion;
3 do not use on the face, axillae, submammary area, and groin;
4 do not use in children under 12 years of age;
5 allow a 1–2 week "drug holiday" between successive full courses of therapy (as is done in intermittent pulsing for maintenance);
6 if using for more than 2 consecutive weeks, consider measuring a.m. plasma cortisol; reduce or stop daily dosing if it is low.

A recent study has shown that 46% of 187 patients receiving oral prednisone with normal basal plasma cortisol levels had blunted responses to human corticotropin-releasing hormone (CRH) [17]. Moreover, there was poor correlation between the CRH response and the daily dose of corticosteroids, duration of administration, and cumulative dose. Therefore, a CRH test may be indicated if the a.m. basal cortisol level is considered borderline or unreliable.

Clinical studies

Combination therapy

Topical corticosteroids are most useful for patients with limited psoriasis (< 10%). Therefore, in patients with more extensive disease the role of steroids as adjunctive therapy with UV light has been explored and reviewed recently [18].

Although the seven studies reported combining UVB phototherapy and topical steroids utilized different methodologies, UVB protocols, topical steroids, and concomitant topical medications, surprisingly little advantage was conferred by the combination in treating psoriasis compared to UVB alone. Only one study reported a significantly improved rate of clearing (2.5 weeks vs 4 weeks) with the addition of clobetasol propionate ointment to UVB and increasing concentrations of anthralin [19]. Most studies showed a more rapid early, but not final clearing. Two of seven reports noted a shorter remission time when UVB was combined with clobetasol ointment or hydrocortisone valerate cream, respectively. In the former, statistical analysis was not reported; in the latter study, both groups received a coal tar gel plus suberythemogenic UVB and active or placebo cream. The time to relapse was 5.9 weeks vs 17.9 weeks. The steroid used in this study is from group IV and would not be expected to be especially beneficial for psoriasis except perhaps for face and intertriginous areas. In only one study was the remission time greater when UVB was combined with a topical steroid (fluocinonide cream 0.05%), 183 days vs 116 days [20]. However, these results did not attain statistical significance.

In conclusion, the combination of topical steroids with UVB phototherapy appears to have no substantial effect on the time to clearing or the percentage of responders. The long-term effects on remission are inclusive and may be detrimental. Therefore, because of potential toxicity discussed above and increased cost, high potency topical corticosteroids should not be used in addition to UVB. However, low-potency steroids for light protected areas and mid-potency lotions for the scalp are probably still warranted.

Five studies were reviewed, which compared psoralen UVA (PUVA) photochemotherapy with and without various topical corticosteroids used with or without occlusion. In general, all studies showed more rapid clearing rates of psoriasis on the sides or in the groups receiving PUVA plus corticosteroid compared to PUVA alone. There were no differences in the percentage of patients clearing in each group, and only one study reported a higher relapse rate in the patients who received fluocinolone acetonide cream or ointment 0.025% under plastic film occlusion until clearing was achieved [21]. The patients who relapsed progressed to a more aggressive form of psoriasis. It cannot be determined from the design of the study whether this was precipitated by the corticosteroid used or the occlusive dressing. PUVA alone was continued for maintenance. Application of the topical steroid prior to initiation of PUVA conferred no advantage. In the two studies where it was reported, the cumulative UVA dose required for clearing on the corticosteroid side was approximately half that required on the placebo-treated side.

In conclusion, an intermediate- to high-potency topical steroid may be used concurrently during PUVA photochemotherapy in order to achieve faster clearing, a lower total UVA dose at clearing, and a lower final UVA dose (Fig. 10.2). With weaning of the topical steroid (decrease frequency of application or decrease potency) and continuous maintenance PUVA, higher relapse rates are unlikely to occur.

In one study [22] combining triamcinolone cream 0.1% with 5% salicylic acid, which probably increases the penetration rate of the steroid,

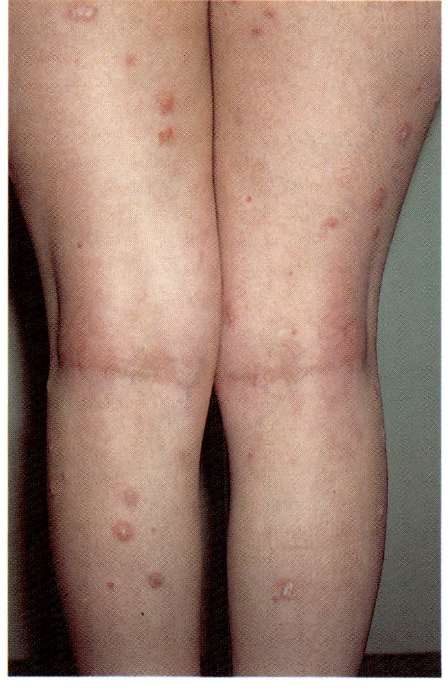

(a)

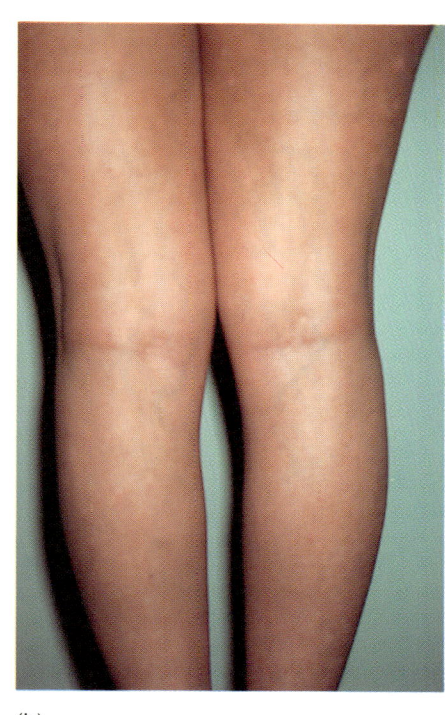

(b)

Fig 10.2 Psoriasis on legs treated with triamcinolone ointment 0.1% and psoralen UVA (a) before and (b) after 5 months.

allowed low-dose oral etretinate to be as effective as higher doses. This helped decrease retinoid-related side effects and reduced the cost of therapy.

In a bilateral paired comparison, combining fluocinonide 0.01% with increasing concentrations of anthralin did not change the final time to clearance. The sides receiving the steroid showed less burning and more staining from the anthralin, but unfortunately a significantly more rapid relapse of psoriasis [23]. It may be advisable to reserve topical steroids for brief stints as "fireman" if intolerable anthralin irritation occurs while reducing the working concentration of anthralin for further treatment.

How much steroid to use

It is disturbing to examine patients in hospital who have just applied their topical steroid and are practically swimming in the stuff so thick that the tracks of their (or the nurse's) fingertips can be seen. It is only necessary to apply a quantity of cream or ointment sufficient to cover the lesion site with a thin, uniform, barely perceptible layer. This is easier said than done. Previous estimations of body surface area (BSA) have used a "hand" as approximately 1%. Long *et al.* [24] have calculated one flat closed hand to represent 0.76 and 0.70% BSA for males and females, respectively. They have further determined that one fingertip unit or FTU (the amount of ointment applied from the distal skin crease to the tip of the palmar aspect of the index finger) of ointment weighs about 0.5 g. One FTU covers about two hand areas. The amount of ointment required to treat each anatomic area twice daily can be estimated (Table 10.1).

The entire body skin treated twice daily requires 28.5 g for 1 day and

Table 10.1 How much steroid to use

Anatomic area	No. FTUs required to cover	Amount required for twice-daily application (g)	Amount required for 1 week of b.i.d. treatment (g)
Face and neck	2.5	2.5	17.5
Anterior trunk	7	7.0	49
Posterior trunk	7	7.0	49
Arm	3	3.0	21
Hand (two sides)	1	1.0	7
Leg	6	6.0	42
Foot	2	2.0	14

FTU, fingertip unit.

200 g of medicine for 1 week. The concept of the FTU should provide a more convenient means for the physician to estimate the quantities to dispense and for the patient to translate lesion size (one hand) into a quantity of medication (0.5 FTU or 0.25 g) to apply with less wastage.

Tachyphylaxis

Tachyphylaxis is defined as the diminishing effect of a pharmacologic agent as it is repeatedly used to achieve a clinical response. This was described for potent steroids when no further vasoconstriction could be elicited after 96 hours [25]. The normal clinical response returned after withdrawal of treatment for 4 days. The mechanism(s) for tachyphylaxis are unknown. All clinicians have had the experience where a previously beneficial topical steroid gradually loses its effectiveness and becomes "no better than Vaseline for the patient." Strategies to avert tachyphylaxis include: (i) apply steroid only once daily and combine treatment with coal tar, anthralin, etc.; (ii) use intermittent courses of therapy (e.g., 2 weeks on, 1 week off) or apply superpotent steroid three times in 36 hours each week; (iii) alternate among different steroids within the same potency class at periodic intervals.

Rebound and pustular flares

It should not be surprising that after abrupt withdrawal of a potent topical steroid a rebound flare may ensue. This is because of the rapid hyperproliferation of the epidermis and stoking of the synthetic machinery of the dermis, which occur within days of stopping the steroid. Since both mechanisms may be involved in the pathogenesis of psoriasis, it is easier to understand why an incompletely treated psoriatic lesion may rebound. It is not uncommon to observe sterile pustules developing within a plaque during therapy. In a rare case, a full generalized pustular flare could occur upon withdrawal of therapy [26]. For this reason, it is advisable to utilize intermittent therapy with potent steroids or continuous therapy with the weakest steroid that is effective; at the same time take care to alternate chemical structures periodically to avoid tachyphylaxis.

Occlusive dressings

The popular use of impermeable polyethylene wraps and plastic sauna suits has declined with the development of potent and superpotent topical corticosteroids and the trend toward outpatient therapy, home UVB units, and psoriasis day-care centers. The group I and II steroids are powerful enough without occlusion. The latter may only enhance local side effects such as atrophy and skin sensitivity while increasing systemic absorption. Occlusive dressings are uncomfortable for patients and may be complicated by sweating, miliaria, and folliculitis [16]. Compliance at home was questionable at best, therefore, supervised use in the hospital setting was favored. Because of the thickness of volar skin and relatively resistant psoriasis there, occlusion of a superpotent steroid on the limited surfaces of the palms and/or soles is tolerable with vinyl examining gloves or Saran wrap.

An alternative occlusive dressing that is elegant and well tolerated is flurandrenolide-impregnated tape ($4\,\mu g/cm^2$), which is only practical for very small lesions and is left in place for 24 hours.

A modification of the hydrocolloid patches developed for wound healing have been marketed for occlusion of localized psoriatic plaques over an intermediate- or high-potency steroid for 48 hours. The patches (Actiderm; Squibb, Convatec) are small (5 × 3.5 inches), self-adhesive, and waterproof. They absorb transepidermal water, keeping the stratum corneum well hydrated and optimal for topical steroid delivery. Maceration and bacterial overgrowth are significantly less with Actiderm compared to plastic film occlusion. Mild folliculitis occurs infrequently. Epilation typically occurs upon removal of the dressing.

Improvement of chronic plaque psoriasis is most rapid and persistent with triamcinolone acetonide (TAC) 0.1% under occlusion with Actiderm compared to TAC and plastic film occlusion or TAC alone [27]. This technique used every third day for palmoplantar pustulosis was more effective than clobetasol propionate cream 0.05% applied b.i.d. (63% vs 21% clear after 4 weeks) [28]. Four weeks after stopping both treatments the lesions returned to their pretreatment status. Excellent results are reported with the weekly application of clobetasol lotion to the lesion, allowing it to dry and then covering it and 0.5–1 cm of surrounding skin with Duoderm or Actiderm occlusive dressing [29]. Nearly 100% of chronic plaques, psoriasis of palms and soles, palmoplantar pustulosis, and skin lesions of Reiter's syndrome obtained complete remission after 1–7 weeks of this treatment. Even more surprising, the majority of patients remained in complete remission at followup visits after 1–8 months after treatment.

Actiderm patches may be ideal as primary therapy for limited plaques of psoriasis on the palms, soles, elbows, knees, and sacrum, for localized pustular psoriasis, and for patients with residual lesions after UV light or systemic therapy. The hydrocolloid patches are expensive but can be obtained without a prescription and can be cut to the desired size; an inexpensive generic ointment such as TAC 0.1% or betamethasone-17-valerate 0.1% can be used with it every 2–3 days. Treatment once per week with the superpotent clobetasol lotion was very effective, and atrophy was not observed in any patient. In frequently traumatized areas, the patches may afford a level of protection (from picking and scratching) that prevents the isomorphic response and allows healing to occur.

Another technique for treating limited or residual psoriasis is intralesional injection of TAC 5 mg/ml. The suspension must be well mixed and the material must be injected into the dermis so that an immediate blanch is seen. There will be a response unless the drug was diluted improperly or injected too deeply. We inject a maximum of 3 ml (15 mg) per month. Atrophy, which usually does not occur at this concentration, is reversible. Healing of plaques may persist for 3 months or longer. This treatment is preferable for patients who are noncompliant with the applications of ointments and patches and who can tolerate the slight discomfort of intradermal injections.

Compounding

It is risky business to compound chemicals with proprietary formulations without knowing the effects on physicochemical stability and skin penetration rate. Ten percent urea caused significant chemical degradation of the active steroid in Topicort, Kenalog, and Westcort creams [30]. On the other hand, frequently used additives such as 0.25% camphor, 0.25% menthol, 0.25% phenol, 2% salicylic acid, or 5% liquor carbonis detergens solution caused no degradation. Salicylic acid 2% enhanced the penetration rate two- to threefold while the others did not. We recommend that extemporaneous compounding be performed by an experienced pharmacist using USP chemicals and petrolatum or Aquaphor as a vehicle. We use TAC USP and hydrocortisone USP most frequently with some of the additives listed above, excluding urea.

Generic formulations of topical corticosteroids

As the patents expire on propietary corticosteroids, generic formulations will proliferate and be marketed for the same indications as the brand name innovator product without the benefit of clinical efficacy studies. Patients (consumers), pharmacists, and physicians have the right to assume that the same chemical at the same concentration, e.g., TAC cream 0.1%, is therapeutically equivalent to Kenalog cream 0.01% (Westwood-Squibb). But would they be correct in that assumption? The bioavailability and rate of release of the corticosteroid is dependent not only on the concentration of corticosteroid in the vehicle but also the composition of the vehicle itself. The design of the vehicle and manufacturing methodology of the final product are not likely to be identical for most brand names and their generic topical corticosteroids.

The vasoconstriction or skin blanching assay has been used as a measure of percutaneous absorption (bioavailability) and potency, that is, clinical efficacy (Table 10.2). The assay has received much criticism [31] and deservedly so (*vide infra*), but it has proven remarkably reproducible when performed by the same experienced observer and by others in completely different settings (location, climate, subjects). The intensity of blanching is dependent on the subject and environmental factors. Comparisons of formulations are valid if obtained on the same group of 30 subjects at the same time. The visual reading of the pharmacodynamic response, the blanching effect, and the grading of it, are highly subjective. There is no objective measurement, no "hard copy" to refer to later for subsequent comparisons, analysis or validation. This is surprising when one considers the technologic advances in other areas of medicine, for example, radiologic imaging techniques, identification and analysis of nanomolar quantities of cytokines, and immunophenotyping and genotyping of cells.

There are many pressures brought to bear upon the prescribing of generic medicines. These are societal, political, and economic but rarely medical pressures. Patients want the best drug that gives the fastest relief from suffering, preferably at low cost or gratis. Physicians usually prescribe what they think will work the best with the least toxicity in a given

Table 10.2 Potency ranking of some commonly used topical corticosteroids based on vasoconstrictor assay and clinical studies in psoriasis

Potency group	Concentration (%)	Generic name	Brand name* (USA)
I Super-high	0.05	Clobetasol propionate	Temovate
	0.05	Halobetasol propionate	Ultravate
	0.05	Betamethasone dipropionate (in optimized vehicle)	Diprolene
	0.05	Diflorasone diacetate (in optimized vehicle)	Psorcon ointment
II High	0.1	Amcinonide†	Cyclocort ointment
	0.05	Betamethasone dipropionate	Diprosone ointment
	0.25	Desoximetasone	Topicort**
	0.05	Diflorasone diacetate	Fluorone ointment
	0.05	Fluocinonide	Lidex
	0.1	Halcinonide	Halog cream
III Intermediate	0.05	Betamethasone dipropionate	Diprosone cream
	0.1	Betamethasone-17-valerate	Valisone ointment
	0.05	Diflorasone diacetate	Maxiflor cream
	0.005	Fluticasone propionate	Cutivate ointment
	0.1	Triamcinolone acetonide	Aristocort A ointment**

Continued on p. 188

Table 10.2 *Continued*

Potency group	Concentration (%)	Generic name	Brand name* (USA)
IV Intermediate	0.025	Fluocinolone acetonide	Synalar ointment
	0.05	Flurandrenolide	Cordran ointment/ tape
	0.1	Mometasone furoate	Elocon cream
	0.2	Hydrocortisone-17-valerate	Westcort ointment
V Intermediate	0.1	Betamethasone-17-valerate‡	Valisone cream
	0.025	Floucinolone acetonide	Synalar cream
	0.05	Fluticasone propionate	Cutivate cream
	0.1	Hydrocortisone butyrate	Locoid cream
	0.2	Hydrocortisone-17-valerate	Westcort cream
VI Low	0.05	Aclometasone dipropionate‡	Aclovate
	0.01	Betamethasone-17-valerate	Valisone cream
	0.05	Desonide	Tridesilon cream
	0.03	Flumethasone pivalate	Locorten cream
	0.01	Fluocinolone acetonide	Synalar cream
VII Very low	0.1	Dexamethasone	Decadron cream
	1, 2.5§	Hydrocortisone	Hytone**

* Product refers to both cream and ointment vehicle unless specified.
† With few exceptions, the ointment formulation of the same concentration of corticosteroid is one class higher in potency than the cream formulation.
‡ Potency rating based on clinical activity in psoriasis, not vasoconstriction assay.
§ Also available without prescription.
** A dose–response curve has not been demonstrated in either vasoconstriction assay or clinical activity for the same formulations of these brands.

situation without regard to rapidity in a chronic incurable condition such as psoriasis and often without regard to price. Pharmacists want to fill prescriptions correctly while following the letter of the law and realizing a legitimate profit. While the cost to the pharmacist is much higher for 30 g of brand name Kenalog ointment 0.1% ($18.98 at the time of publishing) [32], the markup on the generic at $3.09 may be much higher, resulting in a similar price to the consumer. Some physicians dispense their own prescriptions. Finally, governments and institutions usually include those drugs on their formularies which can be obtained at the lowest wholesale price, regardless of generic or brand name status.

The first comparison of the vasoconstrictor assay between popular brand name topical corticosteroids and several manufacturers of their generic equivalents, namely TAC 0.1%, betamethasone valerate 0.1%, and fluocinolone acetonide 0.25% creams was published by Stoughton [33]. Using a slightly different vasoconstrictor assay Jackson *et al.* [34] confirmed that Valisone (Schering) and Kenalog (Westwood-Squibb) 0.1% creams were significantly more potent than at least some generic formulations. The Food and Drug Administration (FDA) contracted with Stoughton to blindly compare again some brand name corticosteroids vs generic formulations made by Fougera & Co [33]. Valisone cream 0.1% was again shown to be superior to generic betamethasone valerate, which was later confirmed by an independent investigator [35]. Stoughton [33] detected significant differences between the brand name and the Fougera products: Synalar cream 0.025% was more potent than fluocinolone acetonide 0.025%, but TAC creams 0.025% and 0.05% were more potent than corresponding Aristocort cream (Lederle Laboratories).

The Center for Drug Evaluation and Research of the FDA acknowledged that the vasoconstrictor (skin blanching) test provides one reliable means of evaluating topical corticosteroids and suggested modifications such as assessment at several time points after drug removal to develop a profile over time analogous to the area under the curve determinations used for oral drug administration [31]. An objective method of quantifying the blanching effect could be achieved with reflectance spectrophotometry, Doppler laser velocimetry, or surface thermography. The FDA recently introduced an *in vitro* method, which measures the diffusion of active drug from the vehicle across a synthetic membrane and into a chamber containing a liquid medium [36]. The fluid is withdrawn at intervals and the active drug is measured using high pressure liquid chromotography. The test will be used in the same way that the FDA now uses dissolution assays to assure batch-to-batch uniformity and bioavailability of capsule and tablet dosage forms. The results will serve as the quality control standard for subsequent batches.

The brand name formulations were not spared scrutiny by the vasoconstrictor assay studies of Stoughton and Wullich [37]. It was shown that higher concentrations of the same corticosteroid in the same vehicle made by the same manufacturer do not necessarily predict higher activity or bioavailability. In most cases no differences in activity were found (Kenalog ointment 0.025, 0.1, 0.5%; Aristocort ointment 0.1, 0.5%; Aristocort cream 0.025, 0.1, 0.5%; Topicort cream 0.05, 0.25%; Hytone cream 1.0, 2.5%). The Fougera generic TAC cream 0.025 and 0.5% were also equivalent. Aristocort A cream 0.1% was more potent than 0.5%, which was equal to 0.025%. Synalar and Valisone creams were exceptional in that there was a dose–response with increasing concentrations of drug. For the others, it may be that the vasoconstrictor response is sigmoidal and plateaus at the lower concentration. A maximal blanching effect does not, however, mean that there is not more drug in the dermis. There may be differences in the rate and extent of blanching activity that are not detectable by a single time-point reading. Moreover, no dose proportionability studies correlating concentration, blanching activity, and clinical efficacy have been reported. Notwithstanding the relative lack of any lasting effect of the aforementioned drugs in psoriasis, the following should be pointed out.

1 Brand name topical corticosteroids are priced according to concentration (e.g., the average cost at the time of publishing of Hydrocortisone 1% and

2.5% to the pharmacist is $5.63 and $9.93, respectively). If the lower concentration is equally potent, prescribe it preferentially. Aristocort A cream 0.5% costs $53.42 for 30 g and is equivalent to 0.025% at $15.34; the more potent 0.1% formulation costs $19.46. In this case the most economic and efficacious choice is obvious.

2 Where generic formulations are equivalent in potency to brand name, prescribe the former because of cost savings. You would have to know which generic company the pharmacist dispenses, however, since the generics are not all the same. Valisone ointment 0.1% (30 g tube) cost the pharmacist $24.84. Some generics (Fougera, URL) are equivalent at $6.31.

3 Until comparative potency labeling of all generic topical corticosteroids is required, it is not feasible to prescribe the most cost-effective generic in all cases. As a general rule, generic ointment formulations are closer to brand names in vasoconstriction assays. Prescribe generic ointments or specify brand name creams if that vehicle is desired.

Generic substitution is common, occurring more than half the time in a recent survey of 12 pharmacies, and it is certainly here to stay. There are a plethora of generic varieties of topical corticosteroids on the market with more to come. Even more frightening than generic substitution is therapeutic substitution. This gives the pharmacist authority to substitute different antibiotics, nonsteroidal antiinflammatory drugs, and topical corticosteroids, for example, because they are all used to treat the same kind of disease ("steroid-responsive dermatosis") within a given drug classification. If the topical steroids are rated within a range of potency, then any drug within that range could conceivably be substituted without regard to the desired vehicle (cream or ointment), unwanted additives in the vehicle, such as preservatives and propylene glycol, or consideration of tachyphylaxis or allergy to the active drug.

TOXICITY

While the effects of systemic absorption, HPA-axis suppression and iatrogenic Cushing's syndrome, are serious concerns with conservative use of the superpotent topical steroids, they may occur with the intermediate to high potency compounds as well. Fortunately, such reports are rare and usually implicate grossly inappropriate use of the medication. While the potential hazards of superpotent steroids are greater, the tendency for abuse of the former is more likely because there are no limitations on quantities dispensed, recommendations for daily dosage and rest periods, prohibitions against occlusive dressings and use in children. Notwithstanding, in practice, it is the local unwanted effects of topical corticosteroids that give the most frequent cause for concern.

Atrophy

The most common adverse effect of topical corticosteroid use is cutaneous atrophy. This atrophy involves both the epidermis with thinning secondary to decreased mitotic activity and DNA synthesis as well as the dermis with decreased fibroblast synthesis of collagen and ground substance. The clinical counterpart to steroid-induced atrophy is increased transparency, shininess of the skin with loss of skin markings, and telangiectasia [3].

Epidermal and dermal atrophy was induced experimentally in normal skin after 3 weeks of clobetasol under occlusion [37]. At this time the viable epidermis was reduced 42% and was clinically evident. The papillary dermis appeared more compact with rearrangement of collagen and elastic fiber networks. By 6 weeks, the alterations were more profound with involvement of the papillary and reticular dermis, synthetically quiescent (shrunken) fibroblasts, and disappearance of mast cells.

After withdrawal of the steroid treatment, the skin recovered rapidly with fine structure of keratinocytes, melanocytes, and fibroblasts within 2 days, normal glycosaminoglycan synthesis by 14 days with a practically normal appearance of epidermis and dermis at 14 days. The return of mast cells and histamine levels to the skin was significantly delayed by up to 3 months after steroid discontinuation. Katz *et al.* [8] have reported that preatrophy can be detected in psoriatic plaques by 8× magnification as delicate networks of horizontally-oriented vascular channels as early as 2 weeks after conventional superpotent steroid treatment (clobetasol and BDOV).

Atrophy is most commonly detected on the face as telangiectasia; however, the telangiectasia may represent normal or preexisting dilated capillaries in the papillary dermis made more obvious by epidermal thinning. Of course, patients with solar elastosis or rosacea may already have preexisting telangiectasia. For this reason, it is advisable to recommend low-potency nonfluorinated topical steroids for psoriatic lesions on the central face such as hydrocortisone, desonide, and hydrocortisone-17-valerate. More potent steroids should not be used on the eyelid skin because of the risk of increasing intraocular pressure (glaucoma). It is often necessary and appropriate, however, to apply intermediate- to high-potency steroids to psoriasis of the ears and scalp. The medications frequently drip off the hairline on to the facial skin or are inadvertently smeared, rubbed, or applied there when it remains on the fingertips. Shower caps worn over annointed scalps at bedtime are helpful. Thorough washing of hands or covering with gloves if they are also under treatment cannot be overemphasized.

Another common adverse effect occurring on the face is a papulopustular reaction usually in a perioral or periocular distribution, particularly in acne- or rosacea-prone individuals. This may have resulted after intentional treatment of facial psoriasis or inadvertent contact. In some cases, patients may have learned by trial and error that the steroid helps incidental acneiform lesions and use it on their own. If a fluorinated steroid is culpable, wean the patient to a nonfluorinated one rather than stopping all steroids abruptly in order to prevent the rebound flare-up which is almost certain to occur. If the steroid in use is nonfluorinated, stop it and give a tapering 4-week course of tetracycline HCl (1 g/day for 1 week; 750 mg/

day for 1 week; 500 mg/day for 1 week; 250 mg/day for 1 week). Low-dose tetracycline may need to be continued to prevent baseline acneiform lesions.

While preatrophy and atrophy of the skin are reversible, striae caused by rupture of connective tissue and stretching of the epidermis are permanent. They may result from the application of medium- to high-potency steroids to flexural or intertriginous areas such as the axillae and groin which are naturally moist and partially occluded (Fig. 10.3). The author has personally observed striae develop on the medial thighs of a man treated for 2 weeks with a proprietary combination of betamethasone dipropionate 0.05% and clotrimazole 1% for tinea cruris. Particular attention to a child's diaper area is called for here where only hydrocortisone should be used. Also in children, particularly, striae can occur on any skin surface that is treated with medium-potency steroid under plastic wrap occlusion (Fig. 10.4).

In mature patients with age-related atrophy and solar elastosis, purpura occur frequently on the backs of the arms and hands after minor or imperceptible trauma even with use of low- to intermediate-potency steroids. Many patients find these annoying and complain about them. Stellate pseudoscars may develop, particularly if shearing of the epidermis occurs.

Topical steroids may mask cutaneous infections with dermatophytes because of a blunted inflammatory response and slower rate of epidermal turnover. Infections of the groin, buttocks, and feet may be inappropriately treated as psoriasis. Bacterial folliculitis may develop in a hairy area with occlusive ointments. These pustules may be confused with localized pustular flares of psoriasis.

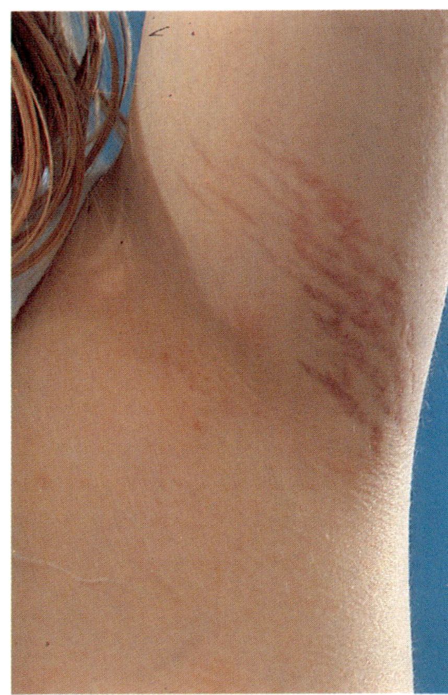

Fig 10.3 Steroid-induced striae in the axilla of a young girl.

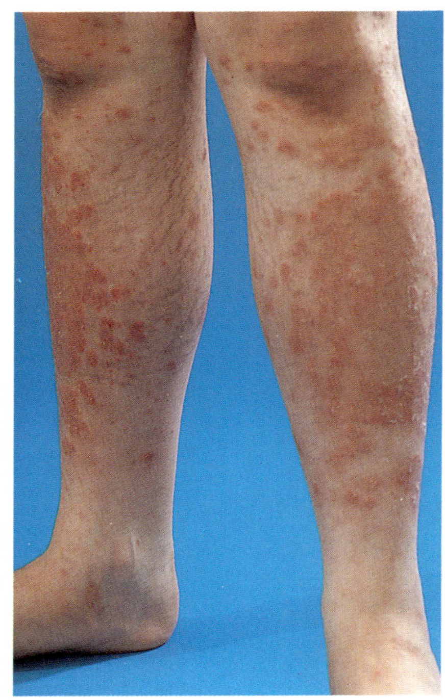

Fig 10.4 Same patient as Fig. 10.3 shows striae on leg where medium potency steroids have been applied under plastic film occlusion.

Allergic contact dermatitis

Hypersensitivity to a topical corticosteroid should be suspected when the skin disease not only fails to respond but worsens during treatment. Allergies to ingredients in the vehicle and to the active corticosteroid itself are not uncommon. A corticosteroid screening series permits patch testing for suspected molecules in a selected way [39], but many problems involving appropriate concentrations and vehicles have arisen. Tixocortol pivalate appears to be an excellent screening compound for contact sensitivity to corticosteroids. Sensitivity to tixocortol pivalate in a large European patch test population was detected at a frequency of 1.9%, which is comparable to parabens, formaldehyde, and ethylene diamine [40]. During the 10-year period 1981–91, 19 patients were identified in the Cleveland Clinic patch test clinic with contact dermatitis to topical corticosteroids; 11 of 19 were allergic to one or more steroids, the others to one or more components in vehicles such as propylene glycol, lanolin alcohol, parabens, and benzyl alcohol. The primary steroids responsible for contact dermatitis were identified as hydrocortisone (five), hydrocortisone-17-valerate (two), amcinonide (three), and clobetasol-17-propionate (one) (L.J. Jagodzinski, J.S. Taylor, personal communication, 1993). Contact dermatitis to corticosteroids must be very uncommon in psoriasis, however, because almost all of the patients reported had underlying chronic eczematous dermatoses or venous stasis ulceration [41].

SYSTEMIC CORTICOSTEROIDS

R. Auerbach has said that "to the extent that one can say 'never' in medicine systemic corticosteroids should never be prescribed for psoriasis." While I do not advocate the use of systemic corticosteroids and have never knowingly prescribed them for psoriasis, we have to deal with their complications when used by other physicians for psoriasis or for concomitant diseases which may overshadow psoriasis in terms of severity, for example, Crohn's disease, rheumatoid arthritis, systemic lupus erythematosus, and renal allograft recipients, to name but a few.

A 1984 survey [42] indicated that 14–18% of dermatologists used systemic corticosteroids for psoriasis at the time, probably in the form of intramuscular TAC suspension, although this was not specified. By contrast, 96% of dermatologists in university settings did not do so. Studies and experience have shown that it is not the systemic steroid treatment *per se* that aggravates psoriasis, but rather the tapering or withdrawal of the drugs. Most cases of psoriasis are initially quite responsive to systemic steroids judging by clearing of the skin during treatment of one of the diseases mentioned above. It is during the taper that the skin disease becomes labile, more inflammatory, spreads, and develops pustulation. In the past, dermatologists who treated psoriasis with prednisone noted that the dose needed to maintain the disease spiraled upward until reaching an uncomfortably high dose that was also ineffective. Upon subsequent tapering and withdrawal of the steroid, a rebound flare, exacerbation, and pustular psoriasis occur unless there is intervention with hospitalization, retinoids, MTX, or cyclosporine. I suspect that these patients accumulate disproportionately at tertiary care centers. Consultation prior to the desperation use of systemic steroids for severe psoriasis may prevent such catastrophes.

In the cases of the patients with psoriasis and serious concomitant systemic diseases, it is imperative to collaborate with the general practitioner or internist in the selection of adjunctive therapy that will help psoriasis but not aggravate the underlying disease, and where possible, the converse. In the examples given, sulfasalazine may benefit Crohn's disease and psoriasis, MTX may improve rheumatoid arthritis, systemic lupus erythematosus, and psoriasis, but antimalarials may aggravate psoriasis; UV light would not be a good choice for psoriasis with lupus, but retinoids may help the cutaneous manifestations of both; many organ transplant recipients receive prednisone along with azathioprine and cyclosporine, which are adequate to maintain psoriasis in check.

NEW DIRECTIONS

The science of developing topical corticosteroids and the art of using them to treat psoriasis has come a long way in 40 years. However, I have noticed a change in trends: from the development of more potent drugs by modification of chemical structures and optimization of vehicles to the development of different chemical structures of equipotency to existing steroids in the same class, extension of product lines by altering concentrations and offering more elegant vehicles, and the proliferation of generically equivalent corticosteroids. There is an effort to create steroids that are less atrophogenic while maintaining clinical efficacy [43]. It has been shown that there can be divergence from the ranking on the vasoconstriction assay and efficacy in psoriasis. Unfortunately, it was in the "wrong" direction for hydrocortisone-17-valerate and aclometasone. Mometasone furoate, which is chlorinated at the C-9 ring position and the C-21 side chain, is a step in the right direction but not the answer. It is as weakly atrophogenic as hydrocortisone and as efficacious as TAC or fluocinolone. It would be desirable if steroids could be developed with an eye toward synergism with other popular antipsoriatic treatments such as coal tar, anthralin, calcipotriol, UV light, and the systemic approaches as opposed to their current weakly additive and sometimes deleterious positions.

The vasoconstriction assay, while a proven valuable tool for evaluating potency, both in efficacy and toxicity, is not sufficiently sophisticated or reproducible to use alone for the next generation of topical corticosteroids. Vasoconstriction and other relevant parameters should be measured objectively and recorded for posterity by changes in light reflectance, color, or temperature.

The generic formulations, while much less expensive than their brand name innovators, are confusing for prescribers, pharmacists, and patients but not governments, institutions, and third-party payors. It is not enough for the FDA to require vasoconstriction assays on 20–30 normal volunteers and an *in vitro* chemical analysis of the substance, which diffuses across a synthetic membrane prior to approval. Labeling of the package with a potency rating would be helpful, but if the gold standard is a test of clinical efficacy in psoriasis, then paired comparisons with 20–30 psoriatic subjects should be performed whatever the cost.

REFERENCES

1 Liem WK, McCullough JL, Weinstein GD. Is topical therapy effective for psoriasis: results of survey of USA dermatologists. *J Invest Dermatol* 1992;98:602(Abstract).

2 Stoughton RB. Enhanced percutaneous penetration with 1-dodecylazacycloheptan-2-one. *Arch Dermatol* 1982;118:474–7.

3 Yohn JJ, Weston WL. Topical glucocorticosteroids. *Curr Probl Dermatol* 1990;2:31–63.

4 Cornell RC, Stoughton RB. Correlation of the vasoconstriction assay and clinical activity in psoriasis. *Arch Dermatol* 1985;121:63–7.

5 Jacobson C, Cornell RC, Savin RC. A comparison of clobetasol propionate 0.05% ointment and an optimized betamethasone dipropionate 0.05% ointment in the treatment of psoriasis. *Cutis* 1986;37:213–20.

6 Jegasothy BV. Clobetasol propionate ointment 0.05% *versus* diflorasone diacetate ointment 0.05% in moderate to severe psoriasis. *Int J Dermatol* 1990;29:729–30.

7 Katz HI, Hien NT, Prawer SE, *et al.* Betamethasone dipropionate in optimized

vehicle. *Arch Dermatol* 1987;123:1308–11.
8 Katz HI, Prawer SE, Mooney JJ, Samson CR. Preatrophy: covert sign of thinned skin. *J Am Acad Dermatol* 1989;20:731–5.
9 Yawalkar S, Wiesenberg-Boettcher I, Gibson JR, *et al.* Dermatopharmacologic investigations of halobetasol propionate in comparison with clobetasol-17-propionate. *J Am Acad Dermatol* 1991;25:1137–44.
10 Mensing H, Korsukewitz G, Yawalkar S. A double-blind, multicenter comparison between 0.05% halobetasol propionate ointment and 0.05% betamethasone dispropionate ointment in chronic plaque psoriasis. *J Am Acad Dermatol* 1991;25: 1149–52.
11 Stoughton RB, Cornell RC. Review of super-potent topical corticosteroids. *Semin Dermatol* 1987;6:72–6.
12 Katz HI, Prawer WE, Medansky RS, *et al.* Intermittent corticosteroid maintenance treatment of psoriasis: a double-blind multicenter trial of augmented betamethasone dipropionate ointment in a pulse dose treatment regimen. *Dermatologica* 1991;183: 269–74.
13 Katz HI, Hien NT, Prawer SE, *et al.* Superpotent topical steroid treatment of psoriasis vulgaris — clinical efficacy and adrenal function. *J Am Acad Dermatol* 1987;16:804–11.
14 Gammon WR, Krueger GG, Van Scott EJ, Kamm A. Intermittent short courses of clobetasol propionate ointment 0.05% in the treatment of psoriasis. *Curr Ther Res* 1987;42:419–27.
15 Watson WA, Kalb RE, Siskin SB, *et al.* Safety of halobetasol 0.05% ointment in treatment of psoriasis. *Pharmacotherapy* 1990;10:107–11.
16 Trozak DJ. Topical corticosteroid therapy in psoriasis vulgaris. *Cutis* 1990;46: 341–50.
17 Schlaghecke R, Kornely E, Senten RJ, Ridderskamp P. The effect of long-term glucocorticoid therapy on pituitary-adrenal responses to exogenous corticotropin-releasing hormone. *N Engl J Med* 1992;326:226–30.
18 Meola T, Soter NA, Lim HW. Are topical corticosteroids useful adjunctive therapy for the treatment of psoriasis with ultraviolet radiation? *Arch Dermatol* 1991;127: 1708–13.
19 Lidbrink P, Johannesson A, Hammar H. Psoriasis treatment: faster clearance when UV-B-dithranol is combined with topical clobetasol propionate. *Dermatologica* 1986;172:164–8.
20 Dover JS, McEvoy MT, Rosen CF, *et al.* Are topical corticosteroids useful in phototherapy for psoriasis? *J Am Acad Dermatol* 1989;20:748–54.
21 Morison WL, Parrish JA, Fitzpatrick TB. Controlled study of PUVA and adjunctive topical therapy in the management of psoriasis. *Br J Dermatol* 1978;98:125–32.
22 Van Der Rhee JH, Tijssen JGP, Herrmann WA, *et al.* Combined treatment of psoriasis with a new aromatic retinoid (Tigason) in low dosage orally and triamcinolone cream topically: a double blind trial. *Br J Dermatol* 1980;102:203–12.
23 Grattan CEH, Christopher AP, Robinson M, Cowan MA. Double-blind comparison of a dithranol and steroid mixture with a conventional dithranol regimen for chronic psoriasis. *Br J Dermatol* 1988;119:623–6.
24 Long CC, Finlay AY, Averill RW. The rule of hand: 4 hand areas = 2 FTU = 1 g. *Arch Dermatol* 1992;128:1129–30.
25 duVivier A, Stoughton RB. Tachyphylaxis to the action of topically applied steroids. *Arch Dermatol* 1975;111:581–3.
26 Tefler NR, Dauber RPR. Generalized pustular psoriasis associated with withdrawal of topical clobetasol-17-propionate. *J Am Acad Dermatol* 1987;17:144.
27 David M, Lowe NJ. Psoriasis therapy: comparative studies with a hydrocolloid dressing, plastic film occlusion, and triamcinolone acetonide cream. *J Am Acad Dermatol* 1989;21:511–14.
28 Kragballe K, Larsen FG. A hydrocolloid occlusive dressing plus triamcinolone

acetonide cream is superior to clobetasol cream and in palmo-plantar pustulosis. *Acta Derm Venereol* 1991;71:540–2.

29 Volden G. Successful treatment of chronic skin diseases with clobetasol propionate and a hydrocolloid occlusive dressing. *Acta Derm Venereol* 1992;72:69–71.

30 Krochmal L, Wang JCT, Patel B, Rodgers J. Topical corticosteroid compounding: effects on physicochemical stability and skin penetration rate. *J Am Acad Dermatol* 1989;21:979–84.

31 Shah VP, Peck CC, Skelly JP. "Vasoconstriction"-skin blanching-assay for glucocorticoids — a critique. *Arch Dermatol* 1989;125:1558–61.

32 Anonymous. Topical corticosteroids. *Med Lett* 1991;33:108–10.

33 Stoughton RB. Are generic formulations equivalent to trade name topical glucocorticoids? *Arch Dermatol* 1987;123:1312–14.

34 Jackson DB, Thompson C, McCormack JR, Guin JD. Bioequivalence (bioavailability) of generic topical corticosteroids. *J Am Acad Dermatol* 1989;20:791–6.

35 Olsen EA. A double-blind controlled comparison of generic and trade-name topical steroids using the vasoconstriction assay. *Arch Dermatol* 1991;127:197–201.

36 Shah VP. Topical corticosteroids: quality control considerations. *Int J Dermatol* 1992;31(Suppl. 1):34–7.

37 Stoughton RB, Wullich K. The same glucocorticoid in brand-name products. *Arch Dermatol* 1989;125:1509–11.

38 Lavker RM, Schechter NM, Lazarus GS. Effects of topical corticosteroids on human dermis. *Br J Dermatol* 1986;115:101–7.

39 Rivera G, Tomb R, Foussereau J. Allergic contact dermatitis from topical corticosteroids. *Contact Dermatitis* 1989;21:83–91.

40 Dooms-Goosens A, Degreef H, Coopman S. Corticosteroid contact allergy: a reality. In Frosch PJ, Dooms-Goossens A, Lachapelle JM, *et al.*, eds. *Current Topics in Contact Dermatitis*. Berlin: Springer-Verlag, 1989:233–7.

41 Wilkinson SM, English JSC. Hydrocortisone sensitivity: Clinical features of 59 cases. *J Am Acad Dermatol* 1992;27:683–7.

42 Baughman RD. Psoriasis practices. *Arch Dermatol* 1987;123:1299–300.

43 Korting HC, Kerscher MJ, Schafer-Korting M. Topical glucocorticoids with improved benefit/risk ratio: Do they exist? *J Am Acad Dermatol* 1992;27:87–92.

eleven

Anthralin

INTRODUCTION

In 1877 the British dermatologist B. Squire reported that the yellow powder extracted from the bark of the Brazilian araroba tree had a therapeutic effect in psoriasis. The active ingredient in Goa powder was a hydroxyanthracene called chrysarobin. When the supply became scarce during World War I, a substitute was synthesized, 1,8-dihydroxy-9-anthrone, called anthralin or dithranol [1].

MECHANISM OF ACTION

In the hairless mouse, a single topical application of anthralin results in depression of mitotic index and DNA synthesis. Repeated application to the mouse tail results in a significant decrease in DNA synthesis, global reduction in protein synthesis, epidermal hyperplasia, and the presence of a continual granular layer. Anthralin and its dimer completely inhibit cell growth and thymidine incorporation in cultured human fibroblasts at concentrations ranging from 0.1 to 1.0 μmol/l.

In cell culture, mitochondrial respiration is sensitive to anthralin. The mitochondria of keratinocytes (KCs) increase in size and the cristae become less well defined. Using ^{14}C-labeled anthralin and high-pressure liquid chromatography (HPLC) for detecting breakdown products, it has been shown that in membrane and cytosolic fractions the primary oxidation products, quinone and dimer, are present. Ultrastructural changes in mitochondria of psoriatic skin treated with anthralin are followed by inhibition of cell respiration. Langerhans cells are more sensitive to these changes than KCs. In summary, anthralin is probably an inhibitor of cell respiration, and the mitochondrial membrane is the primary site of action. During the oxidation reaction anthralin is irreversibly degraded and the mitochondria are inactivated.

Polymorphonuclear leukocyte (PMNL) but not monocyte chemotaxis *in vitro* is inhibited by concentrations of anthralin likely to be encountered in skin [2]. Superoxide anion production of both cell types is inhibited by anthralin, but monocytes appear to be 100 times more sensitive to this effect [3]. The increased chemotactic activities of both monocytes [4] and PMNLs [5] in psoriatics were normalized after 3–4 weeks of anthralin therapy. The chemotaxis-enhancing effects of plasma from psoriatic patients returned to normal after 2 weeks of treatment [4]. Tumor promotion caused by phorbol ester in mouse skin was reduced by anthralin [6].

CLINICAL USE OF ANTHRALIN

Efficacy

In studies of *in vitro* effects of pharmacologic concentrations of anthralin on cultured normal human KCs, KC proliferation was inhibited by 98% at an anthralin concentration of 10 ng/ml compared to only 9% inhibition of lymphocyte proliferation [7]. Cell viability was not affected. No cell-cycle-specific growth arrest was observed in the anthralin-treated KCs, but they showed large reductions in transforming growth factor-α (TGF-α) expression and epidermal growth factor receptor binding. In active psoriatic plaques TGF-α and its receptor are overexpressed. It would be of interest to perform similar experiments with cultured psoriatic KCs or KCs from psoriatic skin treated *in vivo* with anthralin. It may not be possible to culture the latter because of the injury to mitochondria.

Anthralin penetrates faster through involved than uninvolved psoriatic skin *in vitro* with large individual variations [8]. The conclusion is that the stratum corneum is the rate limiting step in normal skin but that in diseased skin the rate of release of drug from vehicle is rate limiting.

Arachidonic acid and metabolite concentrations are increased in the suction blister fluid of normal volunteers receiving 0.3% anthralin in petrolatum. By contrast, anthralin was a potent inhibitor of leukotriene B_4 formation by stimulated PMNLs *in vitro*. Topical application of 1% indomethacin gel, a prostaglandin-synthetase inhibitor, had no effect on irritancy due to anthralin [9]. In patients treated with anthralin and oral indomethacin 25 mg t.i.d. or placebo, there was a trend toward a more rapid increase in anthralin concentration and less time to clearance in the indomethacin group [10]. However, in a larger double-blind comparison of oral indomethacin 25 mg t.i.d. and placebo in 50 psoriatic patients undergoing a standard Ingram regimen, no significant differences were found between the two groups in the reduction of plaque severity or body surface area of involvement [11]. There were no significant differences in tolerance of anthralin between the two groups based on the final therapeutic concentrations achieved at 6 weeks: the majority of patients in both groups tolerated the 2% strength (maximum for this study). The authors concluded that a standard dose of indomethacin has no significant harmful effects on patients receiving the Ingram regimen, nor does it positively influence their tolerance to anthralin.

Clinical studies

Anthralin USP is available as a yellow powder, soluble in organic solvents. Anthralin may be dissolved in chloroform and added to petrolatum. The chloroform is allowed to evaporate off, leaving the suspension in petrolatum. Anthralin soft paste contains varying concentrations of anthralin (0.1–5%) in Lassar's paste, which contains zinc oxide 25%, starch 25%, and salicylic acid 2% in petrolatum. Paraffin 5–10% may be added to make a hard anthralin paste. Anthralin sticks (suspended in beeswax) for directed application to limited lesions are available in the UK. Anthralin ointments, creams, and scalp solutions are commercially available in concentrations ranging from 0.1 to 1.0%.

Ingram method

The traditional use of anthralin was developed by Ingram in 1953. The use of anthralin paste was combined with the Goeckerman regimen. The current Ingram method consists of a bath for 15–30 min with a coal tar solution (e.g., Balnetar, Polytar, Zetar, etc.) followed by suberythemogenic doses of UVB starting with one-third or one-half minimal erythema dose (MED) exposure and increasing by this amount each treatment provided no burning occurs. The anthralin paste is then applied with a spatula or tongue depressor to psoriatic plaques at an initial concentration of 0.1% sparing normal surrounding skin. This can be increased every 2–3 days until irritation occurs. The paste is powdered with talc conveniently dabbed on to the treated area with a ball made from a cheesecloth filled with talcum powder. This procedure absorbs moisture from the paste and prevents staining of clothing. The whole body may be covered with a stocking net and worn for 6–24 hours. This type of treatment is most suitable for an outpatient psoriasis day-care situation or for a hospital inpatient.

Prior to repeating the cycle of tar bath and UVB exposure, the hardened paste must be removed by rubbing light mineral oil or baby oil on to it. Adherent scales are removed along with the paste. The rate of increase of UVB dose and anthralin paste concentration is flexible and based on therapeutic response and whether burning or irritation occurs. Some patients improve dramatically with low concentrations, while others need 4% or greater to achieve excellent responses. The therapy may be simplified by omitting the tar bath and suberythemogenic UVB. Alternatively, lower nonirritating concentrations of anthralin (0.01–0.05%) may be combined with sub-erythemogenic UVB irradiation. Because anthralin shows an absorption maximum at 350–360 nm, UVA irradiation may give additional benefit. The combination of PUVA with anthralin gave better results than either regimen alone. The combination of crude coal tar 2% for 30–60 min, anthralin 1–10% for 15–60 min, followed by phototherapy from high-pressure metal halide lamps (consisting of UVA and UVB) three to four times weekly was as efficacious as PUVA or conventional psoriasis day-care therapy for moderate to severe disease [12]. Clearance of psoriasis by the Ingram method allows maintenance of the remission by PUVA given once weekly for 4–5 months, then every other week for 4–5 months, then every third week for a mean dose rate of 28.6 J/cm^2 per month [13].

Short contact anthralin therapy

It is possible to reduce the side effects of anthralin while maintaining efficacy. It is not necessary to produce irritation/erythema in order to obtain the beneficial therapeutic effects of anthralin (Fig. 11.1). Clinical studies indicated that short contact anthralin therapy (SCAT) 1–3% for 10–30 min was equivalent [14] or superior to standard overnight anthralin therapy [14,15]. Contact times of 5–20 min daily are sufficient to clear psoriatic plaques in 22 days (2% anthralin, 0.5% salicylic acid) [16]. Short contact with hard anthralin paste for 2 hours in the Ingram regimen was more effective than 30 min and equal to the standard 24-hour application [17]. However, short contact anthralin 0.3–3% and salicylic acid 2% in petrolatum for 10–30 min yielded only modest improvement in a minority of patients when combined with outpatient UVB phototherapy [18]. The overall shorter times needed for application and cleansing of anthralin in petrolatum and/or Lassar's paste are more acceptable and practical for patients and nursing staff. Physicians and patients should be aware that irritation and staining of skin and clothing can still occur with SCAT. Short contact treatment with a new microencapsulated anthralin formulation (Micanol) did not improve psoriasis as rapidly as anthralin in petrolatum but produced less erythema, burning and staining of skin and clothing [19].

Washing off anthralin (0.2–1.6%) with aqueous 1% potassium hydroxide following application periods of 40 min significantly reduced

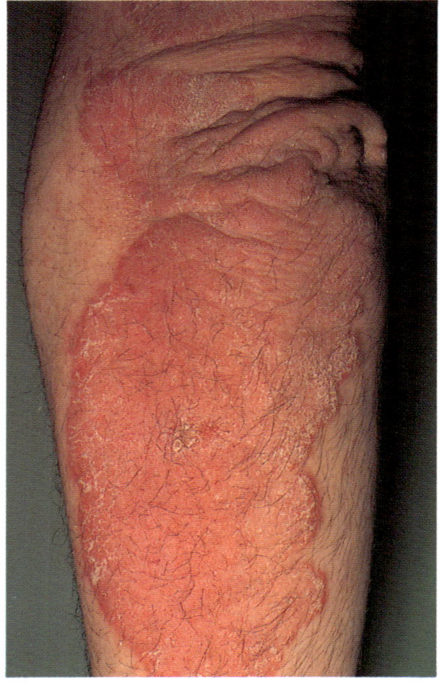

(a)

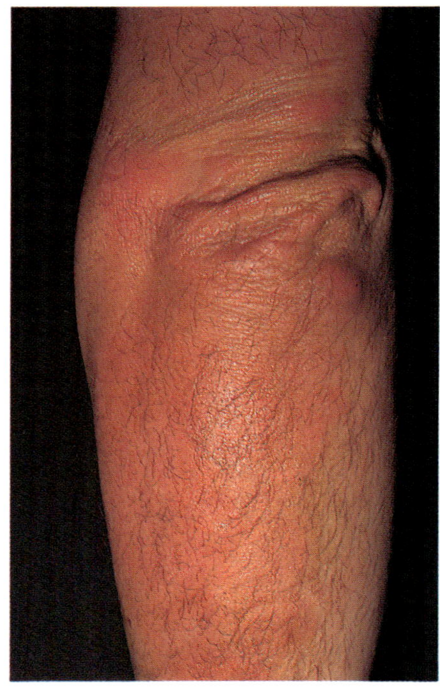

(b)

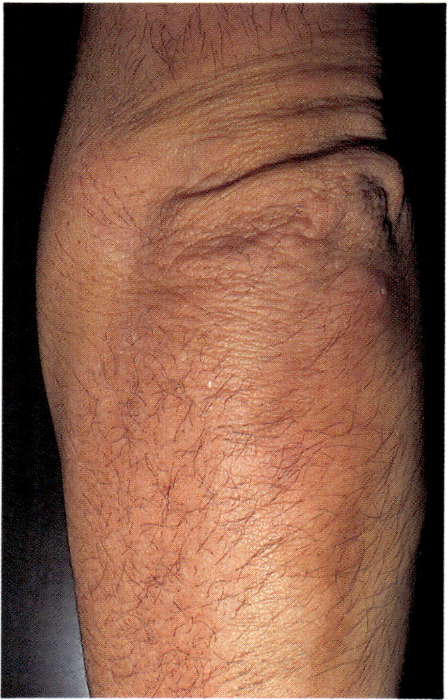

(c)

Fig 11.1 Psoriasis on the arm treated with anthralin ointment 1% for 2 hours daily (a) before treatment, (b) after 1 week, and (c) after 2 weeks.

inflammation without sacrificing therapeutic efficacy [20]. Anthralin-induced perilesional inflammation can be significantly reduced while maintaining clinical efficacy of SCAT if a cream containing 10% triethanolamine is applied to skin following anthralin application [21]. This has been marketed as Cura Stain Spray by Young Pharmaceutical. The authors believe that potassium hydroxide enhances the oxidation of anthralin to inactive products, and that triethanolamine increases the solubility and removal of anthralin.

How to use anthralin at home

Although anthralin is still not well-accepted by patients and is not widely used by dermatologists in the USA, SCAT has allowed use of this important topical agent at home in selected patients with plaque-type psoriasis.

1 Patients start with 0.1 or 0.25% concentrations and increase to 1.0% as tolerated. Most of our compliant patients settle on the 0.5% ointment. If required, concentrations higher than 1.0% should be compounded by the pharmacist.

2 Anthralin cream or ointment is applied to lesions and left on for 20–60 min. If possible, no clothing or else loose-fitting old garments should be worn during treatment.

3 The anthralin is then washed off with liquid soap in the bath or shower.

4 Anthralin stains of white fabrics can be removed by a 10 min soak in full-strength chlorine rinse followed by a water rinse and air drying [22]. Color fabrics should be bleach-safe. A white plastic shower curtain should be cleaned within 5 min with 95% ethyl alcohol followed by a water rinse.

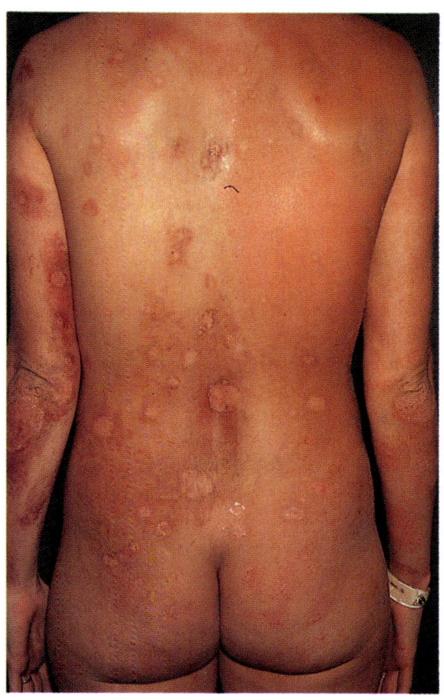

Fig 11.2 Note anthralin-induced inflammation and staining of uninvolved skin surrounding psoriatic plaque on the left side of the body.

TOXICITY

The most important side effects of anthralin are brown staining and irritation of uninvolved skin [23]. The erythema reaction peaks 3 days after the first application and subsides after 4–5 days, even if one continues to apply the same anthralin concentration.

The erythema reaction is not related to skin type. Westerhof and coworkers [24] showed that there was no statistically significant difference in anthralin irritation between vitiligo and normally pigmented skin. Moreover, there is less anthralin-induced inflammation in the skin of a psoriatic plaque than in surrounding uninvolved skin. The violet-brown discoloration of uninvolved skin is caused by uncharacterized anthralin metabolites arising from extensive oxidation and melanin pigmentation (Fig. 11.2). It is dose-dependent and fades a few weeks after treatment is stopped. Other acute side effects include itching, stinging, burning, folliculitis, and rarely conjunctivitis. A few cases of contact allergy to anthralin have been reported. No systemic toxicity due to anthralin has been reported in humans.

REFERENCES

1 Shroot B. Anthralin. In Roenigk HH Jr, Maibach HI, eds. *Psoriasis*, 2nd edn., New York: Marcel Dekker, Inc., 1991:481–99.

2 Schroder JM, Kosfeld U, Christophers U. Multifunctional inhibition by anthralin in non-stimulated and chemotactic factor-stimulated human neutrophils. *J Invest Dermatol* 1985;85:30–4.

3 Mrowietz U, Falsafi M, Schroder J-M, Christophers E. Inhibition of human monocyte functions by anthralin. *Br J Dermatol* 1992;127:382–6.

4 Ternowitz T. The enhanced monocyte and neutrophil chemotaxis in psoriasis is normalized after treatment with psoralens plus ultraviolet A and anthralin. *J Am Acad Dermatol* 1987;16:1169–75.

5 Langner A, Chorzelski TP, Fraczykowska M, *et al.* Effect of anthralin on stratum corneum antigenicity and polymorphonuclear leukocyte chemotaxis. *Br J Dermatol* 1981;105(Suppl. 20):62–3.

6 DeYoung LM, Helmes CT, Chao WR, *et al.* Paradoxical effect of anthralin on 12-O-tetradecanoylphorbal 13-acetate-induced mouse epidermal ornithine decarboxylase activity proliferation, and tumor promotion. *Cancer Res* 1981;41:204–8.

7 Gottlieb AB, Khandke L, Krane JF, *et al.* Anthralin decreases keratinocyte TGF-2 expression and EGF-receptor binding *in vitro*. *J Invest Dermatol* 1992;98:680–5.

8 Wang JCT, Patel BG, Ehmann CW, Lowe N. The release and percutaneous permeation of anthralin products, using clinically involved and uninvolved psoriatic skin. *J Am Acad Dermatol* 1987;16:812–21.

9 Lawrence CM, Shuster S. Mechanism of anthralin inflammation. I. Dissociation of response to clobetasol and indomethacin. *Br J Dermatol* 1985;113:107–15.

10 Shall L, Marks R. The effects of concomitant administration of oral indomethacin with topical dithranol treatment in psoriasis (Letter). *Br J Dermatol* 1987;116:739.

11 Sheehan-Dare RA, Goodfield MJD, Rowell NR. The effect of oral indomethacin on psoriasis treated with the Ingram regime. *Br J Dermatol* 1991;125:253–5.

12 Swinehart JM, Lowe NJ. UVABA therapy for psoriasis. *J Am Acad Dermatol* 1991;24:594–7.

13 Van de Kerkhof PCM, Mali JWH. Low-dose PUVA maintenance in psoriasis following Ingram therapy. *Br J Dermatol* 1981;104:684.

14 Jones SK, Campbell WC, Mackie RM. Out-patient treatment of psoriasis: short contact and overnight dithranol therapy compared. *Br J Dermatol* 1985;113:331–7.

15 Runne U, Kunze J. Short-duration ("minutes") therapy with dithranol for psoriasis: a new out-patient regimen. *Br J Dermatol* 1982;106:135–9.

16 MacDonald KJS, Marks J. Short contact anthralin in the treatment of psoriasis: a study of different contact times. *Br J Dermatol* 1986;114:235–9.

17 Ryatt KS, Statham BN, Rowell NR. Short-contact modification of the Ingram regime. *Br J Dermatol* 1984;111:455–9.

18 Boer J, Smeenk G. Effect of short-contact anthralin therapy on ultraviolet B irradiation of psoriasis. *J Am Acad Dermatol* 1986;15:198–204.

19 Volden G, Bjornberg A, Tegner E, *et al.* Short-contact treatment at home with Micanol. *Acta Derm Venereol* 1992;172(Suppl.):20–2.

20 Lawrence CM, Shuster S, Collins M, Bruce JM. Reduction of anthralin inflammation by potassium hydroxide and Teepol. *Br J Dermatol* 1987;116:171–7.

21 Lawrence CM, Ramsay B, Bruce JM, Shuster S. Triethanolamine reduces inflammation in short contact anthralin therapy without loss of therapeutic effect. *J Invest Dermatol* 1989;92:468.

22 Wang JCT, Krazmien RJ, Dahlheim CE, Patel B. Anthralin stain removal. *J Am Acad Dermatol* 1986;15:951–5.

23 Fiore M. Practical aspects of anthralin therapy. *Cutis* 1990;46:351–4.
24 Westerhof W, Buehre Y, Pavel S, *et al*. Increased anthralin irritation response in vitiliginous skin. *Arch Dermatol Res* 1989;281:52–6.

twelve

UVB Phototherapy and Coal Tar

UVB PHOTOTHERAPY

Phototherapy is not as efficient as radiotherapy but is of value. Its use is not followed by any deleterious effects on the skin. Alderson suggests using an air-cooled lamp and giving treatments twice weekly. He first removes the scales with a keratolytic ointment and follows with short exposures at a 16-inch distance. The object is to produce a mild reaction and pigmentation [1].

Introduction

The earliest reported experimentation with UV light and psoriasis was by Alderson and later embellished by Goeckerman in the 1920s. Elucidation of the erythema action spectrum and the therapeutic action spectrum of psoriasis in 1981 by Parrish and Jaenicke [2] has made possible the development of modern bulbs, which emit virtually monochromatic light capable of clearing psoriasis with less risk of burning. Short-wave UVB (290–320 nm) light is now widely used in the treatment of psoriasis as monotherapy, with emollients, or with crude coal tar (CCT; the Goeckerman regimen). The treatments can be delivered in the office, hospital, day-treatment center, or at home (by the patient).

There are basically three types of UVB sources that are practical for the office: the hot quartz Alpine lamp, high-pressure metal halide lamps, and fluorescent sunlamps (UVB bulbs) [3].

The hot quartz or high-pressure mercury vapor lamps (available from Hanovia and Sperti) were used by the pioneers in phototherapy. The spectral power distribution (SPD) is discontinuous with wavelength peaks of emission including 254, 263, 297, 303, and 366 nm [4]. Sixty percent of the UV emissions are between 250 and 320 nm [5]. The advantages of the hot quartz lamp include: inexpensive, small size for less storage space, mounted on pole with wheels for portability to bedside, ideal for treating limited areas of involvement such as palms, soles, elbows, knees, and scalp.

It can also be used for photopatch testing. The disadvantages are that the relatively small field size requires up to six exposures to treat the entire body skin, 3 min warm-up time, ozone production when first ignited causing delay (10–15 min) in treating the first patient and need for adequate ventilation, and heat production during treatment.

The high-pressure metal halide lamp system consists of five lamps stacked in a column, which deliver a continuous spectrum of UV wavelengths (Dermalight Systems). The selection of UVA or UVB is done by opening and closing filter doors. The advantage of the system is the capability to deliver intense UVA for use with psoralen UVA (PUVA) or the combination of UVA and UVB if unfiltered light is given, potentially shorter treatment times, and no claustrophobia from enclosed cabinets [6]. The disadvantages are that: it is very expensive to purchase and operate; three columns are needed to give a single even exposure; excessive heat production; there is the possibility of wavelength selection errors if both filter doors are left open.

The workhorse in most offices for UVB phototherapy is the fluorescent sunlamp manufactured by Westinghouse (FS series, available as 2-, 4-, and 6-foot tubes) and Philips (TL-12). The glass tube is coated on the inside with a phosphor, which emits a continuous spectrum primarily from 280 to 350 nm. About 60% of the radiant energy is emitted at wavelengths below 320 nm [5] falling into the therapeutic action spectrum for psoriasis, which peaks at 300–305 nm. The therapeutic and erythema action spectra parallel each other from 290 to 365 nm, but wavelengths shorter than 290 nm are far more erythemogenic than therapeutic [7]. The sunlamps can be mounted in open banks or in enclosed cabinets. The output decreases to 70–80% of the original output after about 500 hours of use. The lamps should be replaced after 1000 hours of use. The advantages include inexpensive lamps, large field size when mounted in banks of four to six bulbs, no warm-up time, low heat production, no claustrophobia in the open design, and highly effective UVB phototherapy for psoriasis. An enclosed cabinet system with 12 or more tubes provides generalized exposure in a relatively short period of time, but the disadvantages include greater expense to purchase and operate, possible need for special ventilation and power sources, risk of claustrophobia, falling, or heat intolerance in elderly or infirm patients. The irradiance from the ends of the tubes may be 10–30% less than the central portion [4]. This can be a problem for the lower regions of the legs, especially in short persons, where psoriasis is ordinarily more resistant to phototherapy. Standing on a slightly raised platform may raise more problems than it solves. Additional exposures to the legs with shielding elsewhere may be the only solution. Moreover, the scalp and soles of the feet are not exposed at all. Sitting while bowing, a balding or shaved head, and obtaining a hand/foot unit addresses these problems.

Clinical use of UVB phototherapy

In a practice with only a few patients eligible for UVB phototherapy, an open system with wheels is recommended. It costs less than $1000 (at the time of publishing) but requires more time for treating all sides of the body, and privacy screens are needed for shielding. The panel of lamps can be stored in one examination room, but the room can be dedicated to all purposes when the unit is not in use. A dermatologic practice which intends to treat 10 or more psoriatic patients per week with a range of severity should invest about $13 000 in a combined UVA/UVB cabinet system (see Appendix, Table 3) with safety features such as timer and automatic shut-off, handrails, protection from bulb breakage, and a window for direct visualization of the patient. In regions that are distant from referral centers, it is advisable for dermatologists in the community to encourage their local hospital's physical therapy department to purchase the necessary equipment and provide treatments based on the doctor's orders who continues to follow the patient in the office on a regular basis. In this way, everyone benefits: patients receive the best modality for their psoriasis closer to home, the hospital recovers expenses by collecting the revenue for treatments, and there is one centralized facility without duplication of resources.

Technicians should receive formal training in the operation of equipment and be supervised by the physician. Even with the safety feature of automatic shut-off, a mishap could occur, for example, if the correct UVA time is keyed in, but the technician turns on the UVB lamp. Requesting dosimetry in terms of radiant energy per unit surface area helps to avoid errors because the typical UVB dose is measured in millijoules per square centimeter compared to UVA in joules per square centimeter. Errors could still occur if UVB dosing is not based on radiometric readings but rather in terms of seconds and minutes estimated on the basis of skin type, sunburn history, or the physician's personal experience with other patients. Separate cabinets for UVA and UVB avoids the issue of confounding the two wavebands but are only warranted for large offices, hospital clinics, and psoriasis day-treatment centers with an adequate volume of patients and the proper amount of space, ventilation, and air conditioning. Hand and foot units for UVA or UVB can be added one at a time to a practice at a cost of $1000–1300 each as the need arises for giving extra doses to palmoplantar psoriasis or as the primary treatment for palmoplantar pustulosis.

Phototherapy should probably be reserved as second-line treatment for those patients with extensive (defined as 20% or more involvement of body surface area) or disabling (defined as involving the face, hands, and feet) psoriasis who have had an insufficient response to aggressive topical regimens including keratolytics, corticosteroids, coal tar, and anthralin.

The physician who has a source of UV light in the office now prepares the patient for phototherapy. Those who do not have the equipment should refer to a facility that does rather than bypass UVB phototherapy and risk potentially more toxic systemic therapies, which are more appropriately reserved for third-line treatment.

There are many reputable suppliers of UV equipment and radiometers (see Appendix, Tables 3 and 4). The selection should be based on the company's accessibility to your office, whether installation and service are provided, the frequency and cost of service and regular maintenance calls, space needs and availability of special power lines, ventilation, and air conditioning.

I recommend that the unit be metered daily so that dosages may be calculated in millijoules. This is important not only for standardization of dosages between different centers and different units in the same center but also so that modifications and improvements of protocols published in the medical literature can be immediately duplicated in practice. Metering helps to compensate for the declining output of bulbs. Be aware that great variability between specifications and quality control exists among manufacturers [8]. Purchase the UVB radiometer recommended by the manufacturer of your system. The radiometers themselves must be recalibrated at least once per year. Use the formula to calculate the time needed to administer a given dose in millijoules per square centimeter:

$$\text{Dose desired (mJ/cm}^2\text{)} \div \text{output measured (mW/cm}^2\text{)} = \text{time (seconds).}$$

For a specific measured output, conversion tables can be derived in increments of 5 mJ/cm^2 for quick reference. Some units are supplied with conversion tables by the manufacturers. Newer UVB cabinets have a built-in panel with a calculator. The UVB output is measured with a UVB light meter and punched into the calculator. Next, the desired UVB dose (mJ/cm^2) is entered. The calculator then computes and displays the treatment time (in minutes and seconds) thus eliminating the need for conversion tables. Some UVB units have a built-in UVB light meter that continuously monitors UVB output while light is being administered. After punching in the desired UVB treatment dose (mJ/cm^2) into the control panel, the treatment time is automatically calculated and delivered.

Another decision to be made is whether the patient should be treated as an outpatient, in the hospital, in a psoriasis day-treatment center, or at home by the patient himself. The final recommendation is usually based on the availability of facilities, the physician's philosophy, and patient (or third party payor) preference.

During the last decade in the USA, there has been a precipitous decline in the number of patients admitted to hospital for the treatment of dermatologic diseases. For example, at the Cleveland Clinic the average daily hospital census was 20 in 1985 compared to 3.5 in 1990. There has been a further decline in admissions and length of stay during the last 2 years. This change has come about in part because of a more aggressive stance by Medicare, the federal government's insurance program, which allows only 8.3 days of hospitalization for patients with major skin diseases. Most private third party insurers approve only the most acute and severe cases for admission such as exfoliative dermatitis and generalized pustular psoriasis. In addition, technologic refinements in drug and physical therapies of psoriasis, particularly etretinate and phototherapy, have made it possible to significantly improve almost every patient in an outpatient setting. Admittedly, in the past some admissions to the hospital were for socioeconomic, educational, or research purposes or simply for the convenience of the patient, physician, or both. Unfortunately, the spiraling cost of health care in the USA can no longer validate such reasons.

Psoriasis day treatment is about half the cost of inpatient treatment, but is very time-consuming for patients and labor-intensive for staff [9]. The clinical improvement at the time of discharge is probably equivalent to hospitalization, but there may be intangible benefits that the hospital setting does not provide, for example, daily education about disease and treatment from specialized staff, socialization with professionals and camaraderie with other patients in all stages of disease, reinforcement of good self-treatment habits and the need for followup maintenance. Familiarity with the treatment site, facilities, and staff encourages followup treatment and assessment. For details of the daily routine in a psoriasis day-treatment center see pp. 215–218.

Clinical studies

The starting dose of UVB can be estimated based on the skin type and increased according to Table 12.1. However, it is preferable to give the first dose based on the results of minimal erythema dose (MED) testing, upon which all subsequent doses are based. Phototherapists should understand, meter and maintain their equipment, keep complete and detailed records of exposures for each patient and be able to provide current and cumulative dosages of UVB received in millijoules per square centimeter if the patient moves to another facility.

MED testing is considered by some to be laborious, time-consuming, and tedious, and in fact may be all of the above. It is performed using a piece of flexible plastic foam large enough to cover the patient's back. Five 1.5-cm squares are cut into the foam and the rest of the skin is shielded with drapes before exposing each test site to varying doses of UVB according to skin type (Table 12.2). After 24 hours, the reactions are graded at each site. The dose which has resulted in a barely perceptible erythema or

Table 12.1 UVB dosimetry

Skin type		UVB dose (mJ/cm^2)	
		Start	Increase per treatment
I	Always burn, never tan	10	5
II	Always burn, sometimes tan	20	5–10
III	Sometimes burn, always tan	30	10
IV	Never burn, always tan	40	10–20
V	Moderately pigmented	50	20
VI	Black people	60	20–30

Table 12.2 Minimal erythema dose testing for UVB

Skin type	mJ/cm^2
I, II	10, 15, 20, 25, 30
III, IV	20, 30, 40, 50, 60
V, VI	40, 50, 60, 70, 80

pinkness is defined as the MED. Because we are aware that breasts and the abdomen are more likely to burn than the back, we recommend starting with the next UVB dose below the MED. The MED result is valid for future treatment courses without the need to reproduce it.

Recent studies have clearly demonstrated that erythemogenic UVB given as an outpatient was effective in 90–100% of patients in clearing psoriasis completely. The only adjunctive treatment was the application of white petrolatum immediately prior to exposure and as needed for dryness at home. Two such treatment protocols gave treatments five times per week [10] or three times per week [11]. In the first protocol the initial exposure was 80% of the MED and subsequent exposures were increased by 17% of the previous dose. The second protocol administered one MED on the first day and increased dosages by 50, 40, 30, 20% on subsequent exposures. (The reader is referred to Tables 1 and 2 of reference 11.) The authors gave additional increments of UVB to the extremities such that by the fifth treatment the arms and legs received 50% more radiation than the trunk [11]. Boer and colleagues [12] recommended against extra UVB doses to resistant plaques on the lower legs because they gave only slight additional improvement (5–10%).

The three-times-weekly treatment protocol, although slightly more complicated to deliver, could theoretically improve patient compliance and reduce the risk of UVB erythema or tenderness that could result in missed treatments [11]. Patients who had tender erythema at the time of a scheduled treatment were not treated and subsequently received a dose one increment lower than the one that apparently caused the burn.

In both protocols, the number of treatments needed for clearance ranged from 20 to 30 [10,11]. The three-times-weekly protocol gave a lower average UVB dose at clearing, but the difference was not statistically significant ($652\ mJ/cm^2$ vs $725\ mJ/cm^2$). In both protocols there is a strong linear correlation between an individual's MED and the corresponding total dose needed for lesions to clear. The total number of treatments needed did not differ significantly according to the MED. The average extent of involvement was 38%, a level of severity that would justify admission to a psoriasis day-treatment center if chronic and resistant to topical therapy or to the hospital if acute and progressive.

The world of busy medical offices and clinics is not ideal, and one should not expect 100% of patients to clear completely as was achieved in the studies cited. Moreover, we have found that increasing the UVB dose by a varying percentage of the previous dose increases the potential for calculation errors. Increasing the dose by a fixed amount at each treatment (Table 12.2) gives equally gratifying results. Outpatient UVB phototherapy is an approach worthwhile attempting because of the dramatic cost savings and avoidance of the generally objectionable appearance, odor, and staining of clothing caused by combining UVB with coal tar.

Maintenance phototherapy

Standard clinical practice includes 2–3 weeks of additional biweekly UVB treatments after clearing at the final clearance dose. Defined as complete resolution of at least 90% of psoriasis present prior to initiation of phototherapy, "clearing" was achieved in 76% of patients. A multicenter study designed to determine the time to flare compared a group of patients receiving maintenance UVB biweekly for 4–8 weeks followed by at least weekly treatments for a total of 4 months to a group receiving no maintenance [13]. The protocol called for a maintenance dose equal to 90% of the patient's final clearance dose. As one might expect, the probability of remaining in remission as defined by this study was significantly higher for those patients receiving UVB phototherapy maintenance. Based on a life table analysis, 60% of maintenance therapy vs 28% of no maintenance patients would still be clear 6 months after initial clearing. In another study [12], clearing was defined less stringently as "at least 80% improved" and this was achieved in 81% of patients with four-times-weekly treatment. Maintenance therapy consisted of an attempt to gradually reduce the frequency of treatments to three, two, then one or less times weekly if possible with the UVB dose equal to the last clearing dose. The authors estimated that the probability of remaining in remission for at least 1 year after clearing was 58%.

It would appear to be cost effective to administer outpatient UVB maintenance phototherapy to patients with moderate to severe psoriasis to prevent a relapse in about 50% of patients for half a year, or at least until the patient can benefit from the next season of ambient sunlight.

The future is bright

The therapeutic action spectrum of psoriasis has been exploited with the development of a fluorescent UVB lamp with a peak narrow band of emission at 312 nm and a minor peak at 305 nm. The Philips TL-01 lamp thereby avoids completely the shorter more erythemogenic and carcinogenic UVB and UVC wavelengths that are emitted by conventional sunlamps (Westinghouse FS and Philips TL-12). In a bilateral paired comparison of widespread symmetric psoriasis, the TL-01 side was slightly better than the TL-12 side at the 20th treatment. The number of burning episodes was significantly less with the TL-01 lamps [14]. The TL-01 side received twice as much cumulative UVB dose owing to the ability to increase the time by 40% if the previous exposure induced no perceptible erythema. If carcinogenicity is a concern, then one must question if omitting wavelengths below 305 nm while doubling the dose of radiant energy delivered provides any protective advantage. A new 100 W version of the TL-01 lamp was significantly more effective than the conventional broad-band UVB source (Sylvania UV6) in 20/23 cases [15]. Exposure times were comparable.

Green and coworkers [16] compared the efficacy and time to relapse of TL-01 phototherapy to etretinate 1 mg/kg per day 2 weeks prior to TL-01 and etretinate prior to PUVA (re-PUVA). Only concomitant emollients were allowed. The clearance rate was 80, 93, and 100% for the three groups. At 6 months' followup, 50, 33, and 50% remained in remission, respectively. The cumulative UVB exposure dose was one-third less in the group receiving etretinate. These studies show that TL-01 phototherapy with or without etretinate is less efficacious than re-PUVA and that etretinate does not extend the remission time of TL-01. The effect of maintenance therapy was not investigated. The long-term safety of cumulative doses of narrowband UVB is unknown.

COAL TAR

The tars probably rank next to chrysarobin in the treatment of psoriasis. It is also necessary to leave the preparation on for several hours, as the tars do not produce prompt reactions [1].

Introduction

Most physicians are familiar with Sir Percival Pott's 1775 article describing scrotal carcinomas in chimney sweepers associated with skin contact with coal tar pitch as well as the therapeutic combination of CCT and UV light used in the treatment of psoriasis as published by Goeckerman in 1925 [17].

Wood tars (including pine tar and oil of Cade) have been used in medicine since antiquity, but coal tar was not available until the second half of the nineteenth century when coal gas production was developed. Coal tar is a byproduct of the processing of coke and gas from bituminous coal [18]. It is chemically complex, consisting of 10 000 different compounds, of which only about 400 have been identified constituting 55–60% of the tar by weight [4]. Some of the major compounds in coal tar include the aromatic hydrocarbons such as anthracene, benzene, benzo[*a*]pyrene, and naphthalene. In therapy, either CCT or coal tar extract dispersed in a suitable vehicle is used. The extracts are produced by extraction with ethanol or surfactants or by distillation.

Clinical use

Efficacy

No method of chemical or biologic standardization of the potency of coal tar products has ever been established, rendering direct comparisons between different products difficult if not impossible. Variability in potency between different products with the same concentration of active ingredient as well as variation between batches of the same product is the rule.

In healthy subjects, CCT 5% in hydrophilic ointment initially caused a transient hyperplasia followed over time by a 20% reduction in epidermal thickness [19]. Thickening of the epidermis including the granular layer due to coal tar has been found in some animal models. Coal tar alone or followed by UVB irradiation suppresses epidermal DNA synthesis significantly in the hairless mouse [20].

Is CCT effective as monotherapy for psoriasis in half-and-half body comparisons with inpatients [21]? Using 1 and 5% or higher concentrations of CCT in yellow soft paraffin, the median whole body psoriasis area and severity index (PASI) score fell by about 50% during a 10-day treatment period. Moreover, the authors determined that the dose–response curve for antipsoriatic effects peaked between 1 and 5% CCT. No benefit was derived from increasing the concentration incrementally to a maximum 25%. In this study, the patient's skin was in contact with tar for 24 hours a day, and UVB was not used. While 1% CCT is lighter and more acceptable for home use, it was not as active as 5% CCT. Neither is it practical for home use 24 hours a day. Thus, CCT remains primarily an inpatient or day-care center treatment.

Combined treatment with coal tar and anthralin significantly inhibited the anthralin erythema/irritation of normal-appearing skin [22]. The mechanism for this may be induction of aryl-hydrocarbon hydroxylase by coal tar, which metabolizes anthralin or its irritant products [23].

> Goeckerman employs crude coal tar as an adjunct to quartz-light treatment. The tar ointment is applied thickly (⅛ inch) to all the patches. At the time of the light treatment the excess ointment is removed with olive oil, leaving a ... brown stain. The treatment is repeated daily and was of particular value in general exfoliative dermatitis secondary to psoriasis [1].

Clinical studies

The use of coal tar for the treatment of psoriasis has been inextricably tied to UV light therapy since Goeckerman popularized this combination [17]. He used the hot quartz (high-pressure mercury vapor) lamp which emits discontinuous UV light bands in the short wave (B) and long wave (A) ranges corresponding to the spectral emission peaks of mercury [5]. It is uncertain whether erythemogenic dosages were used. As currently employed by the Mayo Clinic, the Goeckerman regimen consists of a 24 hour per day program of frequent 3–5% CCT application in petrolatum or Lassar's paste to the entire body [24]. Excess tar is then physically wiped away with the aid of cottonseed or corn oil followed by erythemogenic doses of UVB.

Tar is a photosensitizer with an action spectrum in the long wave UV region (UVA: 320–400 nm). Some of the constituents of CCT that define the action spectrum for photosensitivity in the long wave UVA and visible range include anthracene, phenanthrene, pyrene, fluoranthrene, and acridine.

The tar distillate liquor carbonis detergens (LCD) alone has only a weak effect on psoriasis. The clearing effect of light alone was obtained at a maximum of 313 nm, which was not enhanced by pretreatment with LCD. A distinctly better healing was seen at 365 nm after the pretreatment. However, a smarting sensation was produced, which was most pronounced at 405 nm [25]. Erythemogenic doses of UVA plus tar gel can be as effective as UVB plus tar gel at healing psoriasis but the former combination is limited by the "smarting reaction" [26].

Phototoxicity from coal tar is probably not a therapeutic mechanism in the Goeckerman regimen. The dose of UVA required to induce smarting of tar-treated skin is much lower than that needed to produce delayed erythema, and "tar smarts" are not experienced by patients undergoing the Goeckerman regimen. Most modern UVB phototherapy sources, including fluorescent sunlamps and the hot quartz lamp, deliver sufficient UVB energy to produce delayed erythema in normal skin before enough UVA is emitted to cause erythema, even in sites previously photosensitized with CCT.

Tar may have a "UVB-sparing" effect, that is, it may allow the therapeutic benefits of tar and lower, suberythemogenic doses of UVB to be additive. Pretreatment with LCD produced a 30–50% higher UVB erythema threshold than petrolatum [25]. Tar gel (5% CCT USP in a hydroalcoholic gel containing 29% alcohol) alone is equally as effective as suberythemogenic UVB at improving psoriatic plaques (about 50%) [27]. The combination was more effective than either one alone. Moreover, the suberythemogenic UVB plus tar gel group received 59% less total cumulative UVB dose than the erythemogenic UVB plus tar gel group. The efficacy of suberythemogenic UVB plus tar oil b.i.d. was roughly equivalent to maximally aggressive UVB plus emollients t.i.w. given on an outpatient basis [28]. The cumulative dose of UVB at clearing, however, was 44% less in the suberythemogenic UVB plus tar oil group. Stern and coworkers [29] found only a modest decrease (9%) in the dose of UVB t.i.w. needed to clear outpatients when tar oil b.i.d. was compared to the oil vehicle. CCT 2% ointment gave no therapeutic advantage to either daily suberythemogenic UVB or maximally aggressive UVB in the time to clear in the hospital, or the time to relapse, but 80% less UVB was used with suberythemogenic UVB [30]. There is a correlation in the hairless mouse model: 1 MED (erythemogenic UVB) maximally suppressed epidermal DNA synthesis, and an equivalent suppression could be obtained with 0.33 MED (suberythemogenic UVB) with the addition of coal tar [31].

Several studies have questioned whether CCT adds much if any therapeutic benefit to UVB irradiation. UVB radiation alone was almost as effective as 1, 5, or 25% CCT plus UVB [32]. Bilateral comparison studies have consistently shown that daily erythemogenic UVB plus white petrolatum or 5% CCT in petrolatum were equally effective [33,34]. Immediate broad spectrum decreases in spectral remittance (reflectance) of psoriatic stratum corneum occur after the application of white petrolatum. It is possible that this vehicle which is also used to formulate the tar increases UVB transmission. Apparently, some of the commonly used emollients including petrolatum and hydrophilic ointment absorb UVB thereby reducing the potential for erythema in uninvolved skin [35]. Fortunately, the peak absorption spectrum for most of these agents is between 270 and 290 nm, which causes erythema but is below the therapeutic action spectrum for psoriasis. Coconut oil, which does not significantly absorb UVB or UVA did not accelerate clearance of psoriasis when applied prior to narrow-band UVB (TL-01) phototherapy or PUVA [36].

PSORIASIS DAY-TREATMENT CENTERS

In order to be considered a Psoriasis Day-Treatment Center, a facility must be equipped with all of the most modern tools, pharmaceuticals, and a trained skilled full-time nursing staff. Hospitalization is still necessary for patients with erythrodermic or pustular psoriasis, severe plaque-type psoriasis with arthropathy, complications of systemic therapy or concomitant illnesses (e.g., diabetes, emphysema, cardiovascular disease) that make out-patient therapy untenable [37]. While the majority qualify for routine or office phototherapy, certain patients have disease significant enough to justify treatment in a psoriasis day-center. Suggested guidelines for admission include [38,39]:

1 psoriasis involves 20% or more of the body surface area, or is disabling by affecting the face, scalp, hands, and feet;

2 psoriasis is recalcitrant to all reasonable attempts at outpatient therapy for 4 weeks or longer;

3 the patient is a candidate for coal tar and UVB phototherapy; PUVA and systemic therapy are not indicated or not desired by the patient or physician at the present time;

4 complications of systemic therapy necessitate a change to safer yet effective therapeutic alternative;

5 the patient is sufficiently medically or emotionally compromised to require assistance and monitoring, but not severe enough to warrant hospitalization.

Requirements

Space

Examination rooms for consultation with physician
Treatment room for application of medicaments
Toilet facilities for men and women
Phototherapy room for UV light cabinets
Bathrooms for tub bath, whirlpool
Recreation/dining room
Quiet room

Equipment

UVB cabinet
UVA cabinet
Hand and foot units

Sink for hair washing (shampoo machine optional)
Tub for bath PUVA
Whirlpool for debriding scales (and for relief of joint pain)

Pharmaceuticals
Emollients (Aquaphor, Petrolatum, Eucerin, etc.)
CCT 3% with and without salicylic acid 3–5%
Anthralin ointments 0.1, 0.25, 0.5, 1.0%
LCD 10 and 20% in petrolatum
Nivea oil with and without salicylic acid 3–5%
Low- and medium-potency corticosteroid creams and ointments and scalp solutions

Sample schedule

The center at the Cleveland Clinic is open Monday through Friday. A sample daily schedule is shown below.

8:00–10:00 a.m.
Examination by physician
Whirlpool bath, p.r.n.
UVB treatment
Shampoo
Application of coal tar and other topicals

10:00 a.m.–1:00 p.m.
Relaxation/work/sleep
Lectures
Lunch

1:00–3:00 p.m.
Tar removal/bath
UVB treatment
Shampoo
Application of anthralin if needed and other topicals

Treatment

UVB
On day 1 treatment is given according to skin type (Table 12.1), and MED testing is done (Table 12.2). On day 2, a suberythemogenic dose (the dose just below the determined MED) is given. Subsequent daily increases are usually 10–20 mJ/cm^2, as tolerated. Half the daily dose is given in a.m. and the other half in p.m. This allows for greater flexibility in proper dosing and helps to prevent burning.

Trunk and extremities
a.m.: CCT 3% in petrolatum applied by nurse in direction of hair follicle growth. Salicylic acid 3–5% is added in cases with severe scaling.
p.m.: emollients (Aquaphor, Eucerin, etc.) are applied, to be repeated by the patient at bedtime. Some patients are instructed in the proper use of anthralin (short contact therapy), to be applied either at the center or in the evening at home, gradually increasing to 1% concentration.

Scalp
a.m.: tar shampoo (Zetar, T-gel, Ionil-T, etc.), followed by tar oil (Doak or the formulation of Zetar emulsion 13%, salicylic acid 3%, Tween-80 4% in Nivea oil) under a shower cap.
p.m.: repeat tar shampoo, followed by application of a fluorinated corticosteroid solution p.r.n. (e.g., fluocinolone 0.01%, betamethasone valerate 0.1%).

Nonfluorinated corticosteroid cream
For example, hydrocortisone with or without iodoquinol, hydrocortisone valerate, desonide — for hairline, ears, face, skinfolds in a.m. and p.m. p.r.n.

Bath treatment
Whirlpool in a.m., p.r.n. for debridement of severe scaling. Very relaxing to patients — many prefer to continue after scaling subsides and patients with arthritis feel better. Tepid emollient bath in p.m. Tar (Balnetar, Zetar emulsion) is added mostly for instructional purposes for eventual outpatient use.

Weekend treatment
This depends on patient's anticipated activities (family/social/work). It varies from simple lubrication/tar bath/shampoo to a full topical psoriasis day-care regimen without the light or with natural sunlight or home UVB unit if available.

Treatment after discharge from the psoriasis day-treatment center

UVB
Three times per week. If possible, decrease every 4 weeks to maintenance frequency of one to two times per week. The starting dose is 70% of the last total daily dose in the center and is increased by 10–20 mJ/cm^2 per treatment. When the skin is cleared, the UVB dose is held at the last daily dose attained.

Trunk and extremities
Emollients or anthralin at highest tolerated concentration, 10% LCD in petrolatum or 3% CCT to active areas for a few hours in evening.

Fluorinated corticosteroid ointments are rarely used because of possible shortened remission time. Tepid tar bath daily.

Scalp
Tar shampoo daily. When flaring, tar oil with shower cap for a few hours in evening, followed by shampoo and application of fluorinated corticosteroid oil (Dermasmoothe F/S) or solution at bedtime. The solution can be reapplied in the a.m., p.r.n. Low-potency corticosteroid cream to hairline, ears, face, skinfolds b.i.d., p.r.n.

Hospital vs postdischarge treatment
Two groups of severe psoriasis patients treated with the Goeckerman regimen in the hospital for 3 weeks or hospital for 2 weeks and ambulatory treatment center for the last week were compared [40]. All patients were encouraged to have maintenance phototherapy after discharge. No differences in the rate of clearing or the probability to remain at least 80% cleared after discharge were detected between the two groups. A review of 300 patients with severe psoriasis receiving all treatment in the Dallas and San Francisco psoriasis day-care centers showed an average time to at least 90% clearing to be 18 days [41]. Ninety percent remained clear for a minimum of 8 months, and 73% were in remission 1 year after discharge. Patients were encouraged to receive regular natural sunlight or artificial UVB exposures for 1 month after discharge. These results compare favorably to those of 123 patients treated with the Goeckerman regimen as inpatients at the Mayo Clinic where a median remission time of 1–1.4 years was reported (range: 0.2–8.0 years) [42,43]. In the Cleveland Clinic Psoriasis Day Treatment Center, 86% of the last 270 consecutive patients achieved an excellent response defined as less than 5–10% body surface area of residual psoriasis (J.W.E. Dijkstra, personal communication 1992). The median length of stay was 15 treatment days. Modest or poor responders are switched to alternative therapy, usually PUVA first, followed by systemic drugs if necessary.

ALTERNATIVES TO OFFICE PHOTOTHERAPY

Home UVB therapy

One of the most contentious issues potentially dividing the dermatologic community today is the use of home UVB (or Goeckerman) therapy. The controversy over prescribing home UVB units has in some instances made the relationship between therapists and patient support groups more adversarial than cooperative.

Home UVB or Goeckerman therapy is effective when prescribed for selected compliant patients who are educated in the use of the topical medications and the lamps, and who receive adequate followup assessments in the office. Notwithstanding, it is not easy to explain to the other patients why they are not candidates for home UVB. There are excellent units designed for home UVB (or Goeckerman) treatment, which are relatively inexpensive and often covered in part or in full by third-party insurers (see Appendix, Table 1). One of these, the Jordan light, was used in a study of the home Goeckerman treatment [44]. All 55 patients were cleared except for the scalp after completing the 6–8-week program. About 80% maintained satisfactory results for over a year with continued treatments, one to three times per week. The Jordan light is supplied with a well-written and illustrated brochure which emphasizes safety, compliance, as well as followup to the prescriber. Other home units are probably equally as effective. Handy individuals can construct their own wall units or cabinets, and purchase the lamps separately.

Opponents of home UVB therapy argue that treatment of psoriasis is difficult and requires experience, so how is it possible for a patient to do as well as the specialist at home? Home UVB should probably only be prescribed to patients who have undergone similar treatments in the hospital, day-treatment or office setting, and have achieved a good result. They have presumably learned how their skin reacts to UVB and the technique of safely increasing or decreasing the dose for their individual case depending on the clearing response of the involved skin and the burning or tanning of uninvolved skin. This assumption may not always be valid, however.

Some clinicians argue that when they write a prescription for a drug, that prescription is valid for only 1 year and must be renewed by the physician. But a prescription for an UV radiation unit is theoretically in force for a lifetime once the unit is purchased, thus exposing the prescriber to liability for misuse or abuse by the patient and possibly by others. The prescription or a letter from the doctor allows patients to request their insurance carriers to pay their share for treatment of the disease and to utilize any out-of-pocket expense as a tax deduction for medical purposes. Physicians certainly have the choice whether to write a prescription but implicit in the choice to do so is the obligation to instruct the patient in its proper use and to monitor them at intervals for progress and safe operation.

Some patients, seemingly unaware of this unwritten contract, charge that their doctors will not prescribe the unit because they fear the loss of revenue generated for the same services performed in their offices. I believe that is probably overstating the case. It is human nature for patients not to return for followup examinations or provide progress reports when they are doing well. Some may become bored with the home light treatment regimens, discontinue them without receiving proper maintenance phototherapy, and revisit the office only when they are flaring. Almost all physicians who refuse to prescribe home UVB units follow that course because they fear patients will be lost to followup care of their psoriasis, including annual examinations for skin cancer, and not because of lost fees.

In 1925 Goeckerman suggested phototherapy at home: "In exceptional instances, indeed, there is no reason why the patient should not install a lamp for his own personal use, and manipulate it with all the skin required [17]." The risk of UV carcinogenesis was not known in 1925. However, the incidence of skin cancer 25 years after receiving Goeckerman therapy for psoriasis [45] or atopic dermatitis [46] in the hospital was the same as expected for the general population. Several large epidemiologic studies comparing thousands of unselected psoriatics treated with the full range of modalities to the general population of their respective countries revealed a relative risk of developing nonmelanoma skin cancer of 1.17–2.5 [47–49].

In long-term PUVA prospective studies in the USA, patients who received more than 260 treatments had an 11-fold risk of squamous cell carcinoma (SCC) and a twofold risk of basal cell carcinoma (BCC) compared to those receiving less than 160 treatments [50]. The statistics were adjusted for exposure to a "high tar dose" and ionizing radiation, which independently increased the risk of SCC [51]. PUVA probably acts both as an independent carcinogen and a cocarcinogen. In the Swedish 7-year followup of 4799 PUVA patients, the risk of SCC was sixfold compared to the general population [52]. In neither the American [53] nor Swedish [52] PUVA cohorts has there been a significantly increased risk of malignant melanoma, which has been associated with residence in latitudes closer to the equator, genetic lack of melanin in the skin (types I and II), and acute sunburns early in life. Stern and colleagues [54] subsequently found that the risk of invasive SCC of the penis and scrotum was increased 95-fold for PUVA-treated men. After controlling for PUVA, "high levels" of UVB exposure to the male genitalia increased the risk of SCC more than fourfold. In the past, all of the patients had also applied coal tar to the genitalia suggesting that PUVA, UVB, and coal tar may act together as cocarcinogens. It is intriguing how we seem to have come full circle back to Pott's discovery.

In the Cleveland Clinic Department of Dermatology there is a divergence of opinion on the issue of home UVB. I favor home UVB phototherapy when the treatment has already been shown to be effective, when the patient is responsible and intelligent enough to follow explicit directions and use common sense when adjusting dosages, and has a working rapport with the prescriber. My colleague does not prescribe the phototherapy units because of perceived gaps in all patients' comprehension of the operation of the unit, medicolegal concerns, and failure of patients to attend for skin cancer surveillance. One might well ask "how many patients can tell the difference between residual psoriasis and Bowen's disease?"

In summary, patients who understand and accept the implicit contract to follow directions and receive followup examinations for monitoring progress and safety concerns and who respond well to natural sunlight or artificial UVB are appropriate candidates for home UVB phototherapy. It is ultimately the physician who decides and retains the right whether or not to prescribe.

Tanning salons

The cosmetic tanning industry has enjoyed astounding growth and profitability in the USA and Europe. It has been estimated that more than one million people per day visit 20 000 tanning salons in the USA with a gross revenue in excess of $1 billion. Most commercial salons employ lamps that emit predominantly UVA radiation, which is touted to be "safer than the sun." In a study of the SPDs of six UVA bulbs or blacklights as they are called, 96–99% of the radiation was emitted in the UVA band, 320–400 nm [5]. Stated another way, only 0.4–3.8% was emitted at wavelengths less than 320 nm which might be expected to improve psoriasis. There are two UV fluorescent lamps that diverge from the group. The Metec Helarium bulb emits about 8% below 320 nm and 30% between 320 and 340 nm, the most effective UVA wavelengths for psoriasis when combined with psoralens [3]. A high intensity lamp has been developed called "UVA-Sun," which emits only UVA wavelengths above 340 nm; all UVB is effectively filtered out [55].

Because of concern over the rampant use of these devices by unsophisticated proprietors and employees, and the theoretical risks of premature aging and carcinogenesis, organized dermatology has induced some municipalities and states to pass legislation which requires metering and changing of bulbs when they reach 70% of their original 100% irradiance. This is highly impractical because the output decreases to 70–85% after only 10–20 hours of use and the average exposure time for a customer is 15–30 min [56]. While this approach may prevent some episodes of burning, I fail to see how it would decrease the cumulative dose of UVA, and it is improbable that such laws can be implemented or enforced if they are passed.

Occasionally, a patient with psoriasis or vitiligo will ask the physician about the merits of exposures in a tanning salon for its therapeutic value. Without knowing the specifications of the unit in question taken together with the unsupervised and undocumented nature of the procedure, it is not possible to give a definite answer. Interestingly, in a questionnaire survey of tanning salon proprietors 80% boldly said that "skin therapy" was an important reason for their clients to visit [57]. In a recent inspection of tanning parlors in North Carolina, only one of 32 facilities was in compliance with all state and federal regulations [58].

Because of the possibility of low emission of UVB between 300 and 320 nm that may give some slight benefit to psoriasis, I would accept a trial of exposures in a tanning salon for use by patients who: (i) live too far away from a bona fide treatment center; (ii) cannot take time off from other responsibilities to travel to the office or clinic; (iii) have little or no health insurance and cannot afford to pay the fees for phototherapy; (iv) are willing to accept the risks involved (see below) for potentially little or no improvement of skin disease and "cosmetic tanning" of uninvolved skin; and (v) spend the relatively small sums of money to attend the tanning bed in their local community. Some of these might use a tanning salon for cosmetic purposes anyway while hoping to obtain concomitant therapeutic benefit. Not surprisingly, the clinical results are usually disappointing and merely serve to convince the patient that phototherapy must be administered by the physician or by the patient with a home UVB unit. An occasional patient will improve, but there are no controlled studies on which to base recommendation of tanning salons for therapeutic purposes.

The use of photosensitizing agents such as coal tar should be discouraged. One study found that tar–UVA photosentization was as therapeutic as UVB plus tar for psoriasis but the high dose of UVA required, long treatment times (up to an hour), and development of the "smarting reaction" makes this approach impractical [25]. The action spectrum of the smarting reaction lies between 340 and 430 nm. Topical and oral psoralens should never be prescribed unless the UVA is to be measured, administered, and monitored by the physician.

There is some evidence that UVA is not as carcinogenic as UVB in highly susceptible animal models, but this is controversial [59]. Some dermatologists may have exaggerated the risks to humans of repeated exposures to high-intensity UVA without substantial scientific proof, presumably with the altruistic notion of protecting the public welfare. Perhaps they have unfairly extrapolated from the long-term effects of the potent photosensitizer 8-methoxypsoralen combined with UVA. At best, the long-term effects of UVA tanning are unknown at present. At worst, UVA is weakly cocarcinogenic with artificial UVB and natural sunlight. It is a laudable goal to prevent the theoretical long-term outcomes of damage to dermal elastic tissue, premature aging of the skin and photocarcinogenesis especially in predisposed individuals with type I or II skin. The UVA exposures in a tanning salon have been compared to the effect of 2 hours of sun exposure wearing a maximally effective UVB sunscreeen [60].

The most important verifiable short-term risks of UVA exposure in a tanning salon include:

1 cutaneous eruptions due to the concomitant ingestion of phototoxic drugs such as some antibiotics, diuretics, psychotropic medications, or photosensitizers (psoralens) [61] in food (celery [62], parsnip, etc.) or in illicit "tan accelerators" [57];

2 the aggravation or unmasking of photosensitive diseases such as polymorphous light eruption, lupus erythematosus, dermatomyositis, and porphyria cutanea tarda;

3 eye injury such as corneal burns if protective goggles are not provided, not worn or removed prematurely;

4 skin infections from improperly cleaned surfaces transferred to subsequent clients such as impetigo, folliculitis, lice, and herpes simplex;

5 proprietor or client error leading to overexposure resulting in tender erythema ("sunburn"); it is conceivable that a UVA burn could Koebnerize or provoke an annular pustular flare of psoriasis [63].

CONCLUSION

By now it should be obvious how difficult it is to draw conclusions because of the existence of so many unreconcilable variables:

1 the plethora of coal tar preparations available contain inherently incon-

sistent active ingredients and different vehicles (creams, ointments, oils, gels);

2 the frequency and duration of application prior to UV exposure;

3 radiation sources and their spectral power distributions;

4 dosimetry;

5 frequency and duration of treatment;

6 inpatient, outpatient, or home treatment;

7 definition of "clearing" and "relapse";

8 maintenance therapy or no maintenance therapy;

9 study designs: bilateral paired comparison or separate treatment cohorts, randomized or selected, prospective or retrospective open or placebo-controlled.

Using the published information available and personal experience, I offer the following recommendations.

1 UVB alone, especially near 313 nm, can clear psoriasis.

2 Erythemogenic doses of UVB given three to five times weekly give the most rapid clearance.

3 Coal tar is weakly active as monotherapy.

4 White petrolatum or Aquaphor in combination with erythemogenic UVB is as effective as CCT in the same vehicle plus UVB.

5 Coal tar improves the time to clearing in suberythemogenic UVB protocols and may lower the total accumulated UVB dose.

6 While certain constituents of coal tar used in industry are known to be potent carcinogens for human skin, e.g., benzo[*a*]pyrenes, there is no convincing evidence that coal tar as it is used in the treatment of psoriasis, with or without UVB, significantly increases the risk of skin cancer. It is prudent, however, not to apply coal tar to the genitalia and to shield them during UV exposures.

7 The risk of developing cutaneous SCC after UVB and tar therapy is enhanced by PUVA, ionizing radiation, and possibly arsenic ingestion.

8 Coal tar is most useful for: (i) patients receiving modified Goeckerman regimens in hospital, day-treatment centers, or at home; (ii) patients limited to using topical regimens at home such as tar baths, ointments, or gels combined with anthralin and /or corticosteroids; (iii) patients using natural sunlight when that is the only source of UV radiation available.

REFERENCES

1 Ormsby OS, Montgomery H. *Diseases of the Skin*. Philadelphia: Lea & Febiger, 1943:289–291.

2 Parrish JA, Jaenicke KF. Action spectrum for phototherapy of psoriasis. *J Invest Dermatol* 1981;76:359–62.

3 Anderson TF. Phototherapy equipment: selection of apparatus. In Lowe NJ, ed. *Practical Psoriasis Therapy*. Chicago: YearBook Medical Publishers, Inc., 1986: 52–67.

4 Harber LC, Bickers DR. *Photosensitivity Diseases. Principles of Diagnosis and Treatment*, 2nd edn. Toronto, BC: Decker Inc., 1989:142–59.

5 Morison WL, Pike RA. Spectral power distributions of radiation sources used in

phototherapy and photochemotherapy. *J Am Acad Dermatol* 1984;10:64–8.
6 Swinehart JM, Lowe NJ. UVABA therapy for psoriasis. *J Am Acad Dermatol* 1991;24:594–7.
7 Gonzalez E, Parrish JA. Ultraviolet phototherapy. In Roenigk HH Jr, Maibach HI, eds. *Psoriasis*, 2nd edn. New York: Marcel Dekker, Inc., 1991:519–32.
8 Diffey BL, Challoner AVJ, Key PJ. A survey of the ultraviolet radiation emissions of photochemotherapy units. *Br J Dermatol* 1980;102:301–6.
9 Bohm M, Voorhees JJ. The role of the ambulatory psoriasis treatment center as a cost effective program for severe psoriasis. *J Am Acad Dermatol* 1985;12:740–7.
10 LeVine MJ, Parrish JA. Outpatient phototherapy of psoriasis. *Arch Dermatol* 1980; 116:552–4.
11 Adrian RM, Parrish JA, Momtaz-T K, Karlin MJ. Outpatient phototherapy for psoriasis. *Arch Dermatol* 1981;117:623–6.
12 Boer J, Hermans J, Schothorst AA, Suurmond D. Comparison of phototherapy (UV-B) and photochemotherapy (PUVA) for clearing and maintenance therapy of psoriasis. *Arch Dermatol* 1984;120:52–7.
13 Stern RS, Armstrong RB, Anderson TF, *et al.* Effect of continued ultraviolet B phototherapy on the duration of remission of psoriasis: a randomized study. *J Am Acad Dermatol* 1986;15:546–52.
14 Picot E, Meunier L, Picot-Debeze MC, *et al.* Treatment of psoriasis with a 311-nm UVB lamp. *Br J Dermatol* 1992;127:509–12.
15 Storbeck K, Holzle E, Schwier, *et al.* Narrow-band UVB (311 nm) *versus* conventional broad-band UVB with and without dithranol in phototherapy for psoriasis. *J Am Acad Dermatol* 1993;28:227–31.
16 Green C, Lakshmipathi T, Johnson BE, Ferguson J. A comparison of the efficacy and relapse rates of narrowband UVB (TL-01) monotherapy vs etretinate (re-TL-01) vs etretinate-PUVA (re-PUVA) in the treatment of psoriasis patients. *Br J Dermatol* 1992;127:5–9.
17 Goeckerman WH. The treatment of psoriasis. *Northwest Med* 1925;24:229–31.
18 Hjort N, Norgaard M. Tars. In Roenigk HH Jr, Maibach HI, eds. *Psoriasis*, 2nd edn. New York: Marcel Dekker, Inc., 1991:473–9.
19 Lavker RM, Grove GL, Kligman AM. The atrophogenic effect of crude coal tar on human epidermis. *Br J Dermatol* 1981;105:77–82.
20 Lowe NJ, Breeding J, Wortzman MS. The pharmacological variability of crude coal tar. *Br J Dermatol* 1983;107:475–80.
21 Williams REA, Tillman DM, White SI, *et al.* Re-examining crude coal tar treatment for psoriasis. *Br J Dermatol* 1992;126:608–10.
22 Shulze HJ, Steigleder GK. Bilateral comparison study on addition of crude coal tar to standard antipsoriatic dithranol ointment. *Z Hautkr* 1983;59:654–6.
23 Lawrence CM, Finnen MJ, Shuster S. Effect of coal tar on cutaneous aryl hydrocarbon hydroxylase induction and anthralin irritancy. *Br J Dermatol* 1984;110:671–5.
24 Gibson LE, Perry HO. Goeckerman therapy. In Roenigk HH Jr, Maibach HI, eds. *Psoriasis*, 2nd edn. New York: Marcel Dekker, Inc., 1991:535–45.
25 Fischer T. Comparative treatment of psoriasis with UV-light, trioxsalen plus UV-light, and coal tar plus UV-light. *Acta Derm Venereol* 1977;57:345–50.
26 Parrish JA, Morison WL, Gonzalez E, *et al.* Therapy of psoriasis by tar photosensitization. *J Invest Dermatol* 1978;70:111–2.
27 Frost P, Horwitz SN, Caputo RV, Berger SM. Tar gel-phototherapy for psoriasis. *Arch Dermatol* 1979;115:840–6.
28 Menkes A, Stern RS, Arndt KA. Psoriasis treatment with suberythemogenic ultraviolet B radiation and a coal tar extract. *J Am Acad Dermatol* 1985;12:21–5.
29 Stern RS, Gange RW, Parrish JA, *et al.* Contribution of topical tar oil to ultraviolet B phototherapy for psoriasis. *J Am Acad Dermatol* 1986;14:742–7.
30 Eells LD, Wolff JM, Garloff J, Eaglstein WH. Comparison of suberythemogenic and

maximally aggressive ultraviolet B therapy for psoriasis. *J Am Acad Dermatol* 1984;11:105–10.

31 Lowe NJ, Wortzman MS, Breeding JH, *et al.* Coal tar phototherapy for psoriasis re-evaluated: erythemogenic versus suberythemogenic ultraviolet with a tar extract in oil and crude coal tar. *J Am Acad Dermatol* 1983;8:781–9.

32 Petrozzi JW, Barton JO, Kaidbey K, Kligman AM. Updating the Goeckerman regimen for psoriasis. *Br J Dermatol* 1978;98:437–44.

33 Belsito DV, Kechijian P. The role of tar in the Goeckerman therapy. *Arch Dermatol* 1982;118:319–21.

34 Anderson TF, Waldinger TP, Voorhees JJ. UV-B phototherapy. An overview. *Arch Dermatol* 1984;120:1502–7.

35 Schleider NR, Moskowitz RS, Cort DH, *et al.* Effects of emollients on ultraviolet-radiation-induced erythema of the skin. *Arch Dermatol* 1979;115:1188–91.

36 George SA, Bilsand DJ, Wainwright NJ, Ferguson J. Failure of coconut oil to accelerate psoriasis clearance in narrow-band UVB phototherapy or photochemo-therapy. *Br J Dermatol* 1993;128:301–5.

37 Bohm M, Voorhees J, Armstrong RB, *et al.* White paper on hospitalization for psoriasis care. *J Am Acad Dermatol* 1984;10:842–51.

38 Menter NA. Psoriasis day-care centers. In Lowe NJ, ed. *Practical Psoriasis Therapy.* Chicago: YearBook Medical Publishers Inc., 1986:116–30.

39 Lowe NJ, Lowe PS, Wasiowich E. Psoriasis ambulatory treatment centers: United States experience. In Roenigk HH Jr, Maibach HI, eds. *Psoriasis*, 2nd edn. New York: Marcel Dekker, Inc., 1991:547–52.

40 Armstrong RB, Leach EE, Fleiss JL, Harber LC. Modified Goeckerman therapy for psoriasis. A two-year follow-up of a combined hospital-ambulatory care program. *Arch Dermatol* 1984;120:313–8.

41 Menter A, Cram DL. The Goeckerman regimen in two psoriasis day care centers. *J Am Acad Dermatol* 1983;9:59–65.

42 Perry HO, Soderstrom CW, Schulze RW. The Goeckerman treatment of psoriasis. *Arch Dermatol* 1968;98:178–82.

43 Muller SA, Perry HO. The Goeckerman treatment in psoriasis: six decades of experience at the Mayo Clinic. *Cutis* 1984;34:265–9.

44 Jordan WP, Clarke AM, Hale RK. Long-term modified Goeckerman regimen for psoriasis using an ultraviolet B light source in the home. *J Am Acad Dermatol* 1981;4:584–9.

45 Pittelkow MR, Perry HD, Muller SA, *et al.* Skin cancer in patients with psoriasis treated with coal tar: a 25-year followup study. *Arch Dermatol* 1981;117:465–8.

46 Maughan WZ, Muller SA, Perry HO, *et al.* Incidence of skin cancers in patients with atopic dermatatis treated with coal tar. A 25-year follow-up study. *J Am Acad Dermatol* 1980;3:612–5.

47 Alderson MR, Clarke JA. Cancer incidence in patients with psoriasis. *Br J Cancer* 1983;47:857–9.

48 Lindelof B, Eklund G, Liden S, Stern RS. The prevalence of malignant tumors in patients with psoriasis. *J Am Acad Dermatol* 1990;22:1056–60.

49 Olsen JH, Moller H, Frentz G. Malignant tumors in patients with psoriasis. *J Am Acad Dermatol* 1992;27:716–22.

50 Stern RS, Lange R, and members of the Photochemotherapy Follow-up Study. Non-melanoma skin cancer occurring in patients treated with PUVA five to ten years after first treatment. *J Invest Dermatol* 1988;91:120–4.

51 Stern RS, Laird N, Melski J, *et al.* Cutaneous squamous cell carcinoma in patients treated with PUVA. *N Engl J Med* 1984;310:1156–61.

52 Lindelof B, Sigurgeirsson B, Tegner E, *et al.* PUVA and cancer: a large-scale epidemiological study. *Lancet* 1991;338:91–3.

53 Stern RS, Lange R. Cardiovascular disease, cancer and cause of death in patients

with psoriasis: 10 years prospective experience in a cohort of 1380 patients. *J Invest Dermatol* 1988;91:197–201.
54 Stern RS and members of the Photochemotherapy Follow-up Study. Genital tumors among men with psoriasis exposed to psoralens and ultraviolet A radiation (PUVA) and ultraviolet B radiation. *N Engl J Med* 1990;322:1093–7.
55 Mutzhas MF, Holzle E, Hofmann C, Plewig G. A new apparatus with high radiation energy between 320–460 nm: physical description and dermatological applications. *J Invest Dermatol* 1981;76:42–7.
56 Bruyneel-Rapp F, Dorsey SB, Guin JD. The tanning salon: an area survey of equipment, procedures, and practices. *J Am Acad Dermatol* 1988;18:1030–8.
57 Beyth R, Hunnicut M, Alguire PC. Tanning salons: an area survey of proprietors' knowledge of risks and precautions. *J Am Acad Dermatol* 1991;24:277–82.
58 Fleischer AB, Lee WJ, Adams DP, Zanolli MD. Tanning facility compliance with state and federal regulations in North Carolina: A poor performance. *J Am Acad Dermatol* 1993;28:212–7.
59 Van Weelden H, de Gruijl FR, van der Putte SCJ, *et al.* The carcinogenic risks of modern tanning equipment: is UV-A safer than UV-B? *Arch Dermatol Res* 1988; 280:300–7.
60 Gange RW. Tanning. *Dermatol Clin* 1986;4(2):189–93.
61 Bickers DR, Epstein JH, Fitzpatrick TB, *et al.* Risks and benefits from high-intensity ultraviolet A sources used for cosmetic purposes. *J Am Acad Dermatol* 1985;12: 380–1.
62 Ljunggren B. Severe phototoxic burn following celery ingestion. *Arch Dermatol* 1990;126:1334–6.
63 Rosen RM. Annular pustular psoriasis induced by UV radiation from tanning salon use. *J Am Acad Dermatol* 1991;25:336–7.

thirteen

Psoralens and Photochemotherapy (PUVA)

Thomas N. Helm and Charles Camisa

THE PSORALENS

Introduction

Psoralens are natural compounds that interact with sunlight to produce biologic effects. Psoralens were initially used for the treatment of vitiligo. The sacred Indian book *Atharva Veda* referred to plants containing psoralen that were useful in correcting pigmentary disturbances [1]. The Arabic medical literature had similar references. In the thirteenth century, Ibn El Bitar treated vitiligo by having patients ingest *Ammi majus* seeds with honey and pellitory root [1]. The patient then sat in the sun and subsequently developed cutaneous blisters. Upon healing, the skin would repigment [1]. The Buddhist literature from AD 200 and the Chinese literature from AD 700 give similar references to the use of psoralen preparations in the treatment of vitiligo [2].

Although the use of psoralen-containing seeds dates back to ancient times, it was not until the 1940s that Egyptian scientists isolated the active ingredients from these plants [2,3]. The photoactive ingredients were found to be isomers of furocoumarins. These compounds can be widely found in nature in such diverse plant families as *Rutaceae*, *Umbelliferae*, *Leguminosae*, and *Moreacea* [4]. Common plants such as parsnip, celery, lemon, lime, fig, parsley, and bishop's weed belong to these families.

Once the active ingredients of the seeds used by the ancient herbalists were identified, clinical trials with the individual reagents were begun. Sunlamp irradiation or natural sunlight combined with oral 8-methoxypsoralen (8-MOP) was found to be an effective treatment for some cases of vitiligo. This form of treatment was well tolerated and the potential benefit of 8-MOP and light treatment for UV-responsive diseases such as psoriasis was suggested [5]. A report at the 1962 American Academy of Dermatology meeting later confirmed that topical 8-MOP and UV light is helpful in the treatment of psoriasis [4].

In 1974, a report by Parrish *et al.* popularized the use of psoralen and UV-light therapy in psoriasis [6]. Oral 8-MOP given at doses corresponding to patients' weights, followed by high-intensity UVA irradiation in the 320–390 nm wavelength range was given to 21 patients with generalized psoriasis vulgaris who had failed conventional therapy with topical outpatient treatment. These patients had greater than 50% of their surface area involved with psoriasis. Sixteen patients had a paired comparison done in which half of the body was treated with 8-MOP and UVA and the other half of the body was treated with conventional UVB light emitted from a light source equipped with Westinghouse FS40 and FS20 "sunlamp bulbs." All of the patients in the paired comparison showed greater improvement in the UVA-treated side, and all 21 patients in the study had clearing of their generalized psoriasis with psoralen and UVA treatment. This form of treatment was found to be well tolerated, except for a low incidence of nausea and pruritus.

Many subsequent reports confirmed that photochemotherapy with 8-MOP and UVA is useful in the treatment of psoriasis. This form of therapy has become widely known as PUVA therapy; the acronym stands for psoralen (P) and ultraviolet A (UVA) light. This type of treatment is much more effective than UV light therapy given with conventional fluorescent bulbs or a xenon source [7]. Some studies show that 85% of patients on outpatient maintenance treatments remain in remission for up to 400 days [7]. Several other large multicenter trials showed that 83–89% of patients cleared, confirming the benefits of PUVA therapy [8–10].

The emphasis of current research is on ways to enhance the efficacy of PUVA while minimizing side effects. Different modes of application such as topical application via lotions, creams, and bathwater delivery are being compared to modalities such as oral dosing. Psoralen therapy has become a mainstay of treatment for psoriasis and has supplanted other modalities such as methotrexate and cytotoxic drug therapy.

THE PSORALENS

Mechanism of action

The psoralens most widely used for psoriasis therapy are 8-MOP, trimethylpsoralen (TMP), and 5-methoxypsoralen (5-MOP) (Table 13.1). Each of these preparations has different photobiologic effects. 8-MOP is the most widely used preparation. Dosages of 0.6 mg/kg are required in the average patient. 5-MOP produces less nausea and gastrointestinal upset than 8-MOP and also produces less photosensitivity when given at the same dosage as 8-MOP. 5-MOP, however, appears less effective in the treatment of psoriasis. TMP shows greater melanocyte stimulation than the other two commonly used preparations. TMP is most often used in the treatment of vitiligo or psoriasis which has not responded to 8-MOP or 5-MOP. The dosage of TMP is approximately 0.2–0.5 mg/kg [4].

Psoralens belong to the group of compounds known as furocoumarins. Furocoumarins are formed by the combination of a furan ring with a

Table 13.1 Psoralens used for oral therapy

Psoralen	Synonyms	Trade name	Approximate dosage (mg/kg)	Characteristics
8-Methoxypsoralen	8-MOP Methoxsalen	8-MOP Oxsoralen-ultra	0.6 mg/kg 0.4–0.5 mg/kg	Most widely used Greatest photosensitivity and nausea
5-Methoxypsoralen	5-MOP Bergapten		1.2–1.6 mg/kg	Less nausea and photosensitivity than 8-MOP
4,5,8-Trimethylpsoralen	TMP Trioxsalen	Trioxsalen Trisoralen	0.2–0.5 mg/kg	Less photosensitivity than 8-MOP Greater melanocyte stimulation than other psoralens

coumarin ring. When the linear structure is formed, the product is known as a psoralen. If an angular structure is formed, it is known as an angelican [11]. The tertiary structure of these compounds dictates how they will react with cellular constituents after photoactivation. The 3–4 bond of psoralen molecules interacts with the 5–6 bond of the thymidine constituents of DNA, even in the absence of light. This is known as a "dark complex." With activation by sunlight, some psoralens are capable of producing cross-linking of DNA strands known as "bifunctional adducts." Differing wavelengths of light change the type of complexes that form. At wavelengths below 250 nm, greater amounts of mono-adducts are formed than at higher wavelengths [12].

For example, if an 8-MOP/DNA complex absorbs radiant energy, the 8-MOP molecule can change into a 3–4 monofunctional adduct or a 4–5 monofunctional adduct. Only the 4–5 monofunctional adduct can later react to cross-link DNA. Many linear psoralens can undergo this type of reaction, but angular-shaped psoralens such as angelican are not able to form double cross-links because of their angular tertiary structure. Even certain types of monofunctional psoralens are unable to form DNA cross-links.

Initial research suggested that DNA cross-linking is responsible for the biologic effect of PUVA therapy in diseases such as psoriasis. Cross-linking of DNA leads to inhibition of DNA synthesis in epidermal basal cells and thereby creates a marked antiproliferative effect. However, many other factors may be involved. Clinically, optimal phototherapeutic action spectra can differ from the wavelengths which show greatest inhibition of DNA synthesis [13]. This may be due to changes in optical properties of psoriatic epidermis or may indicate that other reactions are occurring after psoralen treatment. Binding to proteins, hemolytic effects, and production of reactive oxygen species have been studied as other mechanisms that may cause the pigment-producing and erythema-producing effects of psoralen therapy [14]. 8-MOP may also combine with receptor DNA complexes on the surface of lymphocytes [15]. Other investigators feel that plasma membranes are the principal target of 8-MOP during PUVA therapy [16]. Cellular changes such as capping and formation of cytoplasmic appendages have been demonstrated in a lymphoblast model during PUVA therapy [16]. It is not necessary for binding of DNA constituents to occur in order to produce phototoxicity. For example, the nonphotosensitizing angular furocoumarin angelican can bind effectively to linolenic acid methyl ester. Although many biologic effects of psoralens are known, the exact mechanism of psoralen therapy remains undetermined.

Three general schemes of PUVA action have been delineated [11]. When psoralens are irradiated with light of 320–400 nm, the electron spin of the surrounding molecules is changed. The absorbed energy can then be released by a variety of different mechanisms including the following.

1 Fluorescence in which light energy is released at a different wavelength than the incident radiation, or phosphorescence in which light energy is released after incident irradiation has stopped.

2 By a direct molecular energy transfer. This type of reaction creates monofunctional and bifunctional adducts with pyrimidine bases.

3 Psoralens can also react with the amino acids of proteins like keratin and albumin; this mechanism of energy transfer requires oxygen as a cofactor and results in the production of reactive species such as superoxide and hydroxyl radicals.

Cell proliferation is inhibited by the production of monofunctional and bifunctional DNA adducts. High quantities of monofunctional adducts lead to cell death. Faulty repair of this type of adduct may give rise to some of the carcinogenic effects that have been attributed to PUVA therapy [11]. The role of monofunctional vs bifunctional adducts in the photobiologic effectiveness of PUVA therapy has not been fully clarified. 8-MOP absorbs radiant energy well at several different wavelengths including 270 nm and again at 310–320 nm. The 8-MOP dark complex, however, seems to have maximal absorption at approximately 313 nm. Wavelengths of 340 nm produce a relatively greater amount of monofunctional 4,5 adducts; whereas, the 260 nm wavelength gives rise to a greater proportion of 3,4 monofunctional adducts. The ratio of monofunctional to bifunctional adducts after initial radiation may not be sufficient to predict the outcome of treatment. Suberythemal UVA doses lead to the production of 8-MOP mono-adducts that lead to erythema upon further UVA stimulation. The mono-adducts that formed and remain in the skin are responsible for these delayed reactions [17]. This type of persistent photosensitivity has practical implications upon the interval of treatment needed for bath PUVA phototherapy (and perhaps for oral PUVA if sufficiently high epidermal concentrations are achieved). Many other structural and immunologic findings have been attributed to PUVA therapy. PUVA therapy might have an effect on the histology of capillaries seen in psoriatic skin [18]. One study demonstrated that PUVA therapy increased the proportion of CD4+ cells in the peripheral blood [19]. TMP bath PUVA depresses immediate contact reactions induced by benzoic acid and methyl nicotinate. Even in nonexposed test sites, allergic contact sensitivity may be suppressed [20]. Mast cell numbers in the skin are decreased by PUVA therapy [21]. A study with monoclonal antibodies to 8-MOP adducts revealed that nuclei in three of five skin biopsies in patients undergoing PUVA therapy contained adducts [22]. Plasma levels of 8-MOP, however, did not correlate with the presence of adducts nor could 8-MOP photoadducts be detected in the DNA from lymphocytes of these PUVA patients. Depression of basal natural killer cell activity has been demonstrated during PUVA therapy [23]. The natural killer cells could be maximally stimulated with interferon because of increased sensitivity to interferon augmentation; however, PUVA does not seem to have a significant deleterious effect on normal immunity. Other immunologic effects of PUVA therapy such as 8-MOP inhibition of phytohemagglutinin-induced DNA synthesis in cultured human lymphocytes [24], decreased interleukin-6 staining on epidermal cell membranes [25], and Langerhans cell depletion [26] have been noted during PUVA therapy and may account for inhibition of delayed cutaneous hypersensitivity.

It is possible that the photosensitizing, Langerhans cell-depleting, and antipsoriatic effects of PUVA therapy are independent of one another. Suberythemal doses of UVA combined with topical 8-MOP application leads to healing of psoriatic lesions without the erythema or the Langerhans cell depletion seen with higher doses of UVA [27]. This observation indicates that skin lesions can be treated without depleting Langerhans cells. As these cells play a role in cutaneous immunoregulation and immune surveillance, it is theoretically advantageous that treatment does not compromise these functions, especially because this may decrease the risk of skin cancer.

Another very interesting effect of PUVA is to increase serum 25-OH vitamin D levels and intestinal calcium absorption [28]. The role of this effect has not yet been determined, but it juxtaposes PUVA with the exciting research on vitamin D and analogs as antipsoriatic therapy.

CLINICAL USE OF PSORALENS

8-Methoxypsoralen

8-MOP is a furocoumarin found in the seeds of the *Ammi majus* plant. Maximum photosensitivity usually occurs 3.9–4.25 hours after ingestion. The 8-MOP binds reversibly to serum albumin and is distributed throughout the body by the circulatory system. The concentration of 8-MOP can be measured in small amounts of fluid by reverse phase high performance liquid chromatography. High pressure liquid chromatography has shown that 8-MOP from different pharmaceutical suppliers may show different peak absorption times. Concomitant administration of food may also affect peak concentrations [29]. The 8-MOP generally causes higher serum levels when taken while fasting rather than with meals [30]. There is great variability from person to person and serum levels from two people of the same size given the same dosage may be quite different [31]. A significant proportion of patients receiving 8-MOP for the first time also have a "first pass effect" [32]. In the case of 8-MOP, the "first pass effect" describes a phenomenon in which the first administration of a medication does not give rise to significant serum levels as expected. This phenomenon is felt to be due to rapid metabolism by liver enzymes [15]. Upon further dosing with 8-MOP, this effect diminishes.

An 8-MOP oral delivery gives peak concentrations 1½ hours after administration; whereas a soft gelatin oral preparation gives a peak level 1 hour after ingestion [33] and levels after ingesting hard gelatin 8-MOP capsules peak at 2–3 hours after ingestion [33]. 8-MOP levels are correlated with blister fluid 8-MOP levels [30]. The skin concentration of 8-MOP seems to approximate one-third of the serum level [34]. Although plasma 8-MOP levels may not correlate with the minimal phototoxic dose (MPD), plasma concentration of 8-MOP correlates with the intensity of an erythema response at a given wavelength [35].

In the USA, the original crystalline form of 8-MOP (Oxsoralen) has been widely replaced by a liquid preparation in a capsule which has a more rapid rate of absorption (Oxsoralen-Ultra). Oxsoralen-Ultra capsules lead to a faster clearing of psoriasis and are also felt to produce a more consistent clearing response [36]. Although this preparation was expected to have a lower incidence of gastrointestinal upset, the incidence of gastrointestinal side effects seems to have actually increased somewhat.

Trimethoxypsoralen

TMP differs from 8-MOP in that it is more effective in stimulating pigmentation. TMP levels peak 2 hours after ingestion and measurable amounts can be detected in the aqueous humor of the eye at this time [37]. Oral TMP is not as potent a photosensitizer as 8-MOP because of its poor solubility and quick metabolism to nonphotosensitizing compounds like 4,8-dimethyl, 5-carboxypsoralen (DMeCP) [38]. Topical application of TMP, a strong photosensitizer, may be helpful in treating psoriasis [38].

5-Methoxypsoralen

5-MOP is a psoralen with comparable efficacy to 8-MOP in treating psoriasis [39]. The 5-MOP causes less phototoxicity than 8-MOP and has a lower incidence of gastrointestinal side effects than 8-MOP. The serum half-life of 5-MOP is about 1 hour [40]. The rapid rate of 5-MOP metabolism keeps undesired photosensitivity after treatment to a minimum. This preparation is most useful for patients who do not tolerate 8-MOP; however, it must be obtained from Europe.

ORAL PUVA (PHOTOCHEMOTHERAPY)

Introduction

8-MOP is the most widely used psoralen in psoriasis treatment. When first-line therapies such as corticosteroid preparations, anthralin, or coal tar have not been effective at controlling psoriasis, and the Goeckerman regimen does not produce clearing of psoriasis after a 2–3-week period of intensive inpatient or outpatient day-care treatment, PUVA therapy may be the next alternative.

A careful history should be taken prior to starting therapy, with special emphasis on photosensitivity diseases. PUVA therapy should be avoided in patients with previous bronchiolar or hypersensitivity reactions to psoralens, systemic lupus erythematosus, some types of porphyria (such as porphyria cutanea tarda and variegate porphyria), and xeroderma pigmentosa (Table 13.2). Pregnant women or women planning pregnancy in the immediate future should also be excluded because PUVA is mutagenic and effects on pregnancy have not been adequately studied, although PUVA does not seem to be a potent teratogen. PUVA exposure in women around the time of conception or pregnancy has been associated with a greater abortion rate than when the male partner is receiving PUVA therapy [41]. Since the lens of the eye shields the retina from incident UVA light, an aphakic patient has greater potential for retinal damage and PUVA therapy should be reserved as a treatment of last resort. The effects of PUVA on children are not well studied, and the use of this modality in children is controversial, although some investigators report a favorable experience. Lasting eye disease attributable to PUVA therapy is very rare. Nevertheless, a baseline eye examination which measures not only visual acuity, but includes slit-lamp examination looking for lenticular opacities is recommended. In this way, lenticular abnormalities which antedate PUVA therapy can be clearly identified and later screening studies can better evaluate changes. If no abnormalities are detected on initial examination, followup examinations

Table 13.2 Contraindications to PUVA therapy

Relative contraindications
Aphakic patients
Children <12 years old
Previous ingestion of trivalent inorganic arsenic
Previous treatment with ionizing radiation
Previous treatment with topical nitrogen mustard
Prolonged therapy with >400 PUVA treatments
Definite contraindications
Hypersensitivity/bronchiolar reactions to PUVA in the past
Pregnancy
Systemic lupus erythematosus
Xeroderma pigmentosa

by the same ophthalmologist at intervals ranging from 6 to 12 months seem to help detect any changes early.

Because hepatic inactivation of psoralens is necessary for clearance, oral psoralen therapy should be used with caution in patients with active liver disease. Liver function tests should be screened prior to beginning PUVA therapy. Although some investigators perform antinuclear and Ro (SSA) antibody tests in addition to a urinary porphyrin screen and complete blood count to ensure that no photosensitive diseases have been overlooked, a careful history and examination usually render these tests unnecessary.

A cumulative dose of UVA light greater than $1000\,J/cm^2$, concomitant ingestion of photosensitizing drugs such as thiazide diuretics, tetracyclines, or nonsteroidal antiinflammatory drugs (like benoxaprofen and piroxicam), previous skin cancer (including basal cell carcinoma, squamous cell carcinoma, or melanoma) or exposure to cancer promoters such as X-ray or trivalent inorganic arsenic are relative contraindications to PUVA therapy. The use of concurrent topical photosensitizers such as tar preparations needs to be avoided.

Because PUVA therapy has been shown to depress the immune system, patients on other immunosuppressive medications such as azathioprine (Imuran), cyclosporine (Sandimmune), or cyclophosphamide (Cytoxan) should be treated with caution if PUVA is used at all. The effects of PUVA therapy on patients with AIDS have not been adequately studied and might prove detrimental to overall health, although a study of PUVA on five HIV-infected patients showed rapid clearing of resistant dermatoses and no obvious detriment to their overall health [42]. UVB has been successfully used to treat eosinophilic folliculitis in HIV-infected patients [43] and extracorporeal photopheresis (which employs psoralen and UVA light) has been reported to improve patients with the AIDS-related complex (ARC) [44]. Extracorporeal photopheresis of psoriatic patients has been associated with decreased skin reactivity to intradermal recall antigens and decreased lymphocyte interleukin-2 production in response to *in vitro* stimulation [45].

Another variable which must be assessed is whether or not a patient is able to cooperate with therapy, stand unassisted for several minutes in a light box, and withstand the cardiovascular stress caused by prolonged vasodilation in the phototherapy unit. (Lie-down units that help avoid some of these problems are available from some companies.) Patients must also be able to comply with the use of photoprotective lenses that need to be worn the remainder of the day of therapy.

Although some physicians have advocated the use of patient consent forms prior to starting PUVA therapy, a careful and fully documented discussion regarding the side effects of PUVA therapy is essential before starting therapy and may obviate the need for standardized consent forms. No consent form can foresee all possible outcomes of therapy and an open discussion is most helpful. (ICN Pharmaceuticals has prepared a patient instruction video on PUVA, which serves as a good adjunct to the physician's discussion.)

Clinical use

For suitable candidates, three treatments per week may be anticipated to control psoriasis and at least 20 treatments must be given before a maximal therapeutic effect can be expected (Figs 13.1, 13.2). Patients are issued wrap-around style glasses, which can be either tinted or clear depending

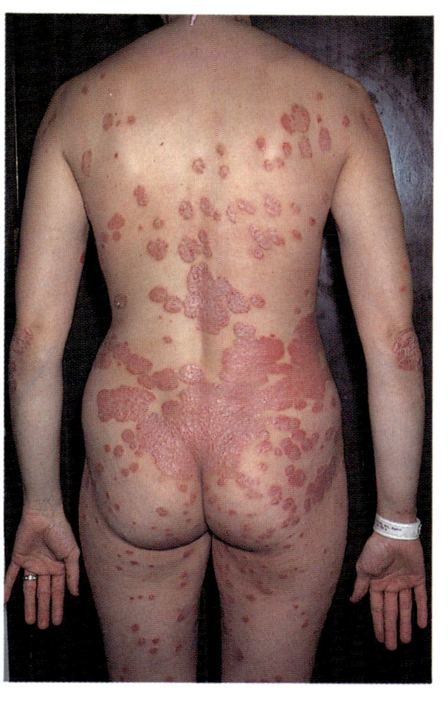

(a)

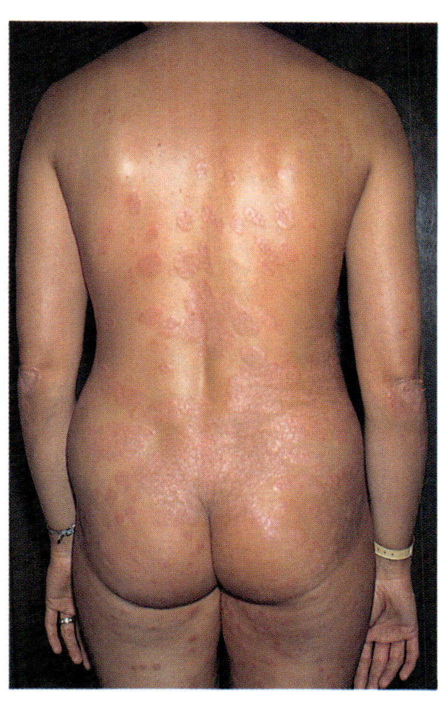

(b)

Fig 13.1 Patient (a) before and (b) after 2 weeks of psoralen UVA.

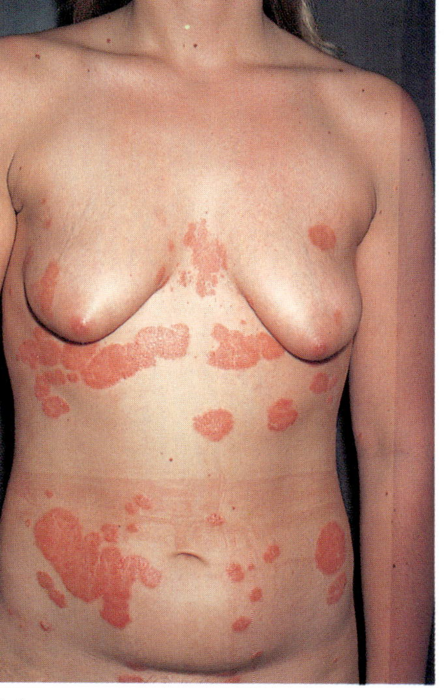

(a)

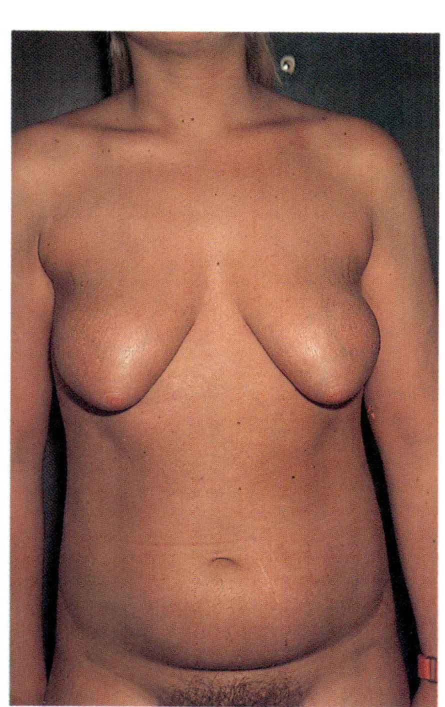

(b)

Fig 13.2 Patient (a) before and (b) after 4 weeks of psoralen UVA.

upon the patient's preference (Fig. 13.3). Some dermatologists have recommended that special eye glasses with impregnated lenses and special coatings be worn instead of wrap-around glasses. Acceptable transmission of light has been reported to be less than 10% at 390 nm, less than 5% at 380 nm, less than 2% at 370 nm, and less than 1% at 360 nm [46]. Table 13.3 lists some sources of acceptable UVA-blocking optical equipment.

Although the wrap-around glasses will block almost all incident UVA, eyeglasses may allow for UVA reflection to penetrate the eye from lateral angles. Admittedly, this reflection is probably only a small amount of UVA. Although wrap-around glasses are more protective than specially coated or treated eyeglasses because scatter from the sides is prevented, it may be better to have a patient obtain a fashionable product that he or she will use rather than a theoretically more protective product which will immediately be discarded after leaving the doctor's office. Clearly, the type of protective eye gear recommended should be individualized for each patient by the physician.

Nevertheless, use of skin type information obtained from patient history can give useful estimates of appropriate starting UVA dosing. A widely used regimen is shown in Table 13.3.

For the initial dose of 8-MOP, patients bring their medication to the office and take their first dose under the supervision of the nurse (Table 13.4). The time of the medication is carefully recorded in the medical record and UVA light is administered $1\frac{1}{2}$–2 hours later. Although higher doses of serum psoralen can be obtained when psoralen is taken on an

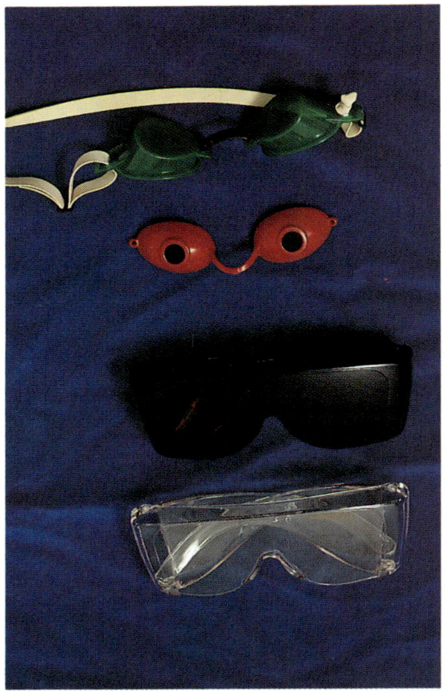

Fig 13.3 The lower two wrap-around glasses are worn for 24 hours after ingestion of 8-methoxypsoralen. The upper two goggles can be worn during the UVA exposure.

Table 13.3 Skin type and UVA dosing

Skin type	History	UVA dose (J/cm^2)
I	Always burn, never tan	0.5
II	Always burns, sometimes tan	1.0
III	Sometimes burns, always tan	1.5
IV	Never burns, always tan	2.0
V	Darkly pigmented	2.5
VI	Black	3.0

Table 13.4 Oral 8-methoxypsoralen PUVA treatment

Begin treatments at intervals of 48 hours or greater (usually Monday, Wednesday, Friday)

Give 0.6 mg/kg Oxsoralen $1\frac{1}{2}$ hours prior to UVA with a standardized light meal

Instruct patient to wear protective UV blocking eyewear immediately after taking medication and for the remainder of the day

Begin UVA exposure as outlined for skin type or at 75–100% of minimal phototoxic dose

If successful, clearing should be noted in 16–20 treatments

empty stomach, the preparations are much better tolerated if they are taken with a small meal. A similar amount and type of food should be taken each time so that serum levels are more likely to remain relatively uniform. In this way, the desired response can be achieved by changing the UVA dosage. If patients do not respond to PUVA at all, it is reasonable to measure serum levels. A level of more than 50 ng is felt to be therapeutic, and the dosage of 8-MOP can be increased until this level is reached.

Although some physicians feel that skin type determined by history can be a rough starting point for UVA dosage, history is often an unreliable indicator of MPD and minimal erythema dose (MED). MPD testing gives an accurate estimate of optimal starting dose. To perform MED testing, the patient ingests psoralen as he or she would prior to a treatment. Instead of irradiating areas affected with psoriasis, small squares on the back or buttock are irradiated with differing amounts of UVA light. An opaque plastic sheet with six 1.5-cm squares is used for this purpose. Each square is irradiated with a different incremental amount of UVA light and in 24–48 hours, the squares are evaluated to find the lowest dose that gives complete erythema of the irradiated area. We usually test in a range of 1–10 J/cm^2. Seventy-five percent to 100% of the MPD can then be given as a starting dose of irradiation and further treatments can be increased by 0.25–1.0 J/cm^2 as tolerated. Aggressive UVA exposure based on weekly MPD testing can greatly reduce total UVA exposure and treatment duration [47]. Patients are cleared quickly by this method at a lower total expense and with what may prove to be a lower risk of skin cancer because of lower cumulative UVA irradiance; however, even the high single dose PUVA regimen used in Europe may cause increased squamous cell carcinomas and basal cell carcinomas [48]. PUVA erythema peaks at 48–96 hours and the dose–response curve is not as steep as in UVB erythema [49].

5-Methoxypsoralen

5-MOP treatment is accomplished in an analogous fashion to 8-MOP treatment. After identical history and laboratory evaluations are performed, patients are begun on a 1.2 mg/kg dose. Unfortunately, 5-MOP is not available in the USA and must be obtained from Europe (Table 13.5). It shows great promise in the therapy of psoriasis because of greater tolerance by patients and lower incidence of unwanted photosensitivity subsequent

Table 13.5 Most widely used psoralens available in USA*

Drug	Unit	Package
8-Methoxypsoralen (methoxsalen USP)	10 mg capsules	30 capsules
Oxsoralen Ultra capsules (methoxsalen USP)	10 mg capsules	50 capsules
Oxsoralen Lotion (methoxsalen USP)	1% lotion	1 oz bottle
Trisoralen Tablets (trioxsalen USP)	5 mg tablets	100 tablets

* This list may not be all inclusive.

to therapy. Oral 5-MOP may also modify circadian rhythm regulation because it stimulates melatonin secretion [50].

Trimethylpsoralen
Oral TMP has limited use in the treatment of common psoriasis. However, if patients fail to respond to 8-MOP or 5-MOP, this modality can be tried before advancing to therapies such as retinoids, methotrexate, or cyclosporine. In the setting of photosensitive psoriasis, TMP PUVA has given excellent results and may be the treatment of choice [51].

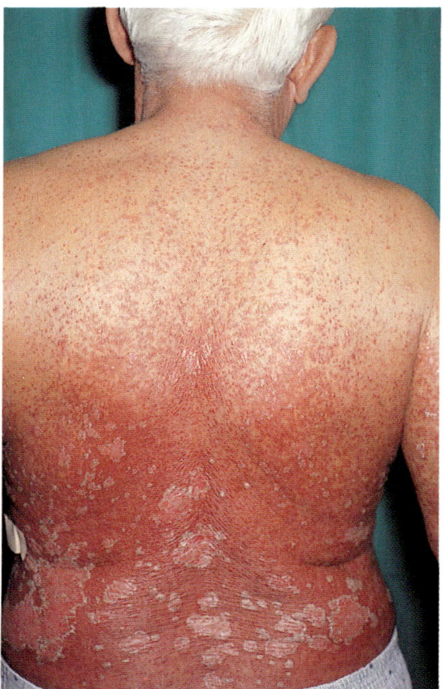

Fig 13.4 Phototoxic reaction to psoralen UVA.

Toxicity

Side effects of PUVA treatment can be divided into acute and chronic effects (Table 13.6). Acute reactions include phototoxicity manifest by erythema (and possibly edema) (Fig. 13.4), nausea which occurs in 20–30% of patients, pruritus, dizziness, flu-like symptoms, headache, and the isomorphic response of Koebner. Chronic side effects include enhanced photoaging, pigmented macules known as "PUVA lentigines," actinic keratoses, squamous cell carcinomas, and possibly anterior cortical cataracts [52]. Elevations of lactic dehydrogenase (LDH) may be seen in approximately one of 23 patients receiving PUVA therapy [53]. Development of fever and liver function test elevation has been reported during PUVA therapy. The liver function abnormalities returned to normal, but with the next PUVA treatment the same reaction occurred [54]. No significant changes, however, have been demonstrated by liver biopsies done before and after PUVA therapy [55]. It seems that psoralens have little or no lasting hepatotoxicity.

The prolonged exertion of standing and thermal exposure during PUVA therapy could conceivably lead to significant cardiovascular stress. A study of 40 patients receiving PUVA therapy, six of whom had cardiovascular disease, did not reveal any significant arrythmias by Holter monitoring although heart rates were found to increase by a mean of 22% over baseline [56]. Blood pressures were not significantly changed and the authors concluded that the PUVA therapy did not subject patients to excessive

Table 13.6 Side effects of PUVA

Acute	Chronic
Erythema	Actinic keratoses
Diarrhea	Basal cell carcinomas
Headache	Cataracts*
Isomorphic reaction	Melanonychia striata
Nausea	Photoaging
Pruritus	Pigmented macules ("PUVA lentigines")
Restlessness	Squamous cell carcinoma (especially
Vesiculation	genital squamous cell carcinoma)

* Documented in laboratory animals only.

cardiovascular stress. When young male patients with mild psoriasis (5% mean body surface area involvement) were exposed to the extreme conditions of a heat exercise test, they showed evidence for heat intolerance with a reduced sweat rate and reduced ability to dissipate extra heat compared to healthy volunteers [57]. PUVA therapy may place some patients with unstable angina at risk for myocardial infarction.

One of the most controversial issues of PUVA therapy is that of carcinogenesis. PUVA therapy has been shown to give rise to microscopic changes such as keratinocyte dysplasia. Epidermal changes similar to actinic keratoses occur during PUVA therapy [58]. The amount of PUVA administered to different individuals does not correlate with these effects and there may be an individual susceptibility to keratinocyte dysplasia from PUVA therapy. Whether or not these changes are permanent is uncertain. Histologic changes such as hyperkeratosis, acanthosis, melanosis, and focal dysplasia in the epidermis occur after PUVA therapy [59]. An increased deposition of acid mucopolysaccharides and a decrease in elastic fibers also occur [50]. Some of these findings may be irreversible because no change was noted on biopsies performed 3 years later.

Melanoma

Two patients developed cutaneous lesions of melanoma during or shortly after PUVA therapy [60].

In the 1380 patients enrolled in the PUVA followup study [61], three melanomas were diagnosed representing an incidence similar to what would be expected in the population at large. At the present time, it would seem that PUVA does not increase the background incidence of melanoma. Further studies are necessary to evaluate the possibility of PUVA-induced melanoma.

Squamous cell carcinoma

A 1.1% incidence of squamous cell carcinoma has been reported in patients undergoing long-term PUVA therapy [8]. Other researchers have noted a skin cancer incidence of 3.1% after PUVA therapy with squamous cell carcinoma representing the greatest proportion of cancers [62]. This is a greater incidence than that expected in the population at large. Patients undergoing high-dose PUVA therapy may have up to a 128 times greater risk of developing squamous cell carcinoma compared to patients receiving a lower cumulative dose [63]. Male patients who have undergone more than 200 PUVA treatments have an incidence of squamous cell carcinoma greater than 30 times that of the population at large [64]. Chuang and colleagues [65] found a sixfold increase in the incidence of invasive squamous cell carcinoma in patients receiving a cumulative UVA dose of more than $1000\,J/cm^2$. Patients in the low-dose group ($< 200\,J/cm^2$) had no more skin cancers than expected. No cases of genital cancer or melanoma were observed. Both men and women who have undergone extensive PUVA therapy may be at higher risk for respiratory cancer, and females may be at greater risk for colonic and renal cancer [64]. The usual relative incidence of one squamous cell for every three basal cell carcinomas is reversed by PUVA therapy. The time interval over which UVA is given, not just the total UVA dose, may be important in carcinogenesis, with longer treatment periods correlating with increased tumor production [66]. These observations, if confirmed, would make aggressive short-term treatment the method of choice for PUVA therapy. These observations may also, in part, explain the discrepancy between the European and American experience with PUVA carcinogenesis; the Europeans have noted a lower incidence of skin cancer and in general do treat their patients more aggressively [67].

Thirteen men in a prospective study of 892 men receiving PUVA therapy developed squamous cell carcinoma of genital skin [68]. These men had not routinely shielded the genital area during treatment; this exposure was hypothesized to explain why the risk of genital cancer in these men was 286 times higher than the incidence expected in an age- and sex-matched population. We have not seen a case of genital carcinoma in our PUVA patients, but we believe it is prudent to recommend genital protection during UV light treatment.

Basal cell carcinoma

The incidence of basal cell carcinoma in PUVA patients without other predisposing risk factors has not been found to be significantly increased over the normal population [64,65].

It would, therefore, seem that the main carcinogenic effect of PUVA therapy is noted as an increased production of actinic keratoses and squamous cell carcinomas, while the effect of PUVA on production of melanoma and basal cell carcinoma still needs to be clarified.

Connective tissue disease

Because PUVA therapy amplifies the effects of sunlight on the skin, many researchers have been concerned that PUVA therapy could cause connective tissue diseases such as lupus erythematosus. PUVA therapy can lead to SSA (Ro) expression in fibroblasts [69]. This may, in part, explain the phenomenon of antinuclear antibody (ANA) development during PUVA therapy [70]. There might be a statistically significant correlation between the duration of PUVA therapy and conversion from a negative to positive ANA test. A study of 1023 patients at 14 centers did not, however, show a higher incidence of ANA in PUVA patients than the population at large [71]. Other studies have suggested that the addition of etretinate could lower the expression of ANAs [72]. Whether connective tissue disease can ever be caused by PUVA is uncertain, but in practice this need not be a major concern. A report of subacute cutaneous lupus erythematosus developing during PUVA therapy likely represents exacerbation of a previously existing condition [73]. Testing for Ro antibodies in addition to the ANA before beginning PUVA can probably prevent such untoward reactions in most cases.

Miscellaneous

Vitiligo and bullous pemphigoid, both considered autoimmune diseases, have been associated with PUVA therapy [74,75]. Other conditions that may represent abnormal clones of epithelium such as disseminated superficial actinic porokeratosis [76], and multiple keratoacanthomas [77] have been reported (Table 13.7). The late onset of neurofibromas during PUVA treatment [78], myelomonocytic leukemia [79], evolution of myelodysplasia to acute myeloid leukemia [80], melanonychia striata [81], zosteriform acantholytic dyskeratotic epidermal nevus [82], and photoonycholysis [83] have also been observed.

The eye

In 1961, a study of guinea pigs injected with methoxsalen documented the development of "cataracts, devascularization of the iris, and abnormal dilatation of the pupil" upon exposure to long wave UV light [84]. Cataracts are opacifications of the lens of the eye. Surgery is needed to correct cataracts because the lens cannot regenerate [85]. To study whether or not 8-MOP binds to the lens in an irreversible fashion and leads to subsequent UV-induced damage to the lens and cataract formation, rat lenses were evaluated after 8-MOP administration [86]. Significant binding of the 8-MOP to the rat lens was noted. UV radiation alone can damage the lens of the eye and 8-MOP may enhance these UV-changes. Subsequent studies showed that free 8-MOP could be detected in human lenses up to 12 hours after a dose of 8-MOP was given [87].

If 8-MOP was exposed to UV light, irreversible binding to the lens occurred. If no photoactivation of the 8-MOP occurred, diffusion from the lens without appreciable binding was noted. The importance of proper UV eye protection therefore becomes obvious. If the lens is shielded from incident UVA exposure, 8-MOP (and presumably other psoralens) simply diffuse away without causing permanent sequelae.

Ordinary eyeglasses give little protection from incident UV radiation as compared to eyeglasses such as Noir, Blak-ray, and Polaroid (see Appendix,

Table 13.7 Rare associated findings of PUVA therapy

Acute myelomonocytic leukemia
Bullous pemphigoid
Disseminated superficial actinic porokeratosis
Hepatitis (elevation in liver function tests)
Keratoacanthoma
Melanoma
Melanonychia striata
Neurofibromas
Photoonycholysis
Subacute cutaneous lupus erythematosus
Vitiligo
Zosteriform acantholytic dyskeratotic epidermal nevus

Table 2) [88]. This table shows sources for UVA protective optical equipment. It is important to stress to patients that outdoor sunlight poses the greatest hazard for inducing lenticular changes during PUVA therapy. Indoor incandescent bulbs or daylight fluorescent bulbs may contribute to UVA exposure, but it is less important to protect lenses from indoor sources than outdoor sources. Some authors have suggested that protection from indoor light sources may even be unnecessary [89].

Adjunctive agents for oral PUVA

Numerous adjunctive therapies have been used with oral PUVA, including topical steroids, anthralin, emollients, methotrexate, etretinate, and UVB. The role of these adjunctive therapies is to hasten clearing of lesions while minimizing side effects.

Topical combination therapy

As soon as oral PUVA therapy became widely used, practitioners attempted to modify standard PUVA protocol to accelerate clearing of psoriasis (see Table 13.4). Topical corticosteroids produce a more rapid clearing, but recurrences of psoriasis may occur sooner (Fig. 13.5). When clobetasol propionate is used in conjunction with PUVA therapy, greater improvement is noted, but the rate and time of relapse is uncertain [90]. Topical coal tar treatment does not seem to reduce the time to clearing and should generally be avoided during PUVA phototherapy because a painful photosensitivity reaction known as "tar smarts" can occur [91]. Anthralin is clinically

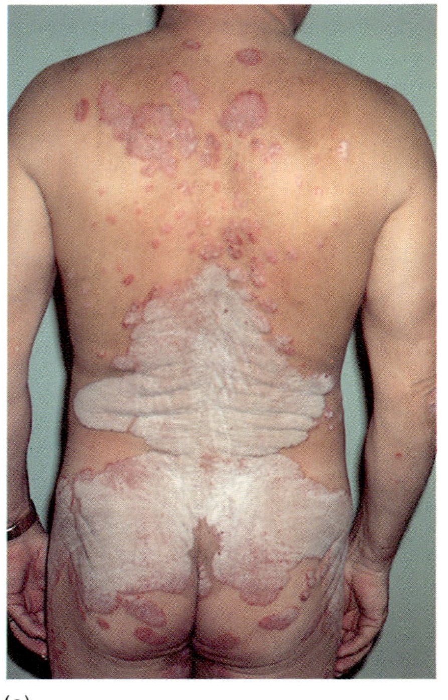
(a)

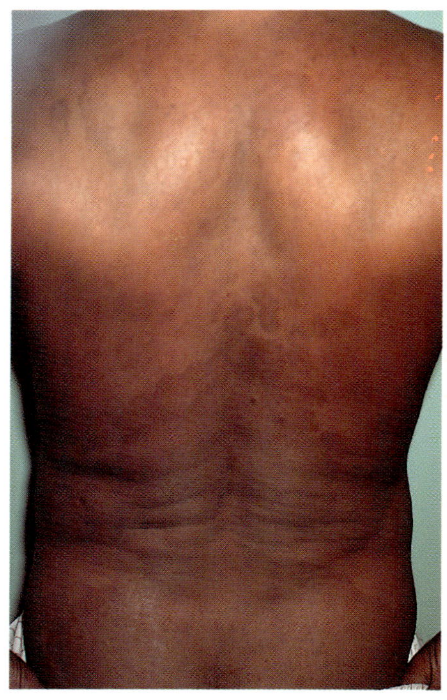
(b)

Fig 13.5 Severe plaque-type psoriasis cleared with topical steroids and psoralen UVA (PUVA) (a) before and (b) 4 months later, receiving PUVA maintenance.

useful [53], but patients are often noncompliant with this form of therapy in the outpatient setting because it is irritating and inelegant.

Systemic combination therapy

Methotrexate has been used to shorten the number of PUVA treatments necessary to clear extensive psoriasis. Methotrexate and PUVA doses can be kept considerably lower when both agents are used together as compared to either modality alone [92]. Whether this effect is additive or synergistic is not known. An interesting side effect noted by this combination therapy is enhanced phototoxicity in some patients. This effect is reminiscent of a UVB-methotrexate type of "recall" reaction. Lack of repigmentation of areas cleared of psoriasis was one of the side effects noted with this form of therapy. Both of these findings suggest that methotrexate may have an effect on normal melanocyte function.

The use of retinoids in conjunction with PUVA [93] (called "re-PUVA" treatment) appears to give the most encouraging results. Both acitretin and etretinate have been studied. All the patients in one study received 50 mg of acitretin or 50 mg of etretinate daily for 2 weeks prior to UVA exposure [94]. PUVA therapy was then started with a dosage of 25 mg of acitretin or 25 mg etretinate daily. UVA light was given three times weekly until remission was noted. Acitretin–PUVA treatment was much superior to placebo–PUVA treatment, and etretinate–PUVA showed some benefit over placebo–PUVA in terms of lesion score. Etretinate reaches peak effects after 3 weeks of therapy with conventional dosage regimens and only slow increases in UVA dosage are then possible because of enhanced phototoxicity. If PUVA and etretinate therapy are given at a dosage of 1 mg/kg per day and are started at the same time, effective doses of UVA for maximal PUVA response can be achieved earlier in treatment [93]. Eighty percent of patients are 100% cleared by the end of the sixth week of therapy by this method. Re-PUVA can reduce the number of treatments needed for clearing by up to one-third and decrease total PUVA cumulative dosage by up to one-fourth of what would be required by simple PUVA therapy alone [95].

5-MOP–oral PUVA has been used with retinoids in an analogous fashion to 8-MOP–PUVA. If etretinate is given at a dose of 0.5 mg/kg per day for 14 days prior to beginning PUVA with 5-MOP at a dosage of 1 mg/kg per day, excellent clearing of psoriasis is seen with a reduction in the total joules needed to achieve clinical remission [96]. This innovation may be superior to 8-MOP–re-PUVA because of the lower radiance of UVA needed to achieve clearance. When cyclosporine and etretinate were studied as adjunctive agents for PUVA therapy, etretinate was found to be more helpful [97].

UVB light has been used in combination with PUVA therapy. UVB light is thought to control the rapid proliferation of keratinocytes in psoriasis by producing thymine dimers in DNA [91]. The thymine dimers may inhibit DNA synthesis much like the photo-adducts formed during PUVA therapy. A study of conventional PUVA therapy and UVB light [98] revealed more rapid clearing of psoriasis on the PUVA–UVB-treated side of the body. Combined UVB and PUVA treatment may reduce total cumulative UV radiation needed to clear psoriasis, although further studies to gauge the side effects of such combination therapy are needed.

Topical PUVA

Topical PUVA has several theoretical advantages over oral PUVA. Small areas can be treated without subjecting uninvolved areas to unnecessary medicines, and systemic adverse effects can be kept to a minimum.

Topical PUVA has been used widely in the treatment of vitiligo. Combinations of the fruits of *Ammi majus* and *Ruta graveolens* were mixed together and applied to vitiligo by ancient Arabs [3]. The first report that topical PUVA was useful for the treatment of psoriasis came from Allyn at the 1962 annual meeting of the American Academy of Dermatology [4]. Unfortunately, this encouraging report was not immediately pursued. The modern use of topical psoralens has been pioneered by researchers in the Scandinavian countries. Vehicles for topical PUVA include cream, lotion, ointment, or bathwater delivery systems. Lotions and creams often give uneven distribution of the psoralen and are, therefore, less widely used than bathwater delivery [99].

Pharmacokinetics of topical psoralens

The degree of photosensitization achieved by a particular psoralen can differ when comparing oral and topical routes. Curiously, 8-MOP causes more photosensitivity than TMP when given orally, but TMP bath delivery leads to greater photosensitivity than 8-MOP bath delivery [100]. This may be due to greater lipid solubility of TMP [101].

After topical application of an alcohol-based 8-MOP solution, the stratum corneum contains 100 times more 8-MOP than the epidermis, indicating a significant barrier effect of the stratum corneum [99]. Nonetheless, topical 1% 8-MOP ointment can give rise to serum levels comparable to that of oral administration [102].

Generally, side effects such as nausea and cataract formation are absent with topical PUVA therapy [103] because of the usually low serum levels.

Mechanism of action of topical psoralens

The mechanism of action of topical PUVA therapy is analogous to oral PUVA. DNA cross-linking occurs and DNA synthesis is inhibited, thereby providing an antiproliferative effect to the skin. Patients seem to show photosensitivity only in the areas treated with the PUVA itself and do not show distant effects. 8-MOP is the most widely used psoralen for topical delivery in the USA. 8-MOP treatment can be given to the whole body by bathtub immersion or to localized areas such as the hands or feet by soaks in basins.

Bath PUVA for extensive psoriasis

Bathwater delivery of 8-MOP can be as effective as oral 8-MOP therapy, but requires up to fourfold less cumulative amounts of UVA dose to achieve clearing [90,104]. The protocol used by Lowe *et al.* involves the use of 8-MOP lotion (Oxsoralen 1% Lotion) [103]. Thirty milliliters of the Oxsoralen 1% lotion is added to 80 liters of bathwater at body temperature. The resultant 8-MOP concentration is 3.75 mg/l [103]. An alternative solution is made when 50 mg of Oxsoralen capsules are solubilized in hot water and added to the bath. The patient bathes for 15 min, is wiped dry, and is then given total body UVA irradiation at doses determined by skin type. Patients with type I skin are given 0.2 J/cm^2 and patients with type II are given 0.5 J/cm^2. UVA irradiation is increased as tolerated with subsequent treatments. Dosage increases are given at the same increments as with oral PUVA to make dosing easier for nursing staff. The maximal dose of UVA needed is usually between 1 and 2 J/cm^2 [105].

One simple method of preparing a psoralen bath is to add 15 ml of the 1% Oxsoralen Solution to 80 liters of bathwater to give a concentration of 1.875 mg/l. Because of this lower concentration, patients need to stay in the bathwater for 30 min to maximize photosensitization. A bathwater concentration of 2.64 mg/l with a 5-min immersion time has also been found to be effective [106].

It is not necessary for patients to wear protective UVA goggles on the day of the treatment. To ensure that the dosage of the clear Oxsoralen Lotion added to the bathwater is uniform, a food coloring dye can be added to the stock solution so that colorimetric indication of correct Oxsoralen Lotion dosing can be visually assessed grossly by nursing personnel.

Our patients have not experienced gastrointestinal side effects from this form of therapy, although erythema and pruritus have been noted by about one-third of patients. An occasional patient will notice a persistent photosensitivity even after 12 hours have elapsed since the time of bathing. Serum levels after local soaks of palmoplantar psoriasis approximated 1/40 the level of oral administration in one study [107]. In another study of 13 patients receiving 8-MOP bath delivery, 8-MOP levels were below the limit of detection of the HPLC assay (< 10 mg/ml) at every time point from 0.5 to 6 hours after treatment [106].

Trimethylpsoralen

Topical trioxsalen may be more effective than topical methoxsalen treatment [108]. The systemic effect of trioxsalen bath preparations is negligible, but histologic studies have shown Bowenoid changes as well as factor XIIIa-positive dendrocytes in the epidermis [109]. A challenge test of 25.2 J/cm^2 on an arm not treated by trioxsalen bath revealed no photosensitivity, nor did facial tanning develop during treatment, arguing against the development of significant systemic psoralen levels. Only one-tenth of the UVA dosage of systemic PUVA treatment is required with the bathwater delivery of

TMP [108]. This form of therapy shows great promise for selected patients with renal or hepatic failure or in those who cannot tolerate long treatment times.

The plasma concentrations after bathwater delivery of trioxsalen could not be detected at significant levels by some researchers [110]. On the other hand, some have noted blood concentrations of TMP after bath delivery, which were similar to those seen after oral dosing [111]. An unusual pattern of phototoxic burning has been reported, presumably from prolonged contact of undissolved TMP crystals with skin and bathtub, a problem resolved by changing positions while soaking and agitating the water [112].

5-Methoxypsoralen
5-MOP has not been used extensively for bathwater delivery of PUVA.

6-Methyl-angelicans
UVA light combined with topical 6-methyl-angelican treatment may prove superior to topical PUVA therapy according to one study. Pigmentation, but no phototoxicity, occurred with this regimen. The absence of phototoxicity was felt to provide a substantial advantage over topical PUVA [113].

Side effects of topical PUVA

The cutaneous side effects of topical PUVA therapy are much the same as oral therapy, although allergic contact or photocontact reactions may occur [114]. Gastrointestinal side effects are not seen, and cataract formation from topical PUVA has not been reported, to our knowledge. Even though systemic absorption may be small, we do not treat pregnant or lactating patients with this therapy.

Bathtubs need to be filled and cleaned, and this makes extensive treatment with bath PUVA impractical for most private practitioners. Bathwater PUVA, however, can be efficiently used in the treatment of localized palmoplantar pustulosis or palmoplantar psoriasis (Fig. 13.6).

Bath PUVA for localized palmar or plantar disease

A simple regimen is to add 0.4 ml of 8-MOP 1% solution (Oxsoralen 1% Lotion) to 1.5 liters of lukewarm bathwater (Table 13.8). The bathwater should have a temperature of approximately 37–38°C. The patient bathes the involved extremity in the resultant 3.7 mg/l 8-MOP solution for 30 min (Fig. 13.7) and then receives UVA with a starting dose of 0.5 J/cm^2 (Fig. 13.8). Alternatively, 1 ml of 1% Oxsoralen Lotion may be dissolved in 2 liters of water and the patient soaks for 30 min [107]. The irradiance is then increased at 0.25 J/cm^2 per treatment as tolerated, until clearing occurs. Treatments are given two to three times weekly. Although a fluorescent light source (F40T12BL) may be used, good results have also been reported with high-pressure metal halide lamps (Dermalight 2001).

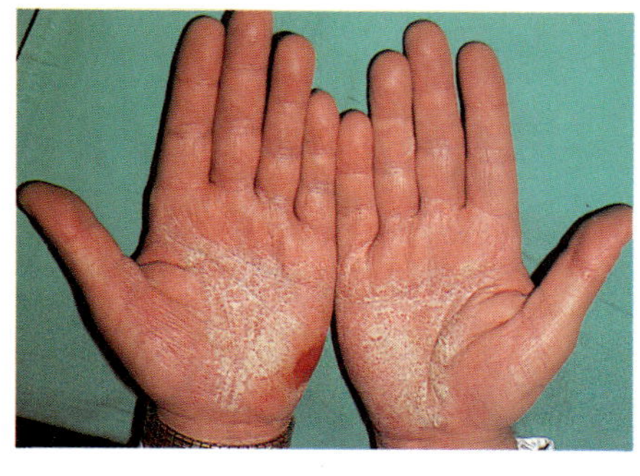

(a)

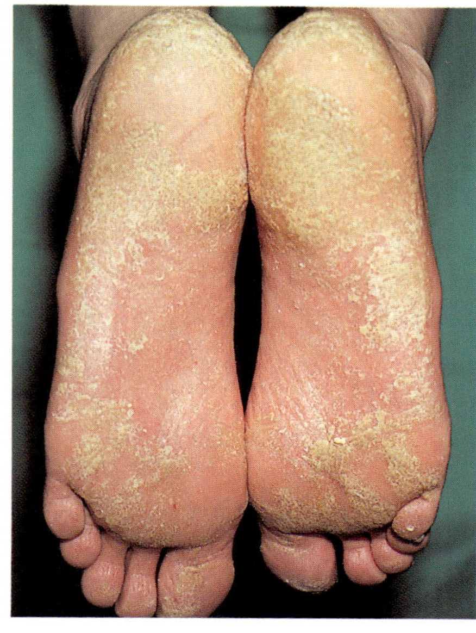

(b)

Fig 13.6 (a) and (b). Palmoplantar psoriasis (same patient), an ideal candidate for bathwater psoralen UVA.

Table 13.8 8-Methoxypsoralen bath water treatment of hand–foot involvement

Add 0.4 ml of 1% 8-methoxypsoralen solution (Oxsoralen 1% lotion) to 1.5 l lukewarm bathwater at 36–38°C.
Soak hands for 30 min
Pat hands dry
Give 1 J/cm^2 and increase by 0.25–0.5 J/cm^2 as tolerated
Two or more light treatments can be given on different occasions after one soak in selected cases, because of persistence of 8-MOP adducts in the skin

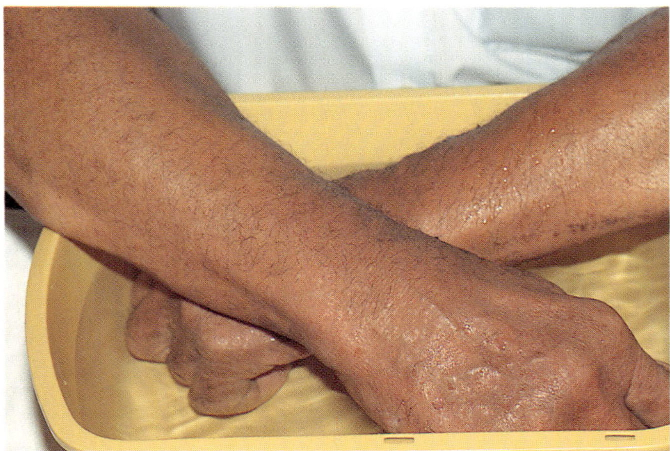

Fig 13.7 Soaking hands in 8-methoxypsoralen solution as part of bathwater psoralen UVA treatment.

If one treatment is missed, the dose is held at the previous irradiance. If two treatments are missed, the dose is decreased by one-half of the initial dose. If three treatments are missed, the UVA is decreased by the amount of the initial dose (unless it is the second treatment in which case the dose

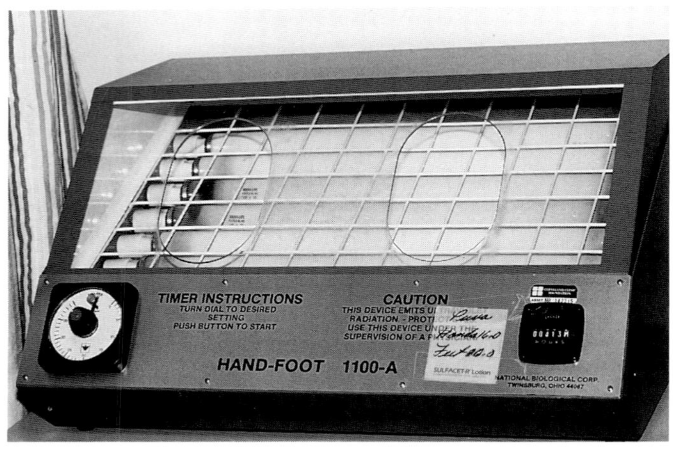

Fig 13.8 Hand/foot unit for localized UVA exposures.

is repeated). If more than three treatments are missed, the physician is reconsulted.

An interesting effect of topical bathwater delivery is that photosensitivity can last for up to 72 hours. Topical PUVA may lead to the production of mono-adducts, which are cleared slowly from the skin. UVA irradiation can still provoke sensitivity days after soaking [115].

This observation suggests that several UVA exposures can be given after one bathwater treatment with psoralens, and this approach has been used in the treatment of a patient with palmoplantar eczema [116]. This method frees up time for the nurses and patients because a 30 min soak can be omitted. The expense of the psoralen solution is also spared. It is likely that similar adjustments in the interval of bathwater delivery will be useful in the treatment of palmoplantar psoriasis. Other dermatologists have used TMP for bathwater delivery of PUVA in cloudy seasons in order to use the greater photosensitization of TMP to hasten clearance. 8-MOP is used at other times when unwanted phototoxic reactions are more likely to occur. Not all researchers have found topical PUVA to be superior to placebo in the treatment of palmoplantar pustulosis [117], but this may depend on the type of topical formulation used.

Combination therapies used with bath PUVA

Just as with oral PUVA, various adjunctive therapies have been used with bath PUVA to speed clearing of psoriasis. Adjunctive agents include emollients, topical steroids, and retinoids. The addition of etretinate at a dosage of 1 mg/kg per day can enhance the effects of bath PUVA [118]. The only side effects noted were redness. The lower UVA dosage needed to attain clearing of psoriasis makes this an excellent treatment for psoriatic lesions. Other authors have noted similar enhanced clearing in patients treated with topical PUVA and etretinate compared to topical PUVA alone [72]. It does not seem to matter whether the retinoid administered is acitretin or etretinate because both give comparable results when used with bath PUVA [119]. Acitretin is theoretically of greater utility because its short half-life

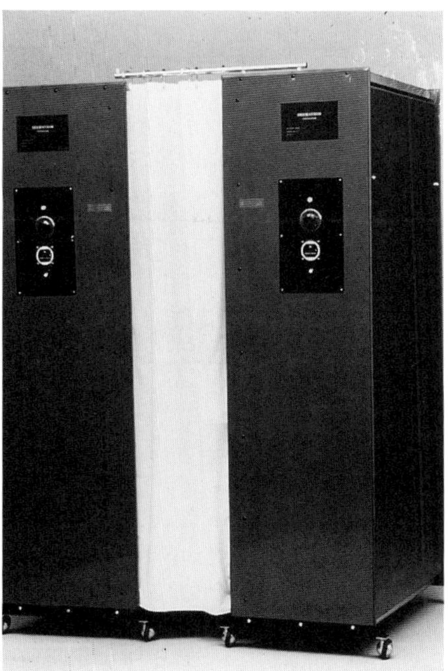

Fig 13.9 Psoralen UVA therapy cabinet.

may make this therapy safe for women who want future pregnancies (as long as they defer pregnancy for at least 2 years after stopping treatment), because the possibility of long-acting metabolites must still be considered.

Light sources

Although the ancient herbalists used psoralens in conjunction with sunlight, one cannot count on a continuing reproducible amount of UVA in most areas. Various artificial indoor light sources are most commonly used to produce UVA. These sources include continuous emission fluorescent sunlamps, black light units, xenon and carbon arcs, and high pressure mercury arc lamps.

The fluorescent sunlamp and black light units use low pressure mercury vapor, which emits 254 nm radiation. Special substances known as phosphors are used to coat the glass tube containing the gas, and these phosphors absorb the emitted radiation and re-emit the radiation at a longer wavelength. The F40 T12 PUVA lamp is a commonly used light source capable of readily inducing a minimally perceptible phototoxic erythema [120]. Most fluorescent UVA systems have a peak emission at 352 nm, but units with peak emission at about 325 nm may prove more effective [121]. One study showed clearing of psoriasis with PUVA at 335 nm to be twice as effective as irradiation at 365 nm [122].

Arc light sources work by ionizing gases between electrodes of different potential. Carbon arcs have the ability to emit various wavelengths of light depending upon which metals have been added to the carbon electrode. Because of their smoke emission and variable output, carbon arcs are not used for PUVA. Mercury and xenon arcs also have a greater risk of causing retinal burns in the unprotected eye. High pressure mercury light sources have limited field sizes and, therefore, have practical limitations for PUVA therapy. High pressure halide light sources have the benefit of relatively high energy output, but have a broad spectrum which may incorporate unwanted wavelengths. Various filters can be used to give irradiance with the desired wavelengths.

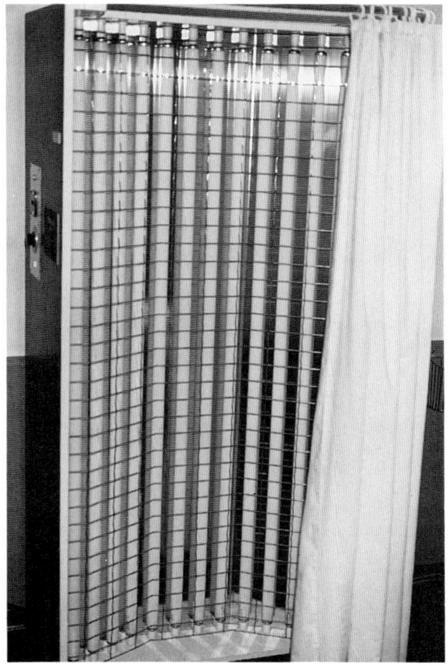

Fig 13.10 Dermatron unit with semicircular configuration.

The type of phototherapy unit needed for a particular office varies not only with the patient volume being seen, but also by the space available. A list of manufacturers is included in the Appendix (Table 3). For the practitioner who sees a substantial number of patients with psoriasis, a phototherapy cabinet allows for rapid and accurate UVA exposure (Fig. 13.9). Units that consist of one panel of lights on coasters may be suitable for practitioners who treat only occasional patients with phototherapy, because in those instances the time needed for the different fields of exposure does not slow the flow of patients through the office (Fig. 13.10). Although some units operate by timers, units that automatically convert settings in joules to the resultant time of irradiance (calculated for the output on that particular unit) allow for easy standardization of therapy. In this way an accurate calculation of the total irradiance a particular patient has received can be maintained, and if the patient goes elsewhere for further treatment, light exposure at a similar irradiance can be continued without fear of a phototoxic reaction.

Many of the small units have similar control panels allowing for dosimetry in joules. Obtaining a unit that can administer both UVA and UVB is most economical for smaller practices with limited space.

Most practitioners feel that fluorescent systems for the delivery of UVA light are of greatest utility, because the fluorescent bulbs are relatively inexpensive, easily exchanged for ones with different phosphors (should a different emission wavelength be desired) and relatively cool. A chart of various UVA fluorescent bulbs available in the USA has been included for review (see Appendix, Table 3).

One of the main problems with fluorescent bulbs is that UV intensity varies with vertical height, with areas near the floor or top of the UV cabinet showing less UV intensity than areas in the center [100]. High pressure mercury halide systems show a greater vertical uniformity than fluorescent systems [123]. If areas on the lower legs are not responding to treatment as expected in a fluorescent UVA cabinet, shorter patients may benefit from standing on a foot stool during treatment in order to increase UVA irradiance to the legs. Radiometry units are available to ensure adequate UVA irradiance (see Appendix, Table 4).

New types of photochemotherapy

Photodynamic therapy is a relatively new treatment modality which uses a photosensitizer and light to produce a photobiologic effect. The most frequently used photosensitizer is a hematoporphyrin derivative. Because cancerous tissues seem to most readily retain this compound [124], photodynamic therapy is most frequently used to combat cancer.

Sn-protoporphyrin has shown usefulness in psoriasis treatment. The authors administered Sn-protoporphyrin followed by UVA light in 10 patients with good response [125,126].

Extracorporeal photopheresis is a newly-developed technique in which the patient ingests psoralens in the usual way and white blood cells are removed from the body, irradiated with UVA, and then returned to the circulation. This treatment is most commonly used for the leukemic phase of cutaneous T cell lymphoma (Sézary syndrome). Extracorporeal photopheresis has also been used to treat patients with psoriatic arthritis. Four of the five patients treated had moderate to slight improvement in their joint disease, but the skin lesions unfortunately did not appear to change [127]. Another patient showed moderate improvement of both skin and arthropathy [128]. A pilot study indicates that extracorporeal photopheresis does have a beneficial effect on cutaneous psoriasis [129]. Because of its expense and complexity of delivery, the practical utility of this therapy for severe psoriasis vulgaris and arthritis will have to await trials with sham-treatment controls.

SUMMARY

PUVA therapy is a safe and effective form of treatment for psoriasis. After conventional topical therapies or UVB light have failed, PUVA therapy should be considered as the next step for treatment of psoriasis. Relative contraindications to PUVA include concomitant photosensitivity diseases, cutaneous squamous cell carcinoma, and cataracts. Bathwater delivery shows much promise for localized disease. Bath treatment for extensive disease is as effective as oral PUVA but is more cumbersome and time consuming. Localized bathwater delivery of PUVA to the palms and soles is the treatment of choice for recalcitrant palmoplantar psoriasis and palmoplantar pustulosis.

CASE STUDIES

Case 1

Long-term PUVA, multiple squamous cell carcinomas, and recalcitrant pustular psoriasis precipitated by wound infections.

A 68-year-old white woman with psoriasis for 40 years was referred to the Cleveland Clinic in November 1990 6 weeks after sustaining a PUVA burn administered at another clinic. She complained of pain from the burn on the skin of her back, shoulders, and chest. She also had a history of a squamous cell carcinoma on the back of the left leg which had been excised and grafted. The past treatments of her psoriasis consisted of the Goeckerman regimen during the 1950s and 1960s. She received methotrexate from 1972 to 1976. PUVA therapy was started in 1979 and used intermittently with fair results. Etretinate was combined with PUVA starting in 1980. Topical corticosteroids have been given with some improvement. She denied ever receiving arsenic compounds or exposure to ionizing radiation.

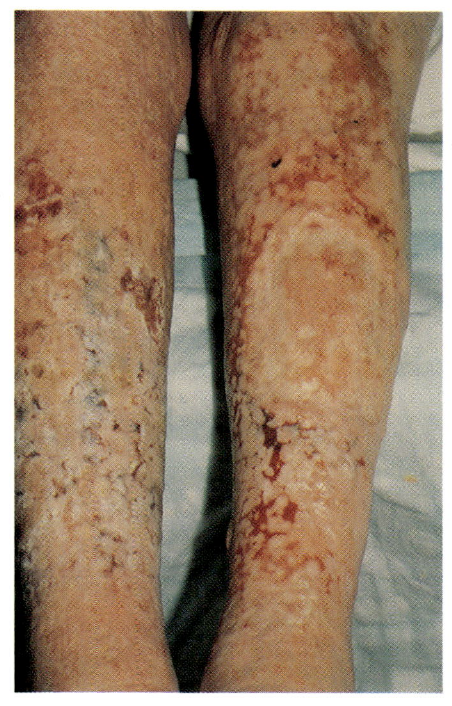

Fig 13.11 Case 1. Cobblestone appearance of shins showing superficially eroded plaques on right and graft site on left.

Examination showed mottled erythema of the extensor surfaces of legs and arms. There was a 5 × 4 cm crusted nodule with ulcerations on the left shin. There were discrete and confluent scaly indurated erythematous plaques distributed over the trunk and extremities. All the nails were dystrophic and pitted. The anterior tibial surfaces had a pebbly appearance. There was a 4 × 3 cm shallow ulceration on the right pretibial area (Fig. 13.11).

A skin biopsy from the dorsum of the left foot revealed mildly active psoriasis. Biopsies from the edges of both tibial ulcerations revealed infiltrating squamous cell carcinoma. Surface wound cultures from the ulcerations revealed Pseudomonas *species and* Staphylococcus aureus *that was resistant to methicillin.*

She was treated with ciprofloxacin 500 mg b.i.d. and intravenous vancomycin 1 g every 24 hours for 2 weeks, daily povidine–iodine whirlpools, 1% ichthammol dressings to the ulcerations and 0.1%

anthralin ointment for the psoriasis. The anthralin caused intolerable irritation of the normal skin and was discontinued. She was then treated with 1% hydrocortisone ointment.

She was readmitted in January 1991. Her psoriasis became steadily worse as she was using only intermediate potency topical corticosteroids. Examination showed confluent yellow crusted papules and erosions of the upper extremities with minute white pustules. There were numerous red papules and erosions of the trunk and weeping erosions and pustules on the back. There were no oral lesions. Cultures of the leg ulcerations continued to show moderate Gram-negative and Gram-positive species. This was considered to be a pustular flare of psoriasis with secondary skin infection. She was given another course of intravenous antibiotics and was started on etretinate 75 mg daily. The pustulation ceased rapidly, and she was then treated with daily povidine–iodine whirlpools, emolliation, and fluocinonide ointment 0.05% to the plaques on the arms and back. The yellow crusts over the psoriatic plaques were gently debrided with warm water baths and aluminum subsulfate compresses three times daily for 1 week. Excisions of both the right and left lower leg tumors were performed by the plastic surgeon. Histopathology revealed in situ *and infiltrating well-differentiated squamous cell carcinomas in both specimens with clear margins. Split-thickness skin grafts were placed over both legs but did not take. The patient developed secondary infection of the wounds with purulent discharge and low-grade fever. More appropriate antibiotics were given.*

During the next 3 months, she continued to have pustular flares. Etretinate was discontinued. She was next treated with wet compresses, mild topical steroids, and PUVA treatments to the arms and trunk three times per week. She tolerated the PUVA treatments well. Calcitriol (vitamin D_3) 0.5 μg at bedtime was started. Another infiltrating squamous cell carcinoma was identified on the right medial calf and was treated as before. This time the graft took well and the psoriasis was well-controlled.

She was discharged and followed in the outpatient clinic where her psoriasis was maintained with PUVA at 4 J/cm^2 three times weekly and later reduced to twice weekly. The reepithelializing areas of the lower legs were not exposed to the UV light. The dose of calcitriol was increased to 0.75 μg daily. The serum calcium remained stable at 9.5 mg%, but the 24-hour urinary excretion of calcium rose from 56 to 200 mg. The serum creatinine increased gradually from a baseline of 1.1 to 1.9 mg%. Calcitriol was discontinued. Subsequent flares of psoriasis have been marked by extensive painful erosions on the trunk and extremities with erythematous weeping papules and scaly plaques on the scalp and dorsal aspects of the feet. Additional skin biopsies have shown epithelial hyperplasia with spongiform pustules consistent with psoriasis. The dose of PUVA was reduced and eventually discontinued. There has been no recurrence or new development of squamous cell carcinoma. The current regimen consisting of 0.1% triamcinolone ointment, dicloxacillin 250 mg daily, zinc oxide *ointment to erosions and oral supplements of iron, zinc, vitamin C, and vitamin E seems to maintain the skin disease and control the pain.*

Comments

1 This patient had five cutaneous squamous cell carcinomas on the legs. She had received tar, and UVB treatments for decades and more than 10 years of PUVA. Thus, while the cumulative dose of UVA could not be calculated, she probably falls into the "high dose" category (>750–1000 J/cm^2) increasing the risk of developing squamous cell carcinoma five to 50 times that of the general population [64,66].

2 After many years of UV exposure and the use of topical corticosteroids, the skin of an elderly person can become quite atrophic, irritable, and recalcitrant to further topical approaches.

3 The cutaneous squamous cell carcinomas were intermingled with biopsy-proven psoriasis. The ulcerations on the legs were probably secondary to the tumors, but erosions elsewhere on the body evolved from pustular lesions of psoriasis.

4 The ulcerations, surgical wounds, and graft sites were often colonized or frankly infected with pathogenic bacteria which might have precipitated the pustular flares.

5 Etretinate at 1.1 mg/kg per day was relatively ineffective at preventing the pustular flares.

6 The empiric use of calcitriol 0.75 μg/day did not provide any benefit, but the dose may have been too low. Pincus and Holick [130] routinely used doses of 1.5–2.0 μg daily without observing any renal toxicity. This patient's urinary calcium excretion increased but remained within the normal range. The cause for the rising creatinine was not determined.

7 After eradication of local squamous cell carcinomas, we were faced with recalcitrant pustular and erosive psoriasis. PUVA was restarted along with conservative local measures and gave an excellent response. The legs, where the cancers had occurred, were not exposed until reepithelialization was complete.

8 The current unconventional combination of topicals, low-dose antibiotic prophylaxis, and oral vitamin and mineral supplements have provided as much relief to the patient as any other treatment previously tried. This provides evidence that creative trial and error approaches, spontaneous remissions and good fortune are sometimes as important in the management of difficult cases of psoriasis as any double-blind study cited in this book.

Case 2

Phototoxic reaction from PUVA combined with doxycycline.

An 86-year-old white woman with a history of chronic lymphocytic leukemia, atrial fibrillation, atherosclerotic disease, and emphysema had a 1½-year history of psoriasis. Her psoriasis was controlled with PUVA

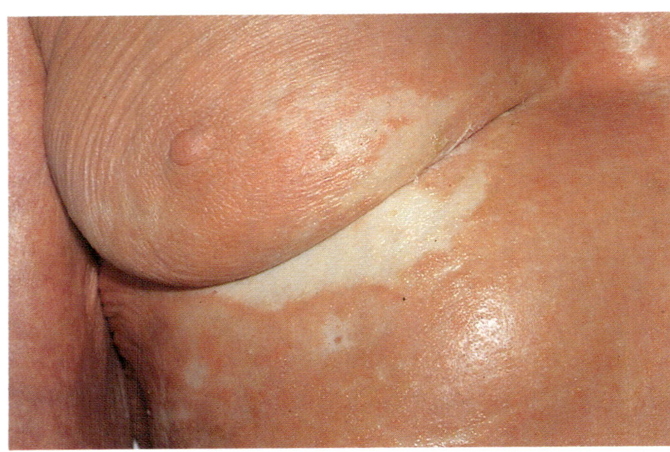

Fig 13.12 Case 2. Phototoxic reaction with sparing of skin under the breast.

treatments given three times weekly. When she developed an upper respiratory infection, her family physician prescribed doxycycline 100 mg twice daily. She did not report her new medication to the technician and her PUVA treatments were continued as per her usual routine. After each of the next three PUVA treatments, she was noted to have increasingly marked erythema of the body skin but did not admit to taking any new drugs even upon direct questioning.

She was admitted to hospital 2 days after the last PUVA treatment. She brought the bottle of capsules disclosing the identity of doxycycline. Examination of the skin showed diffuse erythroderma with sparing of body folds and the submammary areas (Fig. 13.12). There was severe pitting edema of the tibia and ankles (Fig. 13.13). She also had bilateral ectropions and conjunctivitis for which she was given erythromycin ophthalmic ointment. She was managed conservatively with twice-daily oilated colloidal oatmeal whirlpool baths, wet saline compresses, 1% hydrocortisone ointment, and leg elevation. Her recovery was slow but otherwise uneventful.

Her psoriasis was subsequently treated with methotrexate at a dosage of 7.5 mg weekly. Fluocinolone acetonide solution 0.01% and coal tar shampoo have been used to control scalp involvement. The use of a broad-spectrum sunscreen (Parsol 1789 and Padimate-0) has been recommended when outdoors. There has been no "recall phenomenon" of the previous phototoxic reaction while taking methotrexate, and except for occasional nausea, she is doing well.

Comments

This case illustrates some pitfalls in communication that can occur when treating a patient with PUVA. An elderly patient with multiple medical problems who was taking many other medications was given doxycycline, one of the most phototoxic drugs in the tetracycline class with an action spectrum in the UVA range. The prescriber did not notify the dermatologic consultant, nor did the patient volunteer this information prior to her next

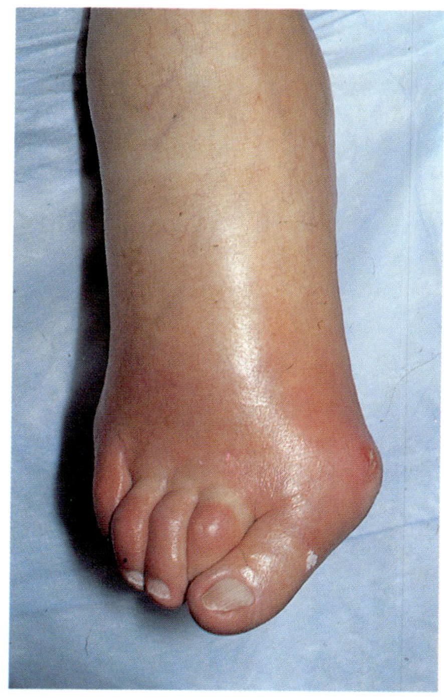

Fig 13.13 Severe edema of dorsum of foot and ankle associated with erythema of forefoot.

PUVA treatment. She did not admit to taking doxycycline upon direct questioning even after she complained of a burn. She apparently believed the prescription to be no more than a "cold medicine."

Phototoxic drugs would theoretically produce a cutaneous reaction in all patients if a sufficient concentration was achieved in skin, which was then exposed to the appropriate wavelengths and intensity of light [131]. Phototoxic reactions to doxycycline have been shown to be dose-related. Of 106 patients being treated for acne, 20% of patients taking 150 mg doxycycline daily developed a rash in a light-sensitive distribution compared to 42% receiving 200 mg daily [132]. Other commonly prescribed drugs that may absorb in the UVA band, besides 8-MOP and the tetracyclines, include the phenothiazines, thiazides, furosemide, quinidine, quinine, piroxicam, sulfonamides, sulfonylureas, and amiodarone [131,133].

REFERENCES

1 El Mofty AM. *Vitiligo and Psoralens*. New York: Pergamon Press, 1968:1–5.
2 Benedetto AV. The psoralens: an historical perspective. *Cutis* 1977;20:469–71.
3 Fahmy IR, Abu-Shady H. The isolation and properties of ammoidin, ammidin, and majudin, and their effect in the treatment of leukoderma. *Q J Pharm* 1948;21: 449–503.
4 Anderson TF, Voorhees JJ. Psoralen photochemotherapy of cutaneous disorders. *Annu Rev Pharmacol Toxicol* 1980;20:235–57.
5 Lerner AB, Denton CR, Fitzpatrick TB. Clinical and experimental studies with 8-methoxypsoralen in vitiligo. *J Invest Dermatol* 1953;20:299–314.
6 Parrish JA, Fitzpatrick TB, Tanenbaum L, Pathak MA. Photochemotherapy of psoriasis with oral methoxsalen and longwave ultraviolet light. *N Engl J Med* 1974;291:1207–11.
7 Wolff K, Fitzpatrick TB, Parrish JA, *et al*. Photochemotherapy for psoriasis with orally administered methoxsalen. *Arch Dermatol* 1976;112:943–50.
8 Roenigk HH Jr, Farber EM, Storrs F, *et al*. Photochemotherapy for psoriasis: a clinical cooperative study of PUVA 48 and PUVA 64. *Arch Dermatol* 1979;115: 576–9.
9 Henseler T, Honigsmann H, Wolff K, Christopher E. Oral 8-methoxypsoralen photochemotherapy of psoriasis. The European PUVA study: a cooperative study among 18 European centres. *Lancet* 1981;i:853–7.
10 Melski JW, Tanenbaum L, Parrish JA, *et al*. Oral methoxsalen photochemotherapy for the treatment of psoriasis. A cooperative clinical trial. *J Invest Dermatol* 1977;68:328–35.
11 Pathak MA. Mechanisms of psoralen photosensitization reactions. *Natl Cancer Inst Monogr* 1984;66:41–6.
12 Shi YB, Hearst JE. Wavelength dependence for the photoreactions of DNA-psoralen monoadducts. 1. Photoreversal of monoadducts. *Biochemistry* 1987;26: 786–98.
13 Kaidbey K. Wavelength dependence for DNA synthesis inhibition in hairless mouse epidermis. *Photodermatology* 1988;5:65–70.
14 Caffieri S, Daga A, Vedaldi D, Dall'Acqua F. Photo-addition of angelicin to linolenic acid methyl ester. *J Photochem Photobiol* 1988;2:515–21.
15 Gasparro FP, Dall'Amico R, Goldminz D, Simmons E, Weingold D. Molecular aspects of extracorporeal photochemotherapy. *Yale J Biol Med* 1989;62:579–93.
16 Malinin GI, Lo HK, Hornicek FJ, Malihin T. Ultrastructural modifications of the plasma membrane in HUT 102 lymphoblasts by long-wave ultraviolet light, psoralen

and PUVA. *J Invest Dermatol* 1990;95:97–103.
17 Ortel B, Gange RW. An action spectrum for psoralen cross-link formation in human skin *in vivo*? *J Invest Dermatol* 1989;92:495A.
18 Trevisan G, Magaton-Rizzi, Dal Canton M. Psoriatic micro-angiopathy modifications induced by PUVA and etretinate therapy. A nail-fold capillary microscopic study. *Acta Derm Venereol* 1989;146(Suppl.):53–7.
19 Kokelj F, Presani G. Evaluation of the serum T cell population variations induced by PUVA therapy. *Acta Derm Venereol* 1989;146(Suppl.):208–10.
20 Larmi E. PUVA treatment inhibits nonimmunologic immediate contact reactions to benzoic acid and methyl nicotinate. *Int J Dermatol* 1989;28:609–11.
21 Toyota N, Kitamura Y, Ogawa K. Administration of 8-methoxypsoralen and ultraviolet A irradiation (PUVA) induces turnover of mast cells in the skin of C57BL6 mice. *J Invest Dermatol* 1990;95:353–8.
22 Yang XY, Gasparro FP, Deleo VA, Santella RM. 8-methoxypsoralen-DNA adducts in patients treated with 8-methoxypsoralen and ultraviolet A light. *J Invest Dermatol* 1989;92:59–63.
23 Viander M, Jansen CT, Eskola J. Influence of whole body PUVA treatments on human peripheral blood NK cell activity. *Photodermatology* 1984;1:23–9.
24 Kruger JP, Christophers E, Schlaak M. Dose effects of 8-methoxypsoralen and UVA in cultured human lymphocytes. *Br J Dermatol* 1978;98:141–4.
25 Oxholm A, Oxholm P, Staberg B, Bendtzen K. Interleukin-6 in the epidermis of patients with psoriasis before and during PUVA treatment. *Acta Derm Venereol* 1989;69:195–9.
26 Moss C, Friedmann PS, Shuster S. How does PUVA inhibit delayed cutaneous hypersensitivity? *Br J Dermatol* 1982;107:511–6.
27 Koulu LM, Jansen CT. Antipsoriatic, erythematogenic, and Langerhans cell marker depleting effect of bath-psoralens plus ultraviolet A treatment. *J Am Acad Dermatol* 1988;18:1053–9.
28 Virvidakis KE, Brokalakis JD, Singhellakis PN, Mountokalakis TD. Effect of PUVA on intestinal calcium absorption. *Br J Dermatol* 1988;118:219–21.
29 de Wolff FA, Thomas TV. Clinical pharmacokinetics of methoxsalen and other psoralens. *Clin Pharmacokinetics* 1986;11:62–75.
30 Herfst MJ, DeWolff FA. Influence of food on the kinetics of 8-methoxypsoralen in serum and suction blister fluid in psoriatic patients. *Eur J Clin Pharmacol* 1982; 23:75–80.
31 Goldstein DP, Carter DM, Ljuggren B, Burkholder J. Minimal phototoxic doses and 8-MOP plasma levels in PUVA patients. *J Invest Dermatol* 1982;78:429–33.
32 Walther T, Haustein U, Quednow B, Meyer FP. Pharmakokinetischer vergleich von drei 8-methoxypsoralen-praparaten und klinische aspekte. *Hautarzt* 1990;41: 317–21.
33 Siddiqui AH, Stolk LML, Cormane RH. Comparison of serum levels and clinical results of PUVA therapy with three different dosage forms of 8-methoxypsoralen. *Arch Dermatol Res* 1984;276:343–5.
34 Stolk LM, Siddiqui AH. Biopharmaceutics, pharmacokinetics, and pharmacology of psoralens. *Gen Pharmacol* 1988;19:649–53.
35 McLelland J, Fisher C, Farr PM, Diffey BL, Cox NH. The relationship between plasma psoralen concentration and psoralen-UVA erythema. *Br J Dermatol* 1991; 124:585–90.
36 Lowe NJ, Urbach F, Bailin P, Weingarten DP. Comparative efficacy of two dosage forms of oral methoxsalen in psoralens plus ultraviolet A therapy of psoriasis. *J Am Acad Dermatol* 1987;16:994–8.
37 Chakrabarti SG, Grimes PE, Minus HR, Kenney JA, Pradhan TK. Determination of trimethylpsoralen in blood, ophthalmic fluids, and skin. *J Invest Dermatol* 1982;79:374–7.

38 Pathak MA, Marciani MS, Guiotto A, Rodighiero G. A study of the relationship between photosensitizing and phototherapeutic activity of 4,5,8-trimethyl psoralen, and its major metabolite 4,8-dimethyl, 5-carboxypsoralen. *J Invest Dermatol* 1983;81:533–9.
39 Tanew A, Ortel B, Rappersberger K, *et al.* 5-methoxypsoralen (Bergapten) for photochemotherapy. *J Am Acad Dermatol* 1988;18:333–8.
40 Herfst MJ, de Wolff FA. Intra-individual and inter-individual variability in 8-methoxypsoralen kinetics and effect in psoriatic patients. *Clin Pharmacol Ther* 1983;34:117–24.
41 Stern RS, Lange R. Outcomes of pregnancies among women and partners of men with a history of exposure to methoxsalen photochemotherapy (PUVA) for the treatment of psoriasis. *Arch Dermatol* 1991;127:347–50.
42 Ranki A, Puska P, Krohn K. Effect of PUVA on immunologic and virologic findings in HIV infected patients. *J Am Acad Dermatol* 1991;24:404–10.
43 Buchness MR, Lin HW, Hatcher VA, Sanchez M, Soter NA. Eosinophilic pustular folliculitis in the acquired immunodeficiency syndrome. Treatment with ultraviolet B phototherapy. *N Engl J Med* 1988;318:1183–6.
44 Bisaccia E, Berger C, Klainer AS. Extracorporeal photopheresis in the treatment of AIDS-related complex: a pilot study. *Ann Int Med* 1990;113:270–5.
45 Vonderheid EC, Bigler RD, Rogers TJ, Kadin ME, Griffin TD. Effect of extracorporeal photopheresis on selected immunologic parameters in psoriasis vulgaris. *Yale J Biol Med* 1989;62:653–4.
46 Jones SK, Moseley H. Clear UV lenses: cosmetically acceptable spectacles for PUVA patients. *Br J Dermatol* 1990;123:58–9.
47 Carabott FM, Hawk JLM. A modified dosage schedule for increased efficiency in PUVA treatment of psoriasis. *Clin Exp Dermatol* 1989;14:337–40.
48 Bruynzeel I, Bergman W, Hartevelt HM, *et al.* "High single dose" European PUVA regimen also causes an excess of non-melanoma skin cancer. *Br J Dermatol* 1991;124:49–55.
49 Cox NH, Farr PM, Diffey BL. A comparison of the dose–response relationship for psoralen–UVA erythema and UVB erythema. *Arch Dermatol* 1989;125: 1653–7.
50 Souetre E, Salvati E, Belugou JL, *et al.* 5-methoxypsoralen as a specific stimulating agent of melatonin secretion in humans. *J Clin Endocrinol Metab* 1990;71:670–4.
51 Ros AM, Wennersten G. PUVA therapy for photosensitive psoriasis. *Acta Derm Venereol* 1987;67:501–5.
52 Gupta AK, Anderson TF. Psoralen photochemotherapy. *J Am Acad Dermatol* 1987;17:703–34.
53 Morison WL, Parrish JA, Fitzpatrick TB. Controlled study of PUVA and adjunctive topical therapy in the management of psoriasis. *Br J Dermatol* 1978;98:125–32.
54 Pariser DM, Wyles RJ. Toxic hepatitis from oral methoxsalen photochemotherapy (PUVA). *J Am Acad Dermatol* 1980;3:248–50.
55 Nyfors A, Dahl-Nyfors BD, Hopwood D. Liver biopsies from patients with psoriasis related to photochemotherapy (PUVA): findings before and after one year of therapy in 12 patients. A blind study and review of literature on hepatotoxicity of PUVA. *J Am Acad Dermatol* 1986;14:43–8.
56 Chappe SG, Roenigk HH Jr, Miller AJ, Beeaff DE, Tyrpin L. Effective photochemotherapy on the cardiovascular system. *J Am Acad Dermatol* 1981;4:561–5.
57 Leibowitz E, Seidman DS, Laor A, *et al.* Are psoriatic patients at risk of heat intolerance? *Br J Dermatol* 1991;124:439–43.
58 Cox AJ, Able EA. Epidermal dystrophy: occurrence after psoriasis therapy with psoralen and long wave ultraviolet light. *Arch Dermatol* 1979;115:567–70.
59 Ingraham DM, Bergfeld WF, Bailin PL, Steck WD, Taylor JS, Tomecki KJ. Long-term or short-term histopathologic changes in the skin after PUVA therapy.

Cleveland Clin Q 1983;50:133–9.

60 Marx JL, Auerbach R, Possick P, Myrow R, Gladstein AH, Kopf AW. Malignant melanoma *in situ* in two patients treated with psoralens and ultraviolet A. *J Am Acad Dermatol* 1983;9:904–11.

61 Gupta AK, Stern RS, Swanson NA, Anderson TF. Cutaneous melanomas in patients treated with psoralens plus ultraviolet A: a case report and the experience of the PUVA follow-up study. *J Am Acad Dermatol* 1988;19:67–76.

62 Salisbury JA, Glover M, Leigh IM, Baker H. The PUVA-associated squamous cell carcinoma: a distinct clinicopathological entity. *Br J Dermatol* 1990;123:65.

63 Stern RS, Laird N, Melski J, *et al.* Cutaneous squamous cell carcinoma in patients treated with PUVA. *N Engl J Med* 1984;310:1156–61.

64 Lindelof B., Sigurgeirsson B, Tegner E, *et al.* PUVA and cancer: a large scale epidemiological study. *Lancet* 1991;338:91–3.

65 Chuang T-Y, Heinrich LA, Schultz MD, *et al.* PUVA and skin cancer. A historical cohort study on 492 patients. *J Am Acad Dermatol* 1992;26:173–7.

66 Stern RS, Lange R and Members of the Photochemotherapy Follow-up Study. Non-melanoma skin cancer occurring in patients treated with PUVA five to ten years after first treatment. *J Invest Dermatol* 1988;91:120–4.

67 Wolff K. Side-effects of psoralen photochemotherapy (PUVA). *Br J Dermatol* 1990;122:117–25.

68 Stern RS and Members of the Photochemotherapy Follow-up Study. Genital tumors among men with psoriasis exposed to psoralens and ultraviolet A radiation (PUVA) and ultraviolet B radiation. *N Engl J Med* 1990;322:1093–7.

69 Wollina U, Beensen H, Kittler L, Schaarschmidt H, Knopf B. PUVA treatment of human cultured fibroblasts from psoriatic skin enhances the binding of antibodies to SSA (Ro). *Arch Dermatol Res* 1987;279:206–8.

70 Kubba R, Steck WD, Clough JD. Antinuclear antibodies and PUVA photochemotherapy. *Arch Dermatol* 1981;117:474–7.

71 Stern RS, Morison WL, Thibodeau LA, *et al.* Antinuclear antibodies and oral methoxsalen photochemotherapy (PUVA) for psoriasis. *Arch Dermatol* 1979;115:1320–4.

72 Takashima A, Sunohara A, Matsunami E, Mizuno N. Comparison of therapeutic efficacy of topical PUVA, oral etretinate, and combined PUVA and etretinate for the treatment of psoriasis and development of PUVA lentigines and antinuclear antibodies. *J Dermatol* 1988;15:473–9.

73 Dowdy MJ, Nigra TP, Barth WF. Subacute cutaneous lupus erythematosus during PUVA therapy for psoriasis. *Arthritis Rheum* 1989;32:343–6.

74 Todes-Taylor N, Abel EA, Cox AJ. The occurrence of vitiligo after psoralens and ultraviolet A therapy. *J Am Acad Dermatol* 1983;9:526–32.

75 Robinson JK, Baughman RD, Provost TT. Bullous pemphigoid induced by PUVA therapy: is this the aetiology of the acral bullae produced during PUVA treatment? *Br J Dermatol* 1978;99:709–13.

76 Hazen PG, Carney JF, Walker AE, Stewart JJ, Engstrom CW. Disseminated superficial actinic porokeratosis: appearance associated with photochemotherapy for psoriasis. *J Am Acad Dermatol* 1985;12:1077–8.

77 Sina B, Adrian RM. Multiple keratoacanthomas possibly induced by psoralens and ultraviolet A photochemotherapy. *J Am Acad Dermatol* 1983;9:686–8.

78 Nishimura M, Hori Y. Late onset neurofibromas developed in a patient with psoriasis vulgaris during PUVA treatment. *Arch Dermatol* 1990;126:541–2.

79 Freeman K, Warin AP. Acute myelomonocytic leukaemia developing in a patient with psoriasis treated with oral 8-methoxypsoralen and longwave ultraviolet light. *Clin Exp Dermatol* 1985;10:144–6.

80 Sheehan-Dare RA, Cotterill JA, Barnard DL. Transformation of myelodysplasia to acute myeloid leukaemia during psoralen photochemotherapy (PUVA) treatment

of psoriasis. *Acta Derm Venereol* 1989;69:262–4.
81 Weiss E, Sayegh-Carreno R. PUVA: induced pigmented nails. *Int J Dermatol* 1989;28:188–9.
82 van der Wegen-Keijser MH, Prevoo RL, Bruynzeel DP. Acantholytic dyskeratotic epidermal naevus in a patient with guttate psoriasis on PUVA therapy. *Br J Dermatol* 1991;124:603–5.
83 Warin AP. Photoonycholysis secondary to psoralen use (Letter). *Arch Dermatol* 1979;115:235.
84 Cloud TM, Hakin R, Griffin AC. Photosensitization of the eye with methoxsalen. *Arch Ophthalmol* 1961;66:689–94.
85 Farber EM. Psoralen and ultraviolet A (PUVA) — a critique. *J Am Acad Dermatol* 1980;2:342–4.
86 Lerman S, Borkman RF. A method for detecting 8-methoxypsoralen in the ocular lens. *Science* 1977;23:1287–8.
87 Lerman S, Megaw J, Willis I. Potential ocular complications from PUVA therapy and their prevention. *J Invest Dermatol* 1980;74:197–9.
88 Wennersten G. Photoprotection of the eye in PUVA therapy. *Br J Dermatol* 1978;98:137–9.
89 Morison WL, Strickland PT. Environmental UVA radiation and eye protection during PUVA therapy. *J Am Acad Dermatol* 1983;9:522–5.
90 Gould PW, Wilson L. Psoriasis treated with clobetasol propionate and photochemotherapy. *Br J Dermatol* 1978;98:133–6.
91 Harber LC, Bickers DR. *Photosensitivity Diseases: Principles of Diagnosis and Treatment*, 2nd edn. Philadelphia: BC Decker Inc., 1989.
92 Morison WL, Momtaz K, Parrish JA, Fitzpatrick TB. Combined methotrexate-PUVA therapy in the treatment of psoriasis. *J Am Acad Dermatol* 1982;6:46–51.
93 Darouti E, Al Rubaie A. Psoriasis treatment with RePUVA in the United Arab Emirates. *Int J Dermatol* 1988;27:593–5.
94 Saurat JH, Geiger JM, Amblard P, *et al.* Randomized double-blind multicenter study comparing acitretin-PUVA, etretinate-PUVA, and placebo-PUVA for the treatment of psoriasis. *Dermatologica* 1988;177:218–24.
95 Fritsch PO, Honigsmann H, Jaschke E, Wolff K. Augmentation of oral methoxsalen photochemotherapy with an oral retinoic acid derivative. *J Invest Dermatol* 1978; 70:178–82.
96 Lane-Brown M. 5-methoxy psoralen, etretinate, and UVA for psoriasis. *Int J Dermatol* 1987;26:655–9.
97 Petzelbauer P, Honigsmann H, Langer K, *et al.* Cyclosporin A in combination with photochemotherapy (PUVA) in the treatment of psoriasis. *Br J Dermatol* 1990; 123:641–7.
98 Park YK, Kim HJ, Koh YJ. Combination of photochemotherapy (PUVA) and ultraviolet B (UVB) in the treatment of psoriasis vulgaris. *J Dermatol* 1988;15: 68–71.
99 Fischer T. Topical psoralen ultraviolet radiation. In Roenigk HH Jr, Maibach HI, eds. *Psoriasis*. New York: Marcel Dekker, Inc., 1985:633–644.
100 Fischer T, Alsins J. Treatment of psoriasis with trioxsalen bath and dysprosium lamps. *Acta Derm Venereol* 1976;56:383–90.
101 Vaatainen N. Phototoxicity of topical trioxsalen. *Acta Derm Venereol* 1980;60: 327–31.
102 Neild VS, Scott LV. Plasma levels of 8-methoxypsoralen in psoriatic patients receiving topical 8-methoxypsoralen. *Br J Dermatol* 1982;106:199–203.
103 Lowe' NJ, Weingarten D, Bourget T, Moy LS. PUVA therapy for psoriasis: comparison of oral and bath water delivery of 8-methoxypsoralen. *J Am Acad Dermatol* 1986;14:754–60.
104 Collins P, Rogers S. Bath-water compared with oral delivery of 8-methoxypsoralen

PUVA therapy for chronic plaque psoriasis. *Br J Dermatol* 1992;127:392–5.
105 Fitzpatrick TB. *Yearbook of Dermatology*. St Louis: Mosby-Yearbook Inc., 1990: 302–3.
106 Thomas SE, O'Sullivan J, Balac N. Plasma levels of 8-methoxypsoralen following oral or bath-water treatment. *Br J Dermatol* 1991;125:56–8.
107 Coleman WR, Lowe NJ, David M, Halder RM. Palmoplantar psoriasis: experience with 8-methoxypsoralen soaks plus ultraviolet A with the use of a high-output metal halide device. *J Am Acad Dermatol* 1989;20:1078–82.
108 Hannuksela M, Karvonen J. Trioxsalen bath plus UVA effective and safe in the treatment of psoriasis. *Br J Dermatol* 1978;99:703–7.
109 Pierard-Franchimont C, Nickels-Read D, Ben Mosbah T, Arrese Estrada J, Pierard GE. Early dermato-pathological signs during bath-PUVA therapy. *J Pathol* 1990; 161:227–31.
110 Fischer T, Hartvig P, Bondesson U. Plasma concentrations after bath treatment and oral administration of trioxsalen. *Acta Derm Venereol* 1979;60:177–9.
111 Ros AM, Wennersten G, Wallin I, Ehrsson H. Concentration of trimethylpsoralen in blood and skin after oral administration. *Photodermatology* 1988;5:121–5.
112 George SA, Ferguson J. Unusual patterns of phototoxic burning following trimethylpsoralen (TMP) bath photochemotherapy (PUVA) (Letter). *Br J Dermatol* 1992; 127:444–5.
113 Cristofolini M, Recchia G, Boi S, *et al.* 6-Methylangelicins: new monofunctional photochemotherapeutic agents for psoriasis. *Br J Dermatol* 1990;122:513–24.
114 Takashima A, Yamamoto K, Kimura S, Takakuwa Y, Mizuno N. Allergic contact and photocontact dermatitis due to psoralens in patients with psoriasis treated with topical PUVA. *Br J Dermatol* 1991;124:37–42.
115 Gange RW, Anderson RR. Topical (bathwater) PUVA therapy. *J Am Acad Dermatol* 1987;16:401–2.
116 Helm TN, Dijkstra JWE. Topical (bathwater) PUVA therapy. *J Am Acad Dermatol* 1991;24:1035.
117 Layton AM, Sheehan-Dare R, Cunliffe WJ. A double-blind, placebo-controlled trial of topical PUVA in persistent palmoplantar pustulosis. *Br J Dermatol* 1991; 124:581–4.
118 Vaatainen N, Hollmen A, Fraki JE. Trimethylpsoralen bath plus ultraviolet A combined with oral retinoid (etretinate) in the treatment of severe psoriasis. *J Am Acad Dermatol* 1985;12:52–5.
119 Lauharanta J, Geiger JM. A double blind comparison of acitretin and etretinate in combination with bath PUVA in the treatment of extensive psoriasis. *Br J Dermatol* 1989;121:107.
120 Cole CA, Forbes PD, Davies RE. Different biologic effectiveness of black light fluorescent lamps available for therapy with psoralens plus ultraviolet A. *J Am Acad Dermatol* 1984;11:599–606.
121 Farr PM, Diffey BL, Higgins EM, Matthews JN. The action spectrum between 320 and 400 nm for clearance of psoriasis by psoralen photochemotherapy. *Br J Dermatol* 1991;124:443–8.
122 Brucke J, Tanew A, Ortel B, Honigsmann H. Relative efficacy of 335 and 365 nm radiation in photochemotherapy of psoriasis. *Br J Dermatol* 1991;124:372–4.
123 Chue B, Borok M, Lowe NJ. Phototherapy units: comparison of fluorescent ultraviolet B and ultraviolet A units with a high-pressure mercury system. *J Am Acad Dermatol* 1988;18:641–5.
124 Russo AR, Mitchell JB, Pass HI, Glatstein EJ. Photodynamic therapy. In Devita VT, Hellman S, Rosenberg SA, eds. *Cancer, Principles and Practice of Oncology*, Philadelphia: JB Lippincott, 1989:2449–59.
125 Emtestam L, Berglund L, Angelin B, Kappas A. Treatment of psoriasis vulgaris with a synthetic metalloporphyrin and UVA light. *Acta Derm Venereol* 1989;146

(Suppl.):107–10.

126 Emtestam L, Berglund L, Angelin B, Drummond GS, Kappas A. Tin-protoporphyrin and long wavelength ultraviolet light treatment of psoriasis. *Lancet* 1989;i: 1231–3.

127 Wilfert H, Honigsmann H, Steiner G, Smolen J, Wolff K. Treatment of psoriatic arthritis by extracorporeal phototherapy. *Br J Dermatol* 1990;122:225–32.

128 DeMisa RF, Azana JM, Harto A, Ledo A. Extracorporeal photochemotherapy in the treatment of severe psoriatic arthropathy (Letter). *Br J Dermatol* 1992;127:448.

129 Vonderheid EC, Kang C, Kadin M, Bigler RD, Griffin TD, Rogers TJ. Extracorporeal photopheresis in psoriasis vulgaris: clinical and immunologic observations. *J Am Acad Dermatol* 1990;23:703–12.

130 Pincus S, Holick M. 1,25-Dihydroxyvitamin D_3: rationale for its use in the treatment of psoriasis. In Roenigk HH Jr, Maibach HI, eds. *Psoriasis*, 2nd edn. New York: Marcel Dekker, Inc., 1991:791–807.

131 Harber LC, Bickers DR. *Photosensitivity Diseases. Principles of Diagnosis and Treatment.* Toronto: BC Decker Inc., 1989:160–202.

132 Layton AM, Cunliffe WJ. Photosensitive eruptions to doxycycline — a dose related phenomenon. *Br J Dermatol* 1992;127(Suppl. 40):31(Abstract).

133 Bickers DR, Epstein JH, Fitzpatrick TB, *et al.* Risks and benefits from high-intensity ultraviolet A sources used for cosmetic purposes. *J Am Acad Dermatol* 1985;12:380–1.

fourteen Retinoids

INTRODUCTION

Retinoids are compounds naturally or synthetically derived from vitamin A (retinol). Their effects on skin are similar to those of vitamin A, namely, antiinflammatory, antikeratinizing, and antiproliferative. Indeed, the systemic toxicity of retinoids, with certain exceptions, is that of hypervitaminosis A. The advent of synthetic retinoids for dermatologic therapy was welcomed by all clinicians with anticipation and excitement. Because the possible modifications of the vitamin A molecule's three main building units (the cyclic end group, the polyene side-chain, and the polar end group; Fig. 14.1) seemed unlimited, the potential for synthesizing retinoids suitable for many diseases existed. Hoffmann-La Roche [1] has screened over 2500 retinoids in mice with the goal of dissociating therapeutic action from the toxic effects of hypervitaminosis A using a chemically induced skin papilloma model.

Retinoid	Chemical structure	Therapeutic index
All-*trans*-retinoic acid (tretinoin)	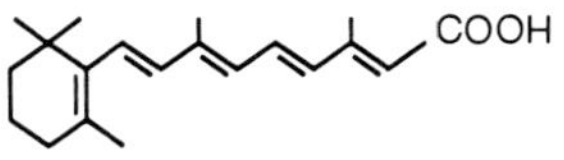 COOH	0.2
13-*cis*-retinoic acid (isotretinoin)	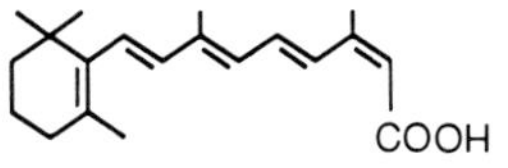 COOH	0.5
Etretinate	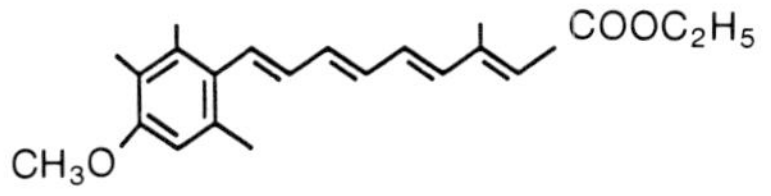 $COOC_2H_5$, CH_3O	2.0
Acitretin	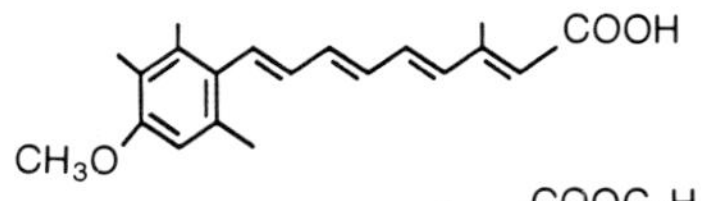 COOH, CH_3O	2.0
Arotinoid ethylester	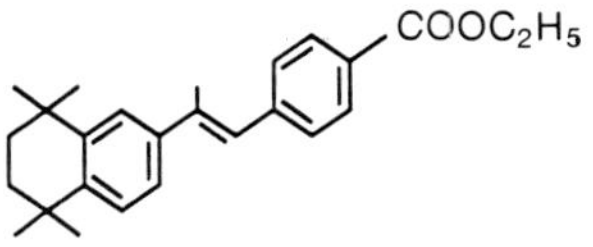 $COOC_2H_5$	2.0

Fig 14.1 Chemical structures and therapeutic indices of selected retinoids.

The "first-generation" of retinoids are those compounds resulting from manipulation of the polar end group of the polyene side-chain, such as all-*trans*-retinoic acid (tretinoin) and 13-*cis*-retinoic acid (isotretinoin). Topical tretinoin cream is modestly effective for psoriasis but is impractical because it irritates the skin. Its most significant efficacy has been found in the treatment of acne, actinic keratoses, and solar lentigines ("liver spots"). Systemic isotretinoin is most effective for severe forms of acne producing longlasting remission in 85% of patients. It also temporarily improves inherited disorders of keratinization such as Darier's disease (keratosis follicularis) and lamellar ichthyosis, but has very limited value in the treatment of psoriasis (*vide infra*). Isotretinoin cream 0.1% did not improve psoriasis in one placebo-controlled trial [2].

The "second generation" of retinoids results from replacing the cyclic end group with a series of ring systems. The best known example is the *p*-methoxytrimethylphenyl ethyl ester analog of retinoic acid (etretinate), which was approved by the Food and Drug Administration (FDA) for psoriasis in 1986. Its first-order metabolite, acitretin, has been intensively investigated for psoriasis and is apparently therapeutically equivalent to etretinate.

The "third generation" of retinoids consists of analogs with various forms of cyclization of the polyene side-chain including the arotinoids or benzoic acid derivatives of retinoic acid. Arotinoid ethyl ester is 8000 times more potent than tretinoin in the papilloma regression assay but also 800 times more active in causing hypervitaminosis A. It has been used successfully to treat recalcitrant psoriasis in limited trials [3,4].

The initial optimism with which the retinoids were received — comparisons to the "corticosteroid era" of medicine were made — has been dampened by problems with teratogenicity in general and a particularly long terminal half-life of etretinate. The therapeutic results with etretinate and acitretin in psoriasis have been good to excellent, especially in combination with other conventional treatments. With the exception of teratogenicity, the side effects, while numerous, are generally not serious. The disappointments have been with monotherapy, lack of a durable remission, and the fact that after more than 20 years of retinoid research, only two systemic drugs have been approved in the USA; only etretinate is indicated for psoriasis. A new *in vitro* assay of retinoid effects on human keratinocyte cultures has been developed that may be more relevant for predicting activity in the treatment of psoriasis [5]. Keratin profiles and the extent of envelope formation are assessed. The order of activity was similar in both assays: arotinoid ethyl ester $\geq$ arotinoid acid $\gg$ all-*trans*-retinoic acid $>$ acitretin $\geq$ etretinate.

MECHANISM OF ACTION

It has not been elucidated how synthetic retinoids improve psoriasis. In order for retinoids to have biologic effects, there must be uptake from the plasma by cells, transport and metabolism in the cytoplasm, and interaction with receptors in the nucleus. Isotretinoin, which is very effective for acne yet weakly active in psoriasis vulgaris, reduces sebaceous gland size and inhibits sebocyte proliferation. Isotretinoin also inhibits the conversion of retinol to dehydroretinol in epithelia. The aromatic retinoids do not exert any of these effects. Neither isotretinoin nor the aromatic retinoids alter plasma retinol levels.

Antiinflammatory effects of retinoids have been demonstrated. For example, they inhibit neutrophil functions *in vitro* such as lysosomal enzyme release, superoxide anion production [6], antibody-dependent cytotoxicity [7], as well as chemotaxis in the skin chamber and Boyden chamber techniques in the presence of serum [8]. Topical and systemic administration of retinoids reduces the intraepidermal accumulation of polymorphonuclear leukocytes after epicutaneous application of leukotriene B_4 (LTB_4) [9]. Systemic administration of acitretin to hairless rats increased epidermal interleukin-1 (IL-1) levels as measured by both the lymphocyte activating factor assay and the stimulation of prostaglandin E_2 (PGE_2) release from dermal fibroblasts [10]. The cytostatic effect of IL-1 seems to be associated with a decrease in ornithine decarboxylase activity. In psoriasis, there is a decrease in epidermal IL-1 and increased polyamine synthesis. Kaplan *et al.* [11] showed that etretinate therapy of psoriasis significantly reduced epidermal polyamine levels after 4 weeks before measuring any significant expected decrease in epidermal DNA synthesis; this action might be responsible in part for the subsequent clinical improvement.

CLINICAL USE

Efficacy

Bioavailability of the 40 mg isotretinoin (Accutane-Roche) capsule is 25%. Peak blood concentrations occur at 2–3 hours after ingestion. The blood concentration profile after oral administration can be described with a linear two-compartment pharmacokinetic model. The terminal elimination half-life ranges from 10 to 20 hours. 4-Oxo-isotretinoin is the major metabolite found in blood and urine of patients on chronic therapy. After 6 hours, blood concentrations of the metabolite exceed those of the parent drug. The apparent half-life of the 4-oxo compound ranges from 11 to 50 hours. Enterohepatic circulation may be a component of isotretinoin pharmacokinetics. Isotretinoin is 99.9% bound to plasma albumin. Tissue distribution of ^{14}C-isotretinoin in rats after oral dosing revealed maximum concentrations in many tissues after 1 hour. In most tissues, radioactivity was undetectable after 24 hours, but low levels remained in the liver after 7 days [12].

Etretinate (Tegison-Roche) has an absolute bioavailability of 40% following oral administration of the capsule that is significantly increased when taken with whole milk or a high lipid diet [13]. Peak plasma concentrations occur at about 4 hours. The carboxylic acid metabolite acitretin is formed by enzymatic hydrolysis of the ester in the gut, liver, and blood. Etretinate undergoes significant first-pass metabolism to acitretin prior to reaching the systemic circulation. Therefore, the first-order metabolite acitretin is detectable in the blood before etretinate and exceeds the concentration of the latter parent drug.

After single-dose oral administration the apparent half-life for elimination of etretinate and acitretin is 6–13 hours; however, during chronic therapy, because etretinate is stored in adipose tissue, the terminal half-life is approximately 120 days. The data are consistent with a linear pharmacokinetic model with a deep peripheral compartment.

Following the oral administration of a single 100 mg dose of ^{3}H-etretinate to human volunteers, 75 and 15% of the radioactivity appeared in the feces and urine, respectively. In the feces, 80% of the radioactivity was unchanged drug (60% of the dose) while the remaining activity was unidentified metabolites. In a study of 47 patients receiving long-term etretinate therapy, seven had detectable serum drug levels (0.5–12 ng/ml) 2.1–2.9 years after discontinuing therapy. For comparison, during a 6-month course of treatment with doses ranging from 25 to 100 mg daily, the maximum serum concentrations ranged from 102 to 389 ng/ml [12]. Patients with a greater amount of body fat tended to have higher serum concentrations and slower elimination of etretinate. Etretinate is more than 99% bound to plasma proteins, mainly lipoproteins, and acitretin is predominantly bound to albumin. Animal studies indicate biliary excretion, enterohepatic circulation, and substantial uptake of etretinate by the liver. Liver concentrations of etretinate in patients receiving the drug for 6 months were generally higher than concomitant plasma concentrations and tended to be higher in livers with moderate or severe fatty infiltration [14].

Acitretin, the main active metabolite of etretinate, was developed to avoid the accumulation in adipose tissue and the slow elimination after discontinuation of the parent drug. The bioavailability of acitretin is 60% and is markedly increased with food intake [15]. Peak plasma concentration is reached 2–6 hours after ingestion. During repeated dosing, the steady state plasma concentration of 13-*cis*-acitretin is higher than all-*trans*-acitretin; the relatively short half-lives of acitretin (about 50 hours) and its 13-*cis*-isomer (75 hours) are such that within 3 weeks of cessation of therapy neither can be detected in plasma (< 5 ng/ml). A new high performance liquid chromatography assay (with a solid phase extraction step) on blood samples taken 8 weeks following the last dose of acitretin detected etretinate in some patients. Hoffmann LaRoche is conducting further studies to elucidate the origin and pharmacologic significance of this startling discovery.

Studies

Both etretinate and acitretin were shown to be significantly superior in efficacy to placebo in the treatment of psoriasis in double-blind studies. In most studies of plaque-type psoriasis, good to excellent (> 50% clearing) results were reported in 70–80% of patients after 4–6 months of continuous treatment [7,11,16–19]. Clinical improvement became significant after 8 weeks of therapy in a dose-dependent fashion. The optimal dose was 0.6–0.7 mg/kg per day, equivalent to 50–75 mg/day. All patients showed mucocutaneous side effects with dose-dependent severity. A maintenance dose is necessary because psoriasis generally relapses 2–3 months after discontinuation of therapy.

The aromatic retinoids are also effective for generalized pustular, palmoplantar pustular [20], and erythrodermic psoriasis [21]. In one study etretinate at 0.75 mg/kg per day was much more efficacious than isotretinoin 1.5 mg/kg per day for chronic plaque psoriasis in achieving moderate to complete control [21]. However, in generalized pustular psoriasis isotretinoin (1.5–2.0 mg/kg per day) was effective in 10 of 11 patients with rapid abatement of pustulation and systemic symptoms. Additional therapy was required to induce complete clearing. In some cases, etretinate has improved symptomatic psoriatic arthropathy with decreased pain and stiffness, such that less antiinflammatory medication was required.

In order to achieve a greater therapeutic effect with lower toxicity, the retinoids have been combined with UVB or psoralen UVA (PUVA). The rationale is that the desquamation and thinning of psoriatic plaques produced by retinoids would bring about a more rapid response to UV radiation. The combination of acitretin 50 mg daily for 12 weeks and suberythemogenic UVB t.i.w. was superior to acitretin alone, which was superior to UVB plus placebo. The UVB plus acitretin-treated group received a lower cumulative UV dose than the UVB plus placebo group [22]. In another trial, more aggressive UVB was combined with a lower dose of acitretin (25–35 mg/day) or placebo [23]. At the end of 8 weeks, 60% of patients in the combination group and 24% in the control group attained 75% clinical improvement. The median cumulative UVB energy received was 6.9 J/cm^2 vs 11.8 J/cm^2, or 40% less in the combination group for the same degree of improvement [23].

Photochemotherapy (PUVA) has been combined with etretinate, acitretin, or isotretinoin as concurrent treatment or with prior retinoid treatment, also known as re-PUVA. Dubertret *et al.* [16] "cleared" 36 of 37 patients with the combination of etretinate 1 mg/kg per day and PUVA t.i.w. in less than 10 weeks. After skin clearing, PUVA was given once weekly for 2 months to two groups who were randomized to receive either etretinate 0.5 mg/kg per day or placebo as maintenance treatment for 1 year. In the event of relapse (> 50% of the initial score), the treatment was stopped. The authors found that six of 16 (38%) relapsed in the etretinate group compared to 15 of 20 (75%) in the control group. They further showed that etretinate maintenance mainly benefited patients who cleared rapidly, i.e., requiring less than 18 PUVA irradiations.

The combination of PUVA–etretinate (0.6 mg/kg per day) was more effective than either PUVA or etretinate alone in recalcitrant palmoplantar pustulosis, clearing 78% of the sites compared to 25 or 17%, respectively [24]. No untreated site cleared. Relapses generally occurred within 1–3 months after stopping treatment. When acitretin 1 mg/kg per day or placebo was given for 5 days alone before initiating PUVA four times weekly and continuing the combination, complete clearing or marked improvement occurred in 22 of 23 (96%) and 20 of 25 (80%) patients, respectively. The acitretin–PUVA group required 29% less exposures and a 42% lower cumulative UVA dose than the placebo–PUVA group [25]. Similarly, when lower dosages of acitretin (50 mg then 25 mg daily) or placebo were given prior to and during PUVA, significantly more patients achieved 75% improvement in the acitretin–PUVA group (70% vs 40%) yet required a lower total UVA dose. The acitretin–PUVA combination was superior to placebo–PUVA in the treatment of severe palmoplantar psoriasis. Acitretin 25 mg/day was given for 3 weeks before starting PUVA and continued. Re-PUVA utilizing isotretinoin 0.5–1 mg/kg per day for 1 week prior to initiation of PUVA may be as effective as etretinate plus PUVA in one study [26] but this conclusion is not supported by another [27].

Ethyl ester plus arotinoid acid

Several successful therapeutic trials with the arotinoid ethyl ester and its metabolite arotinoid acid have been reported for psoriasis. These drugs may have pronounced antiinflammatory effects on psoriatic arthropathy and do not seem to produce significant elevations of serum lipids. Two patients experienced complete clearing of severe generalized psoriasis and improved joint function after 8 weeks of treatment with arotinoid ethyl ester 1–2 μg/kg per day [3]. The efficacy of etretinate 10–50 mg daily was compared to arotinoid ethyl ester 0.06–0.1 mg daily in the same group of 17 psoriatics; good to excellent results were initially achieved in 76% vs 65%, respectively [28]. Typical retinoid mucocutaneous side effects required reduction of the arotinoid dose and therefore reduction in efficacy. Psoriatic arthropathy was not improved.

Subsequently, 32 patients with psoriasis were treated in an open uncontrolled trial with arotinoid ethyl ester at a starting dose of 1 μg/kg per day [5]. Again, 66% of patients achieved a good to excellent response, but the joints of three patients with active psoriatic arthropathy improved. The main metabolite of arotinoid ethyl ester, arotinoid acid, is intriguing because it has the highest affinity for human skin retinoic acid binding protein. In the treatment of 12 psoriatics with arotinoid acid as monotherapy, seven patients improved and there was no change in five [29]. At therapeutic doses, it seemed more likely to cause retinoid dermatitis than cheilitis or peeling of palms and soles. Arotinoid acid also improved three patients with psoriatic arthropathy.

In the studies reported with arotinoids, there have been no significant alterations of serum triglycerides or cholesterol including 10 patients treated for 33–130 weeks. Diffuse idiopathic skeletal hyperostosis (DISH)-like changes of the spine developed in one patient after maintenance treatment with arotinoid ethyl ester for 2 years. However, the patient also had fusion of the sacroiliac joints and prior treatment with etretinate suggesting other possible etiologies for the skeletal changes. It appears that the arotinoids exert similar therapeutic effects in psoriasis and psoriatic arthritis at tolerable doses as etretinate and acitretin. However, there seems to be an even more narrow margin in the dosage of arotinoids between efficacy and mucocutaneous toxicity. Confirmation that long-term skeletal toxicity may occur is lacking. The chief advantage to these compounds is the apparent dissociation between mucocutaneous effects and alterations of lipid metabolism, but more controlled studies with larger numbers of patients are needed to confirm this. Unfortunately, because the daily dose in milligrams is 1000 times less than the aromatic retinoids, the technical problems inherent in analyzing such small quantities of arotinoids and their metabolites in body fluids make determination of elimination half-lives difficult if not impossible [30]. Without such information, use in women of child-bearing potential is not practical.

Conventional emollients and topical therapy may enhance the efficacy of systemic retinoids, allowing a reduction in dosage and dose-related mucocutaneous toxicity. The effect of etretinate and anthralin was additive in patients who were previously resistant to anthralin [31]. Etretinate 0.5–0.66 mg/kg per day combined with triamcinolone 0.1% and salicylic acid 5% cream was superior to either agent alone [32]. Retinoids may facilitate penetration of anthralin and corticosteroids.

HOW TO USE SYNTHETIC RETINOIDS

Retinoids are complex and potent drugs. They should only be prescribed by physicians who are experienced in the treatment of moderate to severe plaque-type psoriasis, localized or generalized pustular psoriasis, and erythrodermic psoriasis. The prescriber must be thoroughly familiar with the standard acute and chronic toxicity of retinoids as well as the special severe adverse reactions outlined in this chapter and in the package inserts. Referral to or consultation with a dermatologist is usually in order.

Etretinate is the only synthetic retinoid which is FDA-approved for psoriasis in the USA. The package insert recommends the use of etretinate only after methotrexate (MTX) and systemic corticosteroids have been tried, but I do not agree with it. While MTX is generally more effective than etretinate as monotherapy, I would select the retinoid before MTX in the appropriate clinical setting because there is no need for liver biopsies with etretinate. Moreover, systemic steroids should probably never be prescribed for psoriasis. If available and practical, however, I would consider using UVB or PUVA before choosing a retinoid and possibly combining the retinoid with UV light.

The patient information brochures published and distributed by Hoffmann-LaRoche are excellent sources and should be read by patients prior to prescribing. A good strategy is to order baseline laboratory studies while the patient reviews the brochure, and discuss results and answer any remaining questions about the drug and treatment plan on the next visit.

RECOMMENDED MONITORING GUIDELINES

Men and infertile women only

The dosages, combination strategies and monitoring guidelines shown here apply to etretinate. However, they are roughly the same for acitretin. If acitretin becomes available in the USA, it will probably supplant etretinate.

1 Baseline complete blood count, liver function tests, 12-hour fasting lipid profile, electrolytes, blood urea nitrogen, creatinine, and urinalysis. Liver biopsy is not ordered.

2 Repeat liver function tests and fasting lipids every 2 weeks until they are stabilized.

3 Repeat full battery every 3 months during therapy.

4 Monitor clinical efficacy monthly until disease has stabilized, then every 2–3 months.

5 Ophthalmologic consultation is not routinely ordered. Reserve for purulent conjunctivitis, corneal opacities, decreased night vision or increased glare, papilledema or suspected pseudotumor cerebri. Only the latter is a contraindication to further retinoid therapy.

6 X-rays are not routinely ordered. Reserve for persistently symptomatic bones or joints. The findings of vertebral osteophyte formation, spinal ligament calcification, or extraspinal tendon or ligament calcifications do not preclude further use of etretinate.

7 Strategies to reduce long-term bony toxicity and the cardiovascular risk of sustained unfavorable low density lipoprotein cholesterol/high-density lipoprotein cholesterol (LDL-C/HDL-C) ratios [33] include intermittent courses of etretinate (6–9 months separated by 1–3 months off drug), reduced maintenance dosage, and concomitant low fat diet and fish oil supplementation.

There has been discussion in the literature regarding the dosing of etretinate, that is, whether to start high and taper [7] or start low and work the dose upward [34]. The latter method is predicated on combining the retinoid with efficacious UV therapy, while the former allows retinoid monotherapy to be effective. I favor a starting dose of 0.75–1.0 mg/kg per day to achieve a maximal response and reduce it gradually. The dose should be taken once daily with the largest meal of the day. Doses below about 0.3 mg/kg per day usually result in recrudescence of psoriasis within 2–3 months. Therefore, we will often prescribe concomitant anthralin (highest concentration tolerated) or group II topical steroids to residual lesions.

The optimal combination is retinoid therapy for 1–2 weeks followed by PUVA or UVB phototherapy. This technique allows clearing to occur earlier and at a lower total energy exposure than the respective light therapy alone. The retinoid can be stopped and the light continued at decreased frequency for maintenance of remission. Re-PUVA (systemic or bath) should be used for recalcitrant palmoplantar pustulosis.

Patients with pustular psoriasis usually respond more rapidly than plaque or erythrodermic psoriasis. It has been recommended to start with a lower dosage of etretinate (0.25–0.33 mg/kg per day) and gradually increase upwards by similar increments for erythrodermic psoriasis. This method is intended to avoid the early development of "retinoid dermatitis," which if superimposed upon erythroderma could worsen both the appearance and symptoms of the disease. The dose needed for maximal improvement, however, is usually the same as for plaque psoriasis.

Women of childbearing potential

1 Do not use etretinate
2 If a retinoid is the next logical alternative, isotretinoin must be used with all of the precautions against pregnancy 1 month before, during, and 1 month after therapy with pregnancy tests performed as outlined in the package inserts. In addition, the same laboratory parameters as for etretinate above should be followed.
3 Isotretinoin may be effective for pustular psoriasis at 1.5–2.0 mg/kg per day, but maintenance with isotretinoin, PUVA, or MTX is necessary.
4 Isotretinoin is not very effective for plaque psoriasis as monotherapy or combined with UVB. Therefore, consider using isotretinoin in a re-PUVA regimen.

Children

1 Exhaust all other therapeutic alternatives before considering long-term retinoid therapy including Goeckerman regimen, PUVA, MTX (especially if associated with arthritis), UVA plus UVB plus anthralin (UVABA) [35], re-PUVA, and re-UVB.
2 Do not use etretinate in female children; use isotretinoin instead.
3 If long-term retinoid therapy is contemplated, it is preferable to select children whose epiphyses have closed, that is, 16–18 years of age. In the case of a child under 16 years, annual radiographs of the knees may be advisable.
4 If used for maintenance, prescribe the lowest dose that is still effective. Give "drug holidays" after every 6–9 months of therapy. There is some indication that chronic etretinate at low to moderate doses is less toxic to bones in children than isotretinoin, but it should only be used in male children.

TOXICITY

As mentioned in the Introduction, the toxicity of retinoids is essentially that of hypervitaminosis A. Side effects are common, and some should be expected in all patients who receive therapeutic doses. Patients should be warned not to take supplementary vitamin A beyond the 5000 units ordinarily supplied in multiple vitamin tablets [36]. Fortunately, most of the unwanted effects such as cheilitis are nuisances made tolerable by emollients or by reducing the dosage, and are completely reversible upon cessation of therapy. Theoretical concerns such as long-term cardiovascular risks may be mitigated by screening for other risk factors, frequent monitoring of blood lipids, and early dietary, medical, and/or dose reduction intervention. The severity of idiosyncratic hepatotoxic reactions may be limited by close monitoring of liver enzymes and early discontinuation of therapy. Finally, the most serious adverse effect of all, teratogenicity, may be completely avoided by simply not prescribing retinoids for women of childbearing potential. In practice, such a conservative stance can be modified with precautions.

Mucocutaneous toxicity

The most common and frequently troublesome side effects of oral retinoids relate to the skin and mucous membranes because of changes in the stratum corneum, decreased sebum production, and increased insensible water loss [37]. For a particular retinoid, some effects may be more prevalent in a large population of patients, or some effects may be more severe. In general, it is safer to assume that any or all of the mucocutaneous side effects listed in Table 14.1 could occur in an individual patient with any degree of severity. Cheilitis is the hallmark of retinoid therapy. Without it, one may assume that the patient is noncompliant or that the dosage prescribed is subtherapeutic. Another problem associated with dry lips not frequently mentioned, especially in older patients with dentures, is angular cheilitis, fissures at the angles of the mouth colonized by *Candida* species. It is for this reason that I recommend frequent emolliation of the lips with petrolatum without hydrocortisone and treatment of the fissures with nystatin ointment or clotrimazole cream. Concomitant oral candidiasis must also be treated with nystatin suspension or clotrimazole troches.

Several cutaneous findings may be explained by ultrastructural or kinetic studies of retinoid-treated skin. About 15–30% of patients complain of a

Table 14.1 Mucocutaneous side effects of retinoids

Mucous membranes
Dry lips/cheilitis
Dry mouth/thirst
Dry nasal mucosa/epistaxis
Skin
Dry skin/xerosis
Pruritus
Palm/sole peeling
Fingertip peeling
Skin fragility
Sticky skin
Dermatitis
Flare of psoriasis
Hair/nails
Hair loss
Change in hair texture
Paronychia
Nail changes

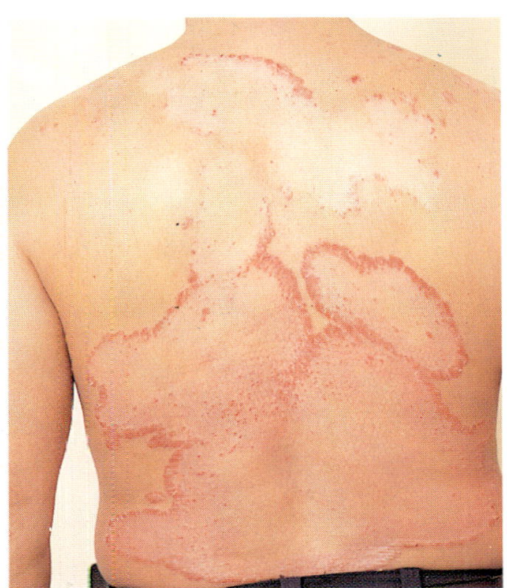

Fig 14.2 Resolution of psoriatic plaque with acitretin monotherapy.

"sticky" or "clammy" feel to their skin. The skin may appear more shiny, pink, and smooth than before treatment. A mucus-like material that is periodic acid–Schiff stain (PAS) positive has been detected in an intra- and intercellular location in the epidermis of etretinate- and arotinoid-treated psoriatics. Increased skin fragility, noted in 20–60% of patients in various studies, may be related to dehiscence of desmosomes between adjacent keratinocytes seen by electron microscopy [38]. It is uncertain whether the family common development of granulation tissue in the nail folds or rare cases of blistering and ulceration [39] represent clinical manifestations of skin fragility.

During the first month of therapy with retinoids, there may be a flare-up of psoriasis seen as expansion of established psoriatic plaques or the appearance of new papulosquamous lesions. There are several possible explanations for this. I believe it was seen more frequently in studies where patients with severe disease were withdrawn from other therapies that had previously maintained stability of their disease. Thus, extension and new lesions could be explained by the natural progression of disease. This phenomenon is observed less frequently in practice because patients whose disease is severe enough to require systemic therapy are not left untreated for 4 weeks and generally are not given retinoids as monotherapy. When chronic plaque psoriasis resolves during etretinate or acitretin therapy, however, it is common to observe central thinning followed by clearing with centrifugal spread of the scaling border, which closely resembles tinea corporis ("ringworm"; Fig. 14.2). The apparent worsening of psoriasis prior to clearing with etretinate may be due to a simultaneous decrease in mitosis in involved skin and an increase in uninvolved skin, which have been demonstrated in cell cultures [40,41]. Another explanation for worsening of psoriasis during retinoid therapy, especially if it occurs later in the course, is the development of an eczematoid eruption that may be confused with psoriasis (Fig. 14.3) [42]. It can occur anywhere but favors the backs of hands and arms. It may be improved with topical steroids or by reducing the retinoid dosage. In my opinion, the development of this so-called "retinoid dermatitis" is highly suggestive of an atopic diathesis. Miscellaneous rare cutaneous complications of etretinate have included erythroderma, toxic epidermal necrolysis, and generalized edema.

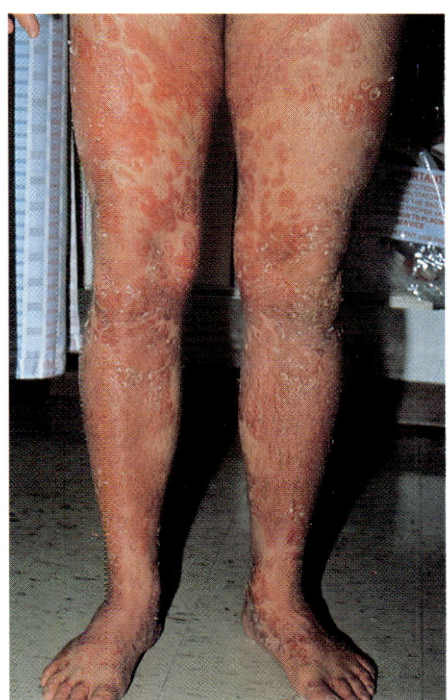

Fig 14.3 The vivid red color and the size of the plaques receded upon discontinuation of a chronic maintenance dose of acitretin (75 mg daily), which seemed ineffective.

Hair loss is definitely more common and more marked at higher dosages in patients receiving the aromatic retinoids than isotretinoin, in the range of 50–70%. It takes several months to evolve and is believed to be a telogen effluvium [43]. The hair loss is not limited to the scalp, but that is where it is most noticeable and distressing, particularly to women. Alopecia is reversible and may be improved by reducing the dose. A smaller percentage of patients notice a change in hair texture. Occasionally straight hair becomes more curly, kinked, or demonstrates pili torti [44]. These latter changes may not be reversible. Chronic paronychia, granulation tissue in the lateral nail folds, and nail dystrophies occur in 10–40% of patients. The latter may include softening of the nail plate, Beau's lines, onychomadesis, proximal onychoschizia, and distal onycholysis if there is also desquamation of fingertip skin [45]. Fingernail growth rates of psoriatic patients, already higher than normal controls, are further increased during etretinate therapy [46].

Ophthalmologic toxicity

Ocular side effects occur in 20–50% of patients in the form of dry eyes, conjunctivitis, or eye irritation probably as a result of changes in Meibomian gland function, an altered lipid layer, and instability of the tear film. Frequent use of artificial tears may decrease irritation, but contact lens users may have to decrease wear time. The dry eye tends to be colonized with *Staphylococcus aureus*, and purulent conjunctivitis may develop. Lid scrubs and ophthalmic antibiotic ointments may be indicated. While corneal opacities usually do not affect vision, it may be prudent to reduce the dose or discontinue treatment if they develop [47]. Synthetic retinoids can cause symptomatic decreased night vision probably as a result of interfering with the visual cycle (rhodopsin dissociated by light to opsin and all-*trans*-retinal). Law and Rando [48] showed that retinoic acid (all-*trans* and 13-*cis*) inhibited the conversion of 11-*cis*-retinol to 11-*cis*-retinal in an *in vitro* frog retina/pigment epithelium system.

Three patients receiving isotretinoin who spontaneously complained of decreased night vision and/or excessive glare problems, especially while driving, were evaluated [49]. All patients had abnormal electroretinograms or dark-adaptation curves while still receiving drug or shortly thereafter. Subjectively, vision gradually returned to normal after stopping treatment. Similar problems have been encountered during therapy with aromatic retinoids [50]. Patients with symptoms of color or night vision dysfunction should be referred to an ophthalmologist. Dark adaptometry may be the preferred test for monitoring night blindness.

Visual disturbances associated with persistent global headaches should alert the physician to the rare occurrence of papilledema or pseudotumor cerebri. The retinoid should be discontinued and treatment undertaken in consultation with the ophthalmologist and/or neurologist. Patients should not receive tetracycline or minocycline in conjunction with retinoids, which may increase the risk of pseudotumor cerebri.

Musculoskeletal toxicity

Muscle cramps and arthralgias are quite common during retinoid therapy. Painless muscle stiffness has been reported for etretinate. A patient with exfoliative dermatitis developed nonspecific myopathy during etretinate therapy. A muscle biopsy indicated segmental muscle necrosis. Three patients developed muscle pain and weakness during etretinate, and the authors concluded that etretinate can induce reversible skeletal muscle damage [51].

Bony changes including demineralization, thinning of the long bones, cortical hyperostosis, periosteitis, and premature closure of epiphyses have been identified in humans suffering from chronic hypervitaminosis A [52].

Since the initial report of a DISH-like syndrome in four patients receiving long-term high-dose isotretinoin [53], it has become clear that small pointed excrescences may develop on the anterior margins of one or more vertebral bodies after only 4 months of therapy [54]. There was generally no correlation between the radiographic finding of small spurs and musculoskeletal signs or symptoms [55].

Similar DISH-like spine involvement was observed in 11 of 38 (29%) patients receiving etretinate (mean dose, 0.8 mg/kg per day) for 5 years. However, extraspinal tendon and ligament calcifications of feet (76%), pelvis (53%), and knees (42%) were more common [56]. About half the patients had no symptoms referable to the site of radiographic abnormality.

Acitretin may produce similar bony changes and ligamentous calcification [57]. Kilcoyne [58] found that 14% of patients showed progression of spinal spurs at two sites after 3 years of therapy. He further enumerated problems with the design of prospective radiographic studies of psoriatic patients. DISH of the spine is usually associated with aging. The psoriatics tend to be older and may have preexisting arthritic changes. There are no control groups consisting of age- and sex-matched normal subjects and psoriatics followed for progressive changes over time without retinoid therapy.

The treatment of children with retinoids is even more complex because of the concern of growth retardation and premature closure of epiphyseal plates which have been reported after sustained high-dose isotretinoin or etretinate for disorders of keratinization [52]. Several authors have not found any skeletal abnormalities after up to 11 years of etretinate treatment in 91 children for disorders of keratinization [56,59]. Glover *et al.* [60] argued that etretinate can be given to children, with low risk of skeletal toxicity so long as patients are monitored using ^{99m}technetium methylene diphosphonate (^{99m}Tc MDP) whole body bone scans and musculoskeletal assessment. While the bone scan provides a lower total dose of radiation, it may not be sensitive enough to detect early epiphyseal closure [52]. Annual bone scans and radiographs of long bone epiphyses with supplemental radiographs of any symptomatic areas have been recommended. In order to avoid unnecessary exposure to radiation, Paige and coworkers performed a baseline selective skeletal survey followed by radiographs of abnormal or symptomatic areas [59]. Similarly, well-established guidelines for monitoring skeletal toxicity in adults are lacking. Some investigators recommend annual radiographs of the lateral spine, of a single lateral ankle, of pelvis and forearms, or only of symptomatic areas.

In summary, it seems likely that many patients will develop vertebral osteophytes and bony bridging during chronic retinoid therapy, but this appears to be more likely with isotretinoin, even at very low doses [61]. DISH-like spinal changes are less frequent with etretinate and acitretin, but extraspinal calcification may be more common. Fortunately, in most cases these changes are not clinically significant and are not contraindications to further treatment. The following strategies may minimize retinoid-induced skeletal toxicity:

1 select alternative therapy for children less than 16 years of age;

2 use the lowest possible dose of retinoid to achieve the desired result;
3 avoid long-term treatment whenever possible;
4 if long-term maintenance with retinoids is required, give a drug-free holiday for 3 months after every 9 months of therapy;
5 order radiographs of symptomatic regions.

Liver toxicity

Elevations of liver function tests, aspartate aminotransferase (SGOT), alanine aminotransferase (SGPT), and lactic dehydrogenase (LDH), occur in about 20% of patients treated with synthetic retinoids. Most of the changes are slight to moderate, are asymptomatic, and normalize during therapy or after it is discontinued. In clinical studies of etretinate in the USA, however, 10 of 652 (1.5%) patients developed evidence of clinical or histologic hepatitis possibly or probably related to the drug. While most cases resolved upon cessation of therapy, sequelae such as chronic active hepatitis [62] and hepatitis-related deaths have occurred. These may represent idiosyncratic reactions to etretinate. It has been suggested that retinoid hepatitis can be devided into four subsets: nonspecific reactive, acute chronic active, and severe fibrosis or cirrhosis [63].

A 3-year prospective study was performed to evaluate histologic alterations of the liver in 20 patients treated with etretinate preselected as high risk because of previous MTX therapy or excessive alcohol intake. After 6 months, 18 of 20 (90%) patients showed no change in the histologic classification of liver biopsy specimens while two deteriorated [14]. After 3 years, 17 patients underwent three or four liver biopsies: nine showed no change, six improved, and two deteriorated. The authors concluded that chronic etretinate therapy did not cause significant damage to the liver in a group of patients preselected for potential hepatotoxicity. It is not necessary to perform liver biopsies on a routine basis in patients treated with long-term etretinate.

Alteration of lipid metabolism

The retinoids cause hyperlipidemia. In the short term, as in isotretinoin treatment of acne or the induction phase of re-PUVA with etretinate or acitretin, reversible laboratory parameters probably have no adverse effect on the risk of cardiovascular disease. However, lipid abnormalities may be clinically significant during long-term therapy of psoriasis, especially if patients have other risk factors such as a personal or family history of a lipid abnormality, obesity, diabetes, smoking, and alcoholism. Etretinate does not alter the insulin requirements of diabetics [7]. Serum triglycerides and cholesterol were elevated in 45–65 and 0–16%, respectively, in patients treated with etretinate or acitretin. Decreases in HDL-C occurred in 30–37% of patients [64].

Experimental evidence seems to support the hypothesis that retinoids induce increased synthesis of apoprotein B (apo B) and triglycerides [65].

Apo B is a major protein component of both very low-density lipoprotein (VLDL) and LDL. Alternatively, degradation of VLDL to intermediate and LDL may be decreased [66]. Strategies to reduce retinoid-induced hyperlipidemia should be implemented if the triglyceride level attains 400 mg%:

1 weight reduction;
2 limit alcoholic intake;
3 cease smoking;
4 reduce simple sugar intake;
5 increase aerobic exercise.

At 600 mg%, reduce the dose or consider discontinuation of therapy. Do not allow triglycerides to reach 800 mg% because of the risk of acute pancreatitis and eruptive xanthomas. It may be necessary to consult a dietician or an endocrinologist if the use of lipid-lowering drugs is contemplated.

Fish oil supplements (3 g of ω-3 fatty acids daily) given to patients receiving etretinate or acitretin significantly decreased triglyceride levels in every patient (mean: 27%). There was a mean increase in HDL-C levels of 11% [67]. Fish oil had no effect on total cholesterol levels although these were increased by retinoid therapy. Fish oil also had no effect on apo B or LDL-C, which were not significantly increased by retinoids. Fish oil supplementation may be a valuable adjunctive measure to ameliorate the lipid changes and potentially reduce the risk of cardiovascular disease in patients receiving long-term retinoid therapy. Phillips [68] reported similar results with Max-EPA fish oil and isotretinoin, except that fish oil did not increase HDL-C. The study also showed that a low-fat isocaloric diet decreased cholesterol and apo B but did not mitigate the increase in triglycerides or the decrease in HDL-C caused by isotretinoin. If these results can be extrapolated to the aromatic retinoids, it would seem that a regimen of a low-fat isocaloric diet supplemented with fish oil concentrate (15 ml daily) combined with an aerobic exercise program could conceivably reverse most of the deleterious retinoid-induced lipid perturbations. Interestingly, Max-EPA contains cholesterol. Therefore, if you use fish oil supplements as a source of ω-3 fatty acids, select the cholesterol-free brands of Max-EPA.

Teratogenicity

Retinoids are known teratogens. Isotretinoin [69,70] and etretinate can cause spontaneous abortions and birth defects when given to women who are pregnant or, in the case of etretinate, even when conception occurred up to 24 months after the drug was discontinued. The anomalies described in the literature include small or absent ears, cleft palate, microphthalmos, micrograthia, central nervous system malformations such as hydrocephalus, conotruncal heart defects and aortic arch abnormalities, retinal or optic nerve abnormalities, and thymic defects [71]. It is possible that a major mechanism of retinoid teratogenesis is a deleterious effect on cephalic neural-crest cell activity at the critical period of embryogenesis. It is estimated that of all fetuses exposed during the first trimester who reach delivery, about 25% will have a major congenital anomaly [64]. To my knowledge, no human teratogenicity has been observed with acitretin, but it is embryotoxic or teratogenic in animal species. Acitretin must be assumed to be teratogenic in humans because it is the active metabolite of etretinate.

All three synthetic retinoids are contraindicated during pregnancy and breast-feeding. In the case of isotretinoin, more fetal exposures and malformations have occurred than for etretinate. Conception is safe one or more cycles after discontinuation of isotretinoin because of its relatively brief elimination half-life. The guidelines for prescribing isotretinoin have been published by Hoffmann-LaRoche and promoted by the FDA and American Academy of Dermatology. It should be mentioned that the only labeled indication for isotretinoin in the USA is severe cystic acne. Notwithstanding, it is currently the only synthetic retinoid available in the USA that should be prescribed for fully informed women of childbearing potential with severe psoriasis and when appropriate in the best judgment of the dermatologic consultant. Briefly, the guidelines are:

1 begin effective contraceptive measures 1 month before and continue until 1 month after therapy;

2 obtain negative serum pregnancy test within 2 weeks of starting isotretinoin;

3 begin therapy on the second or third day of the next normal menstrual period;

4 repeat serum pregnancy test monthly during therapy and obtain negative result before refilling the prescription.

As discussed earlier, etretinate is stored in the adipose tissue and released slowly for months or years after discontinuation of therapy. Low levels of etretinate were detected in the blood of five of 47 patients up to 2.9 years after therapy [72]. Three of 37 pregnancies occurring within 24 months of concluding etretinate therapy resulted in congenital anomalies. There is probably an etretinate blood level below which the risk of fetal malformations is equivalent to the background rate, but until that level is known, I do not recommend the use of etretinate in any fertile woman.

Much of the work done that proved acitretin to be superior to placebo and as efficacious as etretinate, either alone or in combination with UV light, was based on the pharmacokinetic premise that acitretin was not stored in the fat and had a short terminal half-life. If proven to be true, it would have allowed acitretin to be prescribed for fertile woman afflicted with severe psoriasis while following the established contraception guidelines for isotretinoin. The unexpected recent finding that etretinate is a metabolite of acitretin has dashed these hopes until further studies are done. C.E. Orfanos (personal communication 1993) now recommends, that conception be delayed 2 years after discontinuation of acitretin. The manufacturer has voluntarily withdrawn their new drug application for acitretin from FDA consideration.

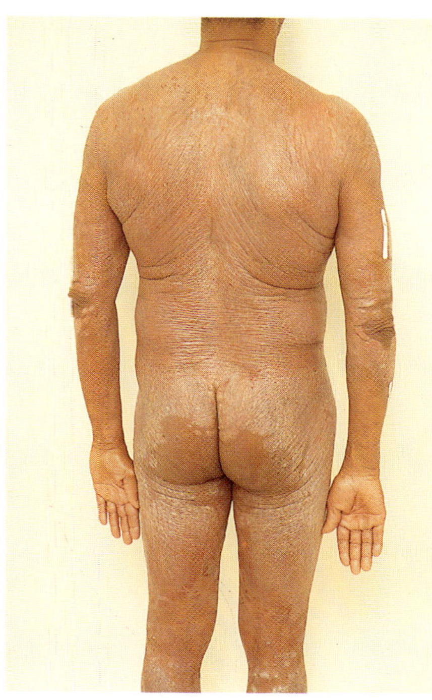

Fig 14.4 Case 1. Severe generalized plaque-type psoriasis.

CASE STUDIES

Case 1

Long-term remission following Goeckerman regimen maintained with etretinate.

A 61-year-old black man had a 13-year history of severe plaque-type psoriasis with arthritis. His current treatment consisting of emollients and UVB t.i.w. was ineffective. Psoriasis affected 88% of the body surface area (Fig. 14.4). He was admitted to hospital for a modified Goeckerman regimen consisting of 3% crude coal tar and 3% salicylic acid ointment, whirlpool, and UVB. Anthralin 0.5% and 50% extra UVB doses were given to resistant plaques on the lower extremities. At baseline his total cholesterol was 195 mg%, triglycerides were 153, and HDL-C was 22 (low). Etretinate was started at 75 mg daily (1 mg/kg per day). The patient had a history of angina. He was discharged after 25 days in an improved condition and continued applying etretinate and anthralin to his legs while at home.

One month after discharge his skin was completely clear, but his cholesterol and triglycerides increased to 268 and 177 mg%, respectively. During the next year, the etretinate dose was gradually reduced to 25 mg daily. Complete remission was maintained with the occasional application of anthralin to isolated lesions. Two years after discharge, the patient complained of decreased night vision. Because his skin was still clear and his cholesterol was elevated (258 mg%), etretinate was discontinued. When last examined, 6 months later, he had one small plaque on his sacrum. His total cholesterol had not changed. His night vision was subjectively improved.

Comment

This patient with extensive plaque disease had a gradual clearing response with the combination of the Goeckerman regimen, anthralin, and etretinate. All treatments except for UVB were new to his psoriasis, and higher UVB doses were required for the legs. This type of combination treatment could now be given in an outpatient day-care setting. The patient was from another state and did not want to stay in a hotel.

The case is somewhat unusual because of the durable remission induced by the Goeckerman regimen and maintained by tapering doses of etretinate and ultimately only the local application of anthralin 1.0%. Case 1 also illustrates the following points.

1 The elevation in total cholesterol of about 25% noted after 1 week on etretinate remained constant despite decreasing the dose and having been off the drug for 6 months. Theoretically, this effect may have increased the cardiovascular risk in a patient with angina, but his triglycerides and HDL-C returned to baseline values.

2 Symptoms of night blindness occur uncommonly during etretinate

therapy (< 1%). Synthetic retinoids may compete with normal retinol binding sites on retinal pigment epithelium or with transport molecules for binding sites on photoreceptor membranes. Detailed evaluation of visual function was performed in four patients during 1 year of etretinate treatment, and no ocular toxicity was found [73].

3 Topical corticosteroids have never been used in this patient, possibly contributing to the long-term remission. The activity of psoriasis usually returns to pretreatment levels 1–3 months after stopping etretinate.

4 Dark-skinned patients respond well to UVB as long as appropriately higher doses for type VI skin are delivered.

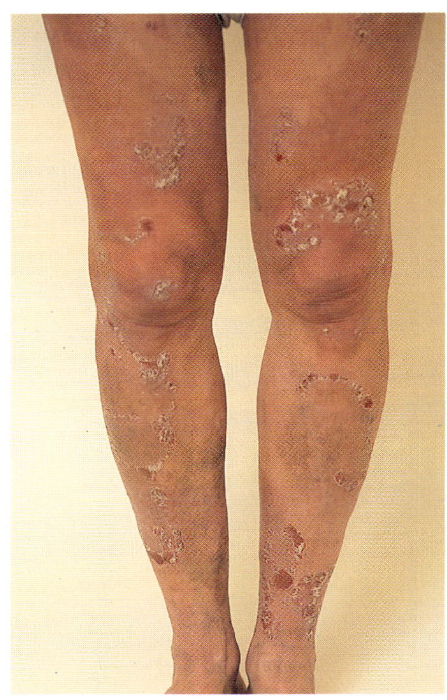

Fig 14.5 Case 2. After 3 months of receiving acitretin 50 mg daily.

Case 2

Long-term acitretin therapy for moderate plaque-type psoriasis is safe and effective.

A 34-year-old white man was first examined in 1985 for moderately severe psoriasis of 10 years' duration. His only prior treatment consisted of fluocinonide cream 0.05%. He volunteered to participate in a double-blind placebo-controlled study of Ro *10–1670 (acitretin), the first-order acid metabolite of etretinate. His plaque-type disease covered 25% body surface area (BSA). During the first 8 weeks of treatment, his psoriasis spread to involve 36% BSA. After breaking the code of the study, it was determined that he was taking 50 mg/day (0.6 mg/kg per day) of the active drug. Adverse experiences included cheilitis, peeling of palms and soles, and generalized hair loss. He desired to continue treatment in the open-label portion of the study and later in the chronic phase (Fig. 14.5). His optimal dose proved to be 75 mg/day (0.9 mg/kg per day), and he gradually improved to 3–6% BSA. He has continued treatment for 7 years with 6-month cycles of treatment followed by a 4-week "drug holiday," during which the psoriasis worsens slightly and the side effects (except for hair loss) disappear completely.*

At the beginning of the study his total cholesterol was 196 mg% and triglycerides were 106; after 7 years of treatment, at the end of a 6-month course, total cholesterol was 221 and triglycerides 154. At 4 weeks off therapy his cholesterol was 213, and his triglycerides were 108. The liver enzymes have remained normal throughout the study. Lateral spine radiographs performed annually have shown that the patient has developed mild loss of disc spaces, anterior osteophytes, and calcification of the anterior longitudinal ligament at the T4–T5 level. These changes are asymptomatic, and the treatment continues.

Comment

Case 2 illustrates the following points:

1 the efficacy and toxicity of acitretin are similar to those of etretinate;

2 in this case, the 10% increase in total cholesterol is probably age-related while the 50% rise in triglycerides is drug-related and reversible;

3 mild skeletal changes and tendon–ligament calcifications occur with either aromatic retinoid, although their clinical significance remains elusive.

REFERENCES

1 Bollag W. The development of retinoids in experimental and clinical oncology and dermatology. *J Am Acad Dermatol* 1983;9:797–805.

2 Bischoff R, DeJong EMGJ, Rulo HFC, *et al.* Topical application of 13-*cis*-retinoic acid in the treatment of chronic plaque psoriasis. *Clin Exp Dermatol* 1992;17: 9–12.

3 Tsambaos D, Orfanos CE. Antipsoriatic activity of a new synthetic retinoid. The arotinoid Ro 13–6298. *Arch Dermatol* 1983;119:746–51.

4 Merot Y, Camenzind M, Geiger J-M, Saurat J-H. Arotinoid ethylester (Ro 13–6298): a long term pilot study in various dermatoses. *Acta Derm Venereol* 1987;67:237–42.

5 West MR, Page JM, Turner DM, *et al.* Simple assays of retinoid activity as potential screens for compounds that may be useful in treatment of psoriasis. *J Invest Dermatol* 1992;99:95–100.

6 Camisa C, Eisenstat B, Ragaz A, Weissmann G. The effects of retinoids on neutrophil functions *in vitro*. *J Am Acad Dermatol* 1982;6:620–9.

7 Ellis CN, Voorhees JJ. Etretinate therapy. *J Am Acad Dermatol* 1987;16:267–91.

8 Dubertret L, Lebreton C, Touraine R. Inhibition of neutrophil migration by etretinate and its main metabolite. *Br J Dermatol* 1982;107:681–5.

9 Lammers AM, van de Kerkhof PCM. Etretinate modulates the leukotriene B4 induced intra-epidermal accumulation of polymorphonuclear leukocytes. *Br J Dermatol* 1987;117:297–300.

10 Schmitt A, Hauser C, Didierjean L, *et al.* Systemic administration of etretin increases epidermal interleukin 1 in the rat. *Br J Dermatol* 1987;116:615–22.

11 Kaplan RP, Russell DH, Lowe NJ. Etretinate therapy for psoriasis: clinical responses, remission times, epidermal DNA and polyamine responses. *J Am Acad Dermatol* 1983;8:95–102.

12 Brazzell RK, Colburn WA. Pharmacokinetics of the retinoids isotretinoin and etretinate. *J Am Acad Dermatol* 1982;6:643–51.

13 DiGiovanna JJ, Gross EG, McClean SW, *et al.* Etretinate: effect of milk intake on absorption. *J Invest Dermatol* 1984;82:636–40.

14 Roenigk HH Jr, Gibstine C, Glazer S, *et al.* Serial liver biopsies in psoriatic patients receiving long-term etretinate. *Br J Dermatol* 1985;112:77–81.

15 McNamara PJ, Jewell RC, Jensen BK, *et al.* Food increases the bioavailability of acitretin. *J Clin Pharmacol* 1988;28:1051–5.

16 Dubertret L, Chastang C, Beylot C, *et al.* Maintenance treatment of psoriasis by Tigason: a double-blind randomized clinical trial. *Br J Dermatol* 1985;113: 323–30.

17 Mahrle G, Meyer-Hamme S, Ippen H. Oral treatment of keratinizing disorders of skin and mucous membranes with etretinate. *Arch Dermatol* 1982;118:97–100.

18 Kingston TP, Matt LH, Lowe NJ. Etretin therapy for severe psoriasis. *Arch Dermatol* 1987;123:55–8.

19 Goldfarb MJ, Ellis CN, Gupta AK, *et al.* Acitretin improves psoriasis in a dose-dependent fashion. *J Am Acad Dermatol* 1988;18:655–62.

20 White SI, Puttick L, Marks JM. Low-dose etretinate in the maintenance of remission of palmoplantar pustular psoriasis. *Br J Dermatol* 1986;115:577–82.

21 Moy RL, Kingston TP, Lowe NJ. Isotretinoin vs etretinate therapy in generalized pustular and chronic psoriasis. *Arch Dermatol* 1985;121:1297–301.

22 Lowe NJ, Prystowsky JH, Bourget T, *et al.* Acitretin plus UVB therapy for psoriasis. Comparisons with placebo plus UVB and acitretin alone. *J Am Acad Dermatol*

1991;24:591–4.
23 Ruzicka T, Sommerburg C, Braun-Falco O, *et al.* Efficiency of acitretin in combination with UV-B in the treatment of severe psoriasis. *Arch Dermatol* 1990;126:482–6.
24 Rosen K, Mobacken H, Swanbeck G. PUVA, etretinate, and PUVA–etretinate therapy for pustulosis palmoplantaris. *Arch Dermatol* 1987;123:885–9.
25 Tanew A, Guggenbichler A, Honigsmann H, *et al.* Photochemotherapy for severe psoriasis without or in combination with acitretin: a randomized, double-blind comparison study. *J Am Acad Dermatol* 1991;25:682–4.
26 Honigsmann H, Wolff K. Isotretinoin–PUVA for psoriasis. *Lancet* 1983;i:236.
27 Roenigk RK, Gibstine C, Roenigk HH Jr. Oral isotretinoin followed by psoralens and ultraviolet A or ultraviolet B for psoriasis. *J Am Acad Dermatol* 1985;13: 153–5.
28 Ott F, Geiger JM. Therapeutic effect of arotinoid Ro 13–6298 in psoriasis. *Arch Dermatol Res* 1983;275:257–8.
29 Saurat J-H, Merot Y, Borsky M, *et al.* Arotinoid acid (Ro 13–7410): a pilot study in dermatology. *Dermatologica* 1988;176:191–9.
30 Goldfarb MT, Ellis CN, Voorhees JJ. Retinoids in dermatology. *Mayo Clin Proc* 1987;62:1161–4.
31 Orfanos CE, Runne U. Systemic use of a new retinoid with and without local dithranol treatment in generalized psoriasis. *Br J Dermatol* 1976;95:101–3.
32 Van der Rhee HJ, Tijssen JGP, Herrmann WA, *et al.* Combined treatment of psoriasis with a new aromatic retinoid (Tigason) in low dosage orally and triamcinolone cream topically: a double blind study. *Br J Dermatol* 1980;102:203–12.
33 Bershad S, Rubinstein A, Paterniti JR, *et al.* Changes in plasma lipid and lipoproteins during isotretinoin therapy for acne. *N Engl J Med* 1985;313:981–5.
34 Debertret L. Etretinate in psoriasis: advantages of low doses progressively increased (Letter). *J Am Acad Dermatol* 1985;13:830–1.
35 Swinehart JM, Lowe NJ. UVABA therapy for psoriasis. *J Am Acad Dermatol* 1991;24:594–7.
36 Wolverton SE. Retinoids. In Wolverton SE, Wilkin JK, eds. *Systemic Drugs for Skin Diseases*. Philadelphia: WB Saunders, 1991:187–218.
37 Shalita AR. Mucocutaneous and systemic toxicity of retinoids: monitoring and management. In Orfanos CE, Stadler R, Gollnick H, eds. *Dermatology in Five Continents*. Berlin: Springer-Verlag, 1988:496–501.
38 Ellis CN, Gold RC, Grekin RC, *et al.* Etretinate therapy stimulates deposition of mucus-like material in epidermis of patients with psoriasis. *J Am Acad Dermatol* 1982;6:699–704.
39 Ramsay B, Bloxham C, Eldred A, *et al.* Blistering, erosions and scarring in a patient on etretinate. *Br J Dermatol* 1989;121:397–400.
40 Krueger GG, Shelby NJ, Hansen CD, Taylor MB. Comparison of labelling indices of skin involved and uninvolved with psoriasis; placebo and oral retinoid Ro 10–9359 vs time. *Clin Res* 1980;28:21A(Abstract).
41 Rusciani L, Massaro P, Orlando P, *et al.* On the effects induced by aromatic retinoid Ro 10–9359 on explants of skin from psoriatic patients. In Orfanos CE, Braun-Falco O, Farber EM, *et al.*, eds. *Retinoids. Advances in Basic Research and Therapy*. Berlin: Springer-Verlag, 1981:139–43.
42 Taieb A, Maleville J. Retinoid dermatitis mimicking "eczema craquelé" (Letter). *Acta Derm Venereol* 1985;65:570.
43 Berth-Jones J, Shuttleworth D, Hutchinson PE. A study of etretinate alopecia. *Br J Dermatol* 1990;122:751–5.
44 Hays SB, Camisa C. Acquired pili torti in two patients treated with synthetic retinoids. *Cutis* 1985;25:466–8.
45 Baran R. Retinoids and the nails. *J Dermatol Treat* 1990;1:151–4.
46 Galosi A, Plewig G, Braun-Falco O. The effect of aromatic retinoid Ro 10–9359 (Etretinate) on fingernail growth. *Arch Dermatol Res* 1985;277:138–40.

47 Fraunfelder FT, LaBraico JM, Meyer SM. Adverse ocular reactions possibly associated with isotretinoin. *Am J Ophthalmol* 1985;100:534–7.

48 Law WC, Rando RR. The molecular basis of retinoic acid induced night blindness. *Biochem Biophys Res Commun* 1989;161:825–9.

49 Weleber RG, Denman ST, Hanifin JM, Cunningham WJ. Abnormal retinal function associated with isotretinoin therapy for acne. *Arch Ophthalmol* 1986;104:831–7.

50 Brown RD, Grattan C. Etretinate and vision (Letter). *Lancet* 1988;i:585–6.

51 Hodak E, David M, Gadoth N, Sandbank M. Etretinate-induced skeletal muscle damage. *Br J Dermatol* 1987;116:623–6.

52 Prendiville J, Bingham EA, Burrows D. Premature epiphyseal closure — a complication of etretinate therapy in children. *J Am Acad Dermatol* 1986;15:1259–62.

53 Pittsley RA, Yoder FN. Retinoid hyperostosis. Skeletal toxicity associated with long-term administration of 13-*cis*-retinoic acid for refractory ichthyosis. *N Engl J Med* 1983;308:1012–4.

54 Ellis CN, Madison KC, Pennes DR, *et al.* Isotretinoin therapy is associated with early skeletal changes. *J Am Acad Dermatol* 1984;10:1024–9.

55 Kilcoyne RF, Cope R, Cunningham W, *et al.* Minimal spinal hyperostosis with low-dose isotretinoin therapy. *Invest Radiol* 1986;21:41–4.

56 DiGiovanna JJ, Peck G. Retinoid toxicity. *Prog Dermatol* 1987;21:1–8.

57 Mark NJ, Kolbenstredt A, Austad J. Efficacy and skeletal side effects of two years' acitretin treatment. *Acta Derm Venereal* 1992;445–8.

58 Kilcoyne RF. The skeletal effects of retinoids and their relationship to DISH. *Fifth International Psoriasis Symposium Proceedings*, San Francisco, July 1991:117.

59 Paige DG, Judge MR, Shaw DG, *et al.* Bone changes and their significance in children with ichthyosis on long-term etretinate therapy. *Br J Dermatol* 1992;127: 387–91.

60 Glover MT, Peters AM, Atherton DJ. Surveillance for skeletal toxicity of children treated with etretinate. *Br J Dermatol* 1987;116:609–14.

61 Tangrea JA, Kilcoyne RF, Taylor PR, *et al.* Skeletal hyperostosis in patients receiving chronic, very-low-dose isotretinoin. *Arch Dermatol* 1992;128:921–5.

62 Weiss VC, Layden T, Spinowitz A, *et al.* Chronic active hepatitis associated with etretinate therapy. *Br J Dermatol* 1985;112:591–7.

63 Sanchez MR, Ross B, Rotterdam H, *et al.* Retinoid hepatitis. *J Am Acad Dermatol* 1993;28:853–8.

64 Cunningham WJ. Side effect profile of retinoids. In Roenigk HH Jr, Maibach HI, eds. *Psoriasis*. New York: Marcel Dekker, Inc., 1991:769–74.

65 Ashley JM, Lowe NJ, Ellis CN. Retinoids and alterations in lipid metabolism. In Roenigk HH Jr, Maibach HI, eds. *Psoriasis*. New York: Marcel Dekker, Inc., 1991:749–54.

66 Marsden J. Hyperlipidaemia due to isotretinoin and etretinate: possible mechanisms and consequences. *Br J Dermatol* 1986;114:407–7.

67 Ashley JM, Lowe NJ, Borok ME, Alfin-Slater RB. Fish oil supplementation results in decreased hypertriglyceridemia in patients with psoriasis undergoing etretinate or acitretin therapy. *J Am Acad Dermatol* 1988;19:76–82.

68 Phillips WG. Is fish oil useful in retinoid hyperlipidaemia? *Fifth International Psoriasis Symposium Proceedings*, San Francisco, July 1991:115.

69 Benke PJ. The isotretinoin teratogen syndrome. *JAMA* 1984;251:3267–9.

70 Robertson R, MacLeod PM. Accutane-induced teratogenesis. *Can Med Assoc J* 1985;133:1147–8.

71 Lammer EJ, Chen DT, Hoar RM, *et al.* Retinoic acid embryopathy. *N Engl J Med* 1985;313:837–41.

72 DiGiovanna JJ, Zech LA, Ruddel ME, *et al.* Etretinate. Persistent serum levels after long-term therapy. *Arch Dermatol* 1989;125:246–51.

73 Pitts JF, Mackie RM, Dutton GN, *et al.* Etretinate and visual function: a 1-year follow-up study. *Br J Dermatol* 1991;125:53–5.

fifteen Methotrexate

INTRODUCTION

Methotrexate (MTX) was first used for psoriasis in 1958. Since then it has become the antimetabolite most commonly prescribed by dermatologists for psoriasis and other skin diseases [1].

MECHANISM OF ACTION

MTX (formerly called amethopterin) is a folic acid antagonist. It competes with folic acid for binding sites on the intracellular enzyme dihydrofolate reductase (DHFR), which converts dihydrofolate to tetrahydrofolate. Tetrahydrofolate is the active form of folic acid necessary for thymidine synthesis and for the donation of methyl groups in purine synthesis. The affinity of MTX for binding sites on DHFR is 100 000 times greater than that of folic acid. The inhibition of folic acid reduction effectively inhibits the DNA synthesis (S) phase of the cell cycle. Psoriatic epidermis is more sensitive to the action of MTX than normal epidermis because of a greater fraction of cells in MTX-susceptible S-phase and a shorter cell cycle in the former [2]. Therefore, if MTX were present in keratinocytes for approximately 36 hours it might be expected to inhibit most of the proliferating psoriatic cells while affecting only about 10% of the normal keratinocytes.

MTX is readily absorbed from the gastrointestinal tract at the doses routinely employed in psoriasis treatment. Intramuscular injections of MTX are rapidly and completely absorbed. The terminal half-life is about 10 hours. Low doses generally between 7.5 and 25 mg weekly can be administered either orally or parenterally to the same patient with the expectation of equivalent efficacy and toxicity. There may be considerable interpatient variability in MTX blood levels based on the rate of absorption, rate of excretion, and exchange between plasma proteins and tissues. MTX is retained in the tissues, particularly the kidneys and liver, for weeks or months presumably bound as polyglutamates to intracellular DHFR [3].

Metabolism of MTX does not seem to occur to a significant degree, and most of the drug is excreted by the kidneys. About 90% of the MTX is excreted unchanged in the urine within 24 hours by glomerular filtration and active tubular secretion. Therefore, renal insufficiency magnifies the toxicity of low doses of MTX.

CLINICAL USE

Efficacy

Double-blind studies have confirmed the superiority of MTX to placebo in improving the skin manifestations, joint symptoms, and function in psoriasis. Good to excellent responses (50–100% clearing of psoriasis) have been reported in 70% of patients with severe disease using a single weekly oral dose of MTX of 20–37.5 mg [4,5]. Complete clearing was obtained in 43–61%. In 204 patients given 25 mg MTX p.o. weekly the estimated mean body surface area (BSA) of involvement decreased from 67 to 5% in 3–6 weeks [6].

It has been suggested that parenteral administration of MTX is safer (perhaps because it bypasses portal circulation) and possibly therapeutically more effective than the oral route. Van Scott *et al.* [7] obtained good to excellent results in 93% of patients with intramuscular injections of MTX every 1–2 weeks, 15–75 mg to outpatients and sometimes higher doses intravenously in hospital. Good to excellent results have been seen in 88% of patients treated with intramuscular MTX 20–150 mg at 1–3 week intervals [8]. Three patients also experienced marked improvement of psoriatic arthritis with MTX. Most of the patients had received short courses of aminopterin orally without a favorable response. Using doses comparable to those recommended today Rees *et al.* [4] (in 1967) obtained good to excellent results in 50% of patients with weekly injections of 15–35 mg. Nausea is the dose-limiting symptom for parenteral MTX.

In 1971, Weinstein and Frost [9] first reported the dosing of MTX 2.5–7.5 mg orally at 12-hour intervals for a total of three doses at weekly intervals. This schedule was based on experimental knowledge of keratinocyte proliferation kinetics and the rationale for chemotherapy with cell cycle-specific drugs. All 26 patients so treated attained good to excellent improvement. In all 11 patients who were previously treated with a single oral or intramuscular weekly dose, a smaller total weekly dose was required with the new schedule in order to achieve at least the same therapeutic effect. The authors also noted that there was less nausea. The Weinstein–Frost regimen was also shown to maintain a serum level for 30–40 hours, albeit very low for the 2.5 or 5 mg dose [10]. Halprin *et al.* suggested increasing and leveling the serum level by administering MTX every 8 hours for a total of four doses in 24 hours. In this way, 88% of their patients were "adequately controlled" or cleared using an average dose of 20 mg weekly. While this method of delivering MTX has not caught on, a recent study confirms a "good to excellent" overall response with a single weekly dose of 5–15 mg in 85% of patients [11].

Clinical studies

Combination therapy

Patients pretreated with MTX followed by combined MTX and UV light generally experienced more rapid clearing with lower doses of UVB or UVA, probably by decreasing scaling and induration of plaques and altering the photooptical properties of skin, making it favorable for UV light penetration.

MTX 15 mg weekly was given for 3 weeks, then UVB t.i.w. was begun. MTX was discontinued when the patient cleared, and UVB was continued at b.i.w. maintenance. All 26 patients cleared with a combination of mean cumulative MTX dose of 112 mg and 12 UVB exposures over 7 weeks [12]. The UVB dose at clearing was less than half that noted in 20 patients treated with UVB alone. Interestingly, the total number of phototoxic episodes was not increased by the combination of MTX with UVB, and MTX recall of UV-induced erythema (photoreaction) was not observed in any patient. In all likelihood, UVB phototherapy will not be able to prevent relapse of psoriasis in patients with the severe aggressive disease usually selected for MTX therapy.

Similarly, MTX combined with PUVA resulted in clearing in 93% of patients with 9.3 PUVA treatments. The final UVA dose was only about one-third of that required for clearing with PUVA alone [13]. The mean cumulative dose of MTX was only 93 mg. PUVA is more likely to maintain clearance alone than UVB. The MTX and PUVA should be used together only in cases previously shown to be failures with UV light alone or who required high final clearance doses, which would then be used for maintenance. A significant adverse effect of combined MTX and PUVA was prolonged phototoxicity.

MTX was given as maintenance treatment to patients with a history of rapid relapse after clearance of psoriasis with an Ingram regimen delivered in hospital. The dose of MTX was 15 mg weekly for 10 months, which was then tapered. The average period of treatment was 29 months with a mean cumulative dose of 1.18 g. The beginning of relapse occurred at 1 year vs 1 month and complete relapse at more than 3 years vs 5 months with MTX maintenance or without it, respectively [14]. If MTX maintenance was required for such a long period, then these patients were probably appropriate candidates for outpatient MTX therapy without the need for admission to hospital after the first rapid relapse or failure of the Ingram regimen.

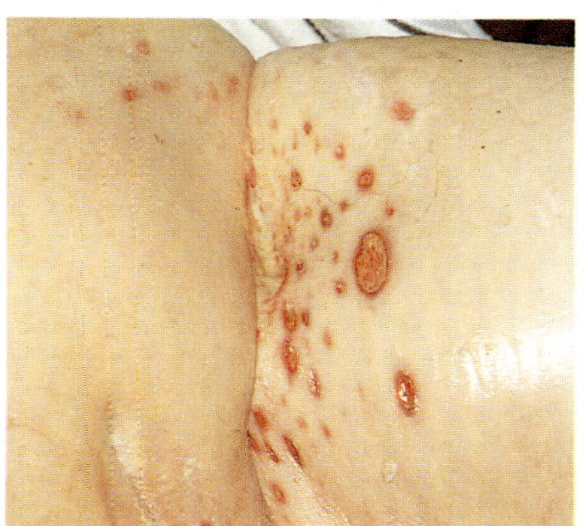

Fig 15.1 Ulcerative skin lesions secondary to the combined toxicity of methotrexate 15 mg/week and etretinate 100 mg daily given for generalized pustular psoriasis.

The combination of MTX and etretinate should be used, if at all, with caution in patients with severe forms of psoriasis, erythrodermic or pustular, who cannot be controlled with either drug alone or in the conversion from one treatment to the other (Fig. 15.1). Additive hepatotoxicity is the main concern, but the toxic hepatitis uncommonly observed with etretinate and fibrosis induced by chronic administration of MTX seem unrelated and due to different mechanisms [15]. Both drugs are bound to albumin in plasma, but free MTX blood levels were similar in one patient with and without concurrent etretinate [16]. In a study of six psoriasis patients treated chronically with the combination of intramuscular MTX and etretinate, the maximal plasma concentration was significantly increased compared to a matched control group receiving only MTX [17]. The levels of etretinate and metabolites were not affected by MTX administration. A patient receiving a slow infusion of MTX (10 mg over 48 hours), a regimen we do not recommend for psoriasis, demonstrated higher, potentially toxic, plasma levels of MTX (0.11 mmol/l) after oral etretinate (30 mg/day) was added [18]. Higher maximal MTX plasma concentrations might predispose patients to hepatic and cutaneous toxicity.

How to treat a patient with MTX

MTX is a very effective treatment for psoriasis, but it has potent effects that can eventually result in death. Before initiating therapy with MTX, consultation with a dermatologist who is well versed in the pharmacokinetics, drug interactions, treatment guidelines, and toxicity monitoring is necessary. There is a frank discussion with the patient regarding the known risks and benefits of MTX compared to the reasonable alternatives. Written material concerning MTX should be given to the patient to read at home and share with family members: e.g., the National Psoriasis Foundation brochure [19], the monograph from Lederle Laboratories [20], or package insert [21] and Methotrexate Patient Instructions from the AAD Guidelines [22].

Patient selection

MTX is indicated for severe or disabling psoriasis that is not responsive to other forms of therapy. Usually the patient has failed topical and UVB phototherapy and is a candidate for systemic treatment. Unless already tried, these would include psoralen UVA (PUVA), etretinate, and MTX. Given the choice, most patients will select simple oral tablets over frequent visits to the clinic or office for UV light. Fear of the liver biopsy and cirrhosis may lead patients away from MTX. We do not prescribe etretinate for women of childbearing potential but would consider MTX.

Indications

1 Extensive plaque-type psoriasis.
2 Psoriatic erythroderma.
3 Pustular psoriasis, generalized.
4 Localized psoriasis preventing employment or activities of daily living (e.g., palmoplantar psoriasis, acrodermatitis continua).
5 Complicated psoriasis, i.e., flaring after systemic corticosteroid withdrawal.
6 Psoriatic arthritis with skin disease (the usual rheumatologic dose, 7.5 mg weekly, is often insufficient for skin disease, and the dose may need to be increased by the dermatologist).

While each patient is evaluated individually with regard to disease severity, symptoms, level of physical and social disability, nail psoriasis or minor plaque disease should not be treated with MTX exclusively for cosmetic benefit, that is, without arthritis or functional impairment. In preselecting a patient for MTX, consider these contraindications and relative contraindications in order to reduce the potential toxicity of MTX.

Contraindications

1 Pregnancy or current desire to become pregnant.
2 Alcoholism.
3 Active hepatitis.
4 Cirrhosis.
5 Active infections.
6 Chronic renal failure.
7 Primary or secondary immunodeficiency.
8 Active peptic ulcer disease.
9 Blood dyscrasias.

Relative contraindications (increase the risk of preexisting liver disease).

1 History of excessive alcohol intake.
2 History of substance abuse.
3 Persistently elevated transaminases.
4 Recent hepatitis.
5 Family history of heritable liver disease.
6 Diabetes.
7 Obesity (also increases risk of complications from liver biopsy procedure).

If in the judgment of an experienced clinician the patient is a candidate for MTX, a complete history and physical examination is performed. Pre-MTX laboratory evaluations include:

1 complete blood count including red cell indices and leukocyte differential;
2 platelet count;
3 kidney function tests;
4 urinalysis;
5 liver function tests;
6 HIV antibody screen (if risk factors can be ascertained);
7 chest X-ray (optional);
8 folic acid level (optional).

We ask our patients to enter into a verbal contract with us that includes a commitment to abstain from alcohol, to take the medicine exactly as prescribed, to inform us of any new medications (over-the-counter and prescription) preferably before it is taken, to keep all followup appointments, and obtain laboratory tests as requested. Finally, they are advised that after 2–4 months of MTX therapy they must have a liver biopsy in order for therapy to continue. During this short period, we can determine whether the patient can tolerate the drug symptomatically and hematologically, whether it is efficacious, and whether the patient is reasonably compliant. We generally do not recommend pretreatment liver biopsies in patients over the age of 60 years [11].

Routine safety monitoring

1 Complete blood count (CBC) after 1 week, then monthly.
2 If significant leukopenia or thrombocytopenia develop, discontinue MTX for 2–3 weeks.
3 Kidney and liver function tests after 1 month, then every 3 months (plan blood test on the day before the next dose of MTX to reduce transaminase levels).
4 More frequent monitoring may be advisable during acute illnesses, when increasing doses, and during concomitant drug therapy.
5 Immediately prior to liver biopsy, obtain CBC, platelet count, prothrombin time and activated partial thromboplastin time.
6 Schedule the biopsy for 1–2 weeks after the last dose of MTX to reduce any acute morphologic alterations. The pathologist should be informed of the clinical situation and be familiar with drug-induced liver abnormalities. The trichrome stain is utilized to detect fibrosis. This grading system should be used [22]:

Grade I: normal; continue MTX
Grade II: fatty infiltration, inflammation; continue MTX
Grade IIIA: fibrosis, mild; continue MTX and repeat liver biopsy in 6 months
Grade IIIB: fibrosis, moderate to severe; discontinue MTX
Grade IV: cirrhosis; discontinue MTX

If the first liver biopsy is grade I or II, the next liver biopsy is planned after an additional cumulative dose of 1.5 g. Use Table 15.1 to prepare the patient for the next biopsy.

If grade IIIA, then the liver biopsy is repeated after 6 months of continuous MTX therapy regardless of cumulative dose. I would not treat patients with grade IIIB or IV with MTX under any circumstances.

HOW TO DOSE MTX

MTX is administered as a single weekly oral or parenteral dose. The oral dosage may be divided over a 24-hour period once weekly. Low daily doses of MTX must never be used for psoriasis. MTX is available as oral 2.5 mg tablets and parenteral isotonic liquid 25 mg/ml with or without preservative. Most patients take the tablets. There is a trend away from

Table 15.1 When to perform a liver biopsy at a given weekly dose of methotrexate

Regular weekly dose (mg)	Months to 1.5 g cumulative dose and next liver biopsy
7.5	50
10.0	38
15.0	25
20.0	19
25.0	15

parenteral therapy [1]. Intramuscular or intravenous bolus injections are reserved for the occasional patient who cannot follow the oral dosing schedule or who is unreliable in keeping followup appointments for laboratory testing. Slow intravenous drips of MTX should never be used for psoriasis. Some patients with erratic absorption of oral MTX demonstrate a better therapeutic response with parenteral MTX and still others have less gastrointestinal symptoms, but this is highly variable and individualized. It is rarely ever necessary to give MTX more than once per week, even for hospitalized patients.

The scientifically elegant Weinstein/Frost method of intermittent dosing over a 24-hour period is utilized by the majority of dermatologists [1]. It seems nevertheless to confer no therapeutic advantage and may be more hepatotoxic than a single weekly oral or parenteral bolus. For consistency we prescribe MTX on Mondays at 8 a.m., 8 p.m., and Tuesday 8 a.m. again on an empty stomach if possible. The doses may be unequal at the different times. Some patients are able to overcome the nausea of a 15 mg dose, for example, by taking 5 mg 12 hours apart or by taking MTX with food, although the latter probably reduces bioavailability of the drug. Folic acid supplementation, 1 mg daily, may be useful at mitigating the toxicity of MTX without altering efficacy during chronic low-dose weekly therapy [23]. The addition of folic acid 5 mg daily relieved gastrointestinal symptoms, particularly nausea, in most patients [24].

Dosage recommendations

After the pre-MTX consultation, education, physical and laboratory examinations are completed (but not necessarily the liver biopsy), initiate MTX with a single oral dose of 7.5 mg. Recheck CBC for an idiosyncratic reaction before the next dose. Continue this dose weekly for 1 month. Increase the dose by 2.5 mg/week each month after checking CBC and other tests as indicated. Dispense only enough MTX for 1 or 2 weeks beyond the next scheduled visit without refills. Monthly intervals between increments in dose allow enough time for a therapeutic response to develop as well as cumulative beneficial effects and dose-related adverse reactions. It is not necessary to induce complete clearing of psoriasis because this could imply overmedicating. We strongly encourage the concomitant use of topicals such as emollients, keratolytics, corticosteroids, anthralin, and tar shampoos for resistant localized plaques. If nausea should become a dose-limiting symptom, begin dividing the weekly dosage into three doses 12 hours apart. Some food with the pills may be added if nausea persists. The goal is to achieve adequate control of psoriasis with the lowest dose possible to overcome the physical and psychosocial disability of psoriasis. The total dose needed usually does not exceed 30 mg weekly: 25 mg or less is sufficient for most, but doses up to 37.5 mg may be needed by a few patients. Elderly patients may require lower mean doses as a function of progressive deterioration in creatinine clearance associated with the natural aging process.

After stability of residual psoriasis (or clearing) is attained, an attempt to taper the dose in monthly 2.5 mg decrements should be made. Increasing the interval between doses of MTX from 7 to 10 or 14 days serves the same purpose but makes for inconsistencies in office practice patterns and changes an established schedule for the patient. The psoriasis may be expected to relapse within weeks to months depending on the type and severity of the disease. There is no "rebound flare-up" of psoriasis as some believe, and no tachyphylaxis is manifest when it is reinstated. A questionnaire survey of American dermatologists completed in 1984 revealed that 60% would take MTX if they had severe psoriasis [1]. A more provocative but unasked question is how many would also agree to undergo the liver biopsies [2].

Topical methotrexate

If systemic MTX is so effective in psoriasis, not appreciably metabolized, and presumably acts directly on proliferating epidermal cells, it is logical to expect that topical MTX would be efficacious for psoriasis if it could penetrate to the basal cell layers. Moreover, the liver would be effectively cut out of the loop, thereby avoiding the most significant toxicity of long-term systemic therapy, hepatic fibrosis.

Concentrations of MTX 0.1–10% formulated in aqueous cream, petrolatum, and dimethyl sulfoxide vehicles were completely ineffective when applied to psoriasis for 7–14 days [25]. Even more surprising, 0.1–1.0% solutions injected intradermally were similarly ineffective. The inactivity of topical MTX was confirmed in 1981 with 0.2–0.5% concentrations applied for 2 or 9 days. Topical MTX 0.5% decreased DNA synthesis and improved the appearance of hyperproliferative skin in essential fatty acid-deficient mice, but it had no effect on DNA synthesis in normal mouse skin or on the clinical appearance of psoriasis plaques [26]. More recently, MTX was formulated with laurocapram (Azone) to enhance percutaneous penetration and applied to psoriasis twice daily for 6 weeks [27]. Fifty-seven percent of lesions were markedly improved compared to 25% with vehicle. No dose–response was detected between 0.1 and 1.0% concentrations, but the authors concluded that it is possible to demonstrate local antipsoriatic effects provided there is adequate percutaneous absorption for a prolonged period of time. At the present time topical therapy with MTX is impractical.

Other folic acid antagonists

Aminopterin and MTX are water-soluble folate antagonists. Aminopterin is no longer in use. The mechanism of hepatotoxicity is unknown but it is believed to be related to the intracellular polyglutamation and prolonged retention of MTX, depriving the hepatocyte of folic acid-dependent one-carbon transfer reaction.

Piritrexim isothionate, a lipid-soluble antifolate that inhibits DHFR as effectively as MTX, is not polyglutamated and therefore not stored in this form within hepatocytes. Because it might be effective in the treatment of psoriasis without the associated risk of late fibrosis or cirrhosis, an open clinical trial was performed [28]. Four different dosage schedules were used; at a dosage of 50 mg b.i.d. four of five patients had good to excellent improvement. Higher doses did not improve results but resulted in leukopenia and elevated transaminases. The laboratory abnormalities normalized with dosage reduction or discontinuation of therapy. Despite this preliminary report of efficacy, further development of piritrexim for psoriasis was suspended because of the need for large numbers of patients followed for long periods of time with liver biopsies in order to assess long-term cumulative toxicity.

Overdosage of MTX

Because of the inherently low doses of MTX used for psoriasis, it is rare to encounter in practice a true overdosage that requires intervention other than decreasing or withholding the next dose and routine laboratory monitoring. The most likely clinical scenarios that may result in overdosage requiring intervention are as follows.

1 A noncompliant patient increases his or her own dose deliberately to improve efficacy or rate of response. He or she may complain of burning or ulceration of psoriasis lesions.

2 A patient develops acute renal failure or an unrelated acute illness with dehydration without reducing the dose of MTX. This may be detected by routine laboratory monitoring or by a call to you from the local emergency room because of leukopenia.

3 The patient is given another drug that increases the serum level of MTX or prolongs the excretion of MTX thereby increasing its toxicity. Trimethoprim-sulfamethoxasole is frequently the "other drug." Patients may complain of sore mouth.

Leucovorin calcium (citrovorum factor, folinic acid) can bypass the metabolic block produced by MTX and supply the active form of folic acid that cells require. It should be readily available in the office or clinic because leucovorin must be given as promptly as possible, preferably within 4 hours of the last dose of MTX. As the time interval between MTX and leucovorin administration increases, the effectiveness of leucovorin as an antidote diminishes, so that by 24 hours it is doubtful that leucovorin will have any effect [22] except in patients with severely depressed creatinine clearance.

In general, if MTX overdose is suspected, give an intramuscular injection of leucovorin equal to the last dose of MTX or 25 mg, whichever is greater. Blood should then be taken to assess hematologic and kidney function parameters and MTX level. In cases of renal impairment repeat the leucovorin dosing every 6 hours until the MTX level is 0.1 μmol/l or less. Neither hemodialysis nor peritoneal dialysis improve MTX elimination. The patient with dehydration should be rehydrated with normal saline and observed. In cases of massive overdosage, admission to hospital is justified for leucovorin rescue. Alkalinization of the urine prevents precipitation of MTX in the renal tubules.

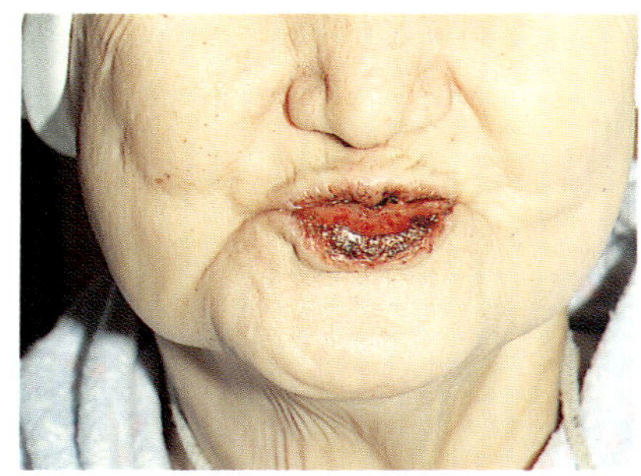

Fig 15.2 Stomatitis secondary to combined toxicity of methotrexate and sulfamethoxasole.

TOXICITY

The most commonly encountered adverse effects of MTX are nausea, anorexia, fatigue, headaches, and alopecia. At the doses normally used in psoriasis treatment oral erosions (ulcerative stomatitis) (Fig. 15.2) and ulcerations of psoriatic lesions generally do not occur and are indicative of toxic serum levels due to drug interactions, dehydration, or deterioration of renal function. Bone marrow depression is more likely to occur under these circumstances.

Leukopenia and thrombocytopenia are the most serious acute side effects of MTX. If the white blood cell count or platelet count drops below 3500 or 100 000/mm^3, respectively, MTX should be discontinued until the cause is found. The nadir for leukocytes and platelets is 8–11 days after the dose. It generally takes about 3 weeks for the bone marrow to recover. It has been suggested that elevated mean corpuscular volume (MCV) is predictive of cytopenia. While this has not been confirmed, elevated MCV is indicative of folic acid deficiency, and low normal pretreatment plasma and red cell folate levels are predictive of future overall toxicity during MTX therapy [29].

MTX has no carcinogenic potential for the skin or viscera. Anecdotal reports, however, have implicated MTX treatment as either teratogenic or abortifacient [30] in pregnant women. It may cause transient infertility in men. MTX should not be used by pregnant women, and pregnancy should be prevented by female patients during MTX therapy and for 3 months after stopping the drug.

The pulmonary complications of MTX are rarely encountered in psoriasis patients. They include acute pneumonitis and diffuse interstitial fibrosis on the basis of hypersensitivity to MTX or as a direct toxic reaction [31]. They are nonresponsive to leucovorin rescue, but corticosteroids may be therapeutically useful [3].

Hepatotoxicity is the primary clinical concern when long-term treatment is planned. Mild elevations (less than twice the upper limit of normal) of transaminases are expected during therapy, but there is no correlation between enzyme levels and hepatic fibrosis. In a study of long-term oral weekly MTX in patients with rheumatoid arthritis, chronic low-grade elevations of serum aspartate aminotransferase (SGOT) after 3–4 years of therapy correlated with increase in the hepatic histologic grade [32]. The AAD has published periodically revised guidelines for the safe use of methotrexate including liver biopsy [22].

Van Scott in 1967 anticipated hepatic fibrosis and cirrhosis with methotrexate [4]: "Balanced against the virtues of this drug are known and unknown perils in its use. ... Many of the possible hazards of chronic effects have not been determined and ... impairments of liver metabolic functions are among these." The incidence of cirrhosis as first reported was probably inflated because pretreatment liver biopsies were not performed, which might have revealed preexisting liver disease [33,34]. The now abandoned regimen of low daily doses of MTX increased the duration of exposure of hepatocytes to MTX thereby increasing toxicity. Other major risk factors for hepatotoxicity that may not have been excluded or minimized include alcoholism, obesity, diabetes, renal insufficiency, and concomitant drugs that increase serum levels or decrease clearance of MTX.

The incidence of cirrhosis occurring in psoriasis patients has been reported at 3–25%, but the risk of it developing below a total cumulative dose of 1.5 g is minimal [35].

It has been said that "MTX-induced cirrhosis appears not be aggressive." The drug has been continued in some patients with cirrhosis without progression and sometimes regression. It is uncertain whether this finding represents regeneration of liver or sampling errors. On the other hand, several patients have been reported who required liver transplantation after developing MTX-induced cirrhosis [36].

The preferred method for assessing pretreatment liver status and monitoring for MTX hepatotoxicity is still the liver biopsy using the Menghini needle. In highly selected patients with acceptable laboratory parameters, the procedure can be safely performed in an outpatient setting. The patient can be monitored for 3 hours and then discharged if stable [37]. Noninvasive alternative methods have been studied. Radionuclide liver scans have been shown to be unreliable [38]. Hepatic ultrasound may be a better screening test for severe toxicity. While the rate of false-positive (with normal histology) and false-negative (with grade IIIA or less severity) studies was high, ultrasound reliably detected grade IIIB or cirrhosis [39] which would interdict further MTX under the current guidelines. On the other hand, dynamic hepatic scintigraphy was very accurate (98.5%) in predicting a normal biopsy but poor for predicting moderate to severe portal fibrosis (25%) [40].

Serum elevations of the aminoterminal propeptide of type III (PIIINP) procollagen are correlated with liver fibrosis or cirrhosis in patients without arthropathy [41]. The authors proposed that PIIINP values be used for screening patients for liver fibrogenesis after the first biopsy at 1.5 g total cumulative dose in order to reduce the number of additional biopsies performed. While this work is promising, independent confirmation is necessary. Moreover, some patients might still prefer confirmation of the diagnosis of liver fibrosis by biopsy before stopping MTX, risking flare-ups and having to undergo changes in their systemic psoriasis therapy. Perhaps a battery of noninvasive tests such as hepatic ultrasound, dynamic scintigraphy and measurement of serum PIIINP would provide data as reliable as a liver biopsy at a somewhat higher cost, but with less risk to the patient.

Drug interactions

MTX toxicity may be increased in cases of folic acid deficiency due to malabsorption or malnutrition. Simultaneous administration of folic acid is usually not necessary during routine psoriasis therapy, but it does not seem to reduce MTX efficacy. Drugs which impair folic acid absorption such as barbiturates and nitrofurantoin should be avoided. Moreover, drugs that inhibit DHFR should not be given concomitantly with MTX: trimethoprim-sulfamethoxazole, triamterene, and pyrimethamine.

Fifty to 70% of MTX is bound to albumin and may be competitively displaced from binding sites by certain drugs including salicylates, sulfonamides, probenecid, and phenytoin, which may increase free MTX. These interactions are usually not clinically relevant in the treatment of psoriasis.

Drugs that also undergo tubular secretion, such as aspirin, probenecid, phenylbutazone, penicillin, ascorbic acid, and sulfonamides may prolong excretion and expose patients to toxic levels of MTX. Toxicity has also been reported with concomitant use of nonsteroidal antiinflammatory drugs (NSAIDs) with higher doses of MTX [3]. Any drug which has the potential to reduce the glomerular filtration rate (i.e., cyclosporine, aminoglycoside antibiotics) should be used with caution in combination with MTX. A small amount of oral MTX is excreted in the feces, proportional to the dosage, probably through the biliary tract. Most MTX excreted in the bile is reabsorbed in the intestine. Oral antibiotics such as tetracycline and nonabsorbable broad spectrum antibiotics may decrease absorption of MTX and interfere with the enterohepatic circulation.

CASE STUDIES

Case 1

MTX to hydroxyurea to MTX to PUVA to Goeckerman to etretinate to MTX, or "all roads lead to methotrexate."

A 43-year-old white man had suffered from severe psoriasis since 1970 (when he was 26). His private dermatologist treated him with methotrexate 50 mg intravenously weekly for about 1 year with good results. His treatment was changed to hydroxyurea 500 mg b.i.d. in 1971. The dose was varied between 500 mg q.d. and 500 mg t.i.d during the next 5 years with almost complete clearing. When taking the highest dose, a modest drop in his white blood cell count occurred. He had a severe relapse in 1976. Hydroxyurea was discontinued, and MTX was restarted at 15 mg orally every 7–10 days with good control until 1985 when he suffered a myocardial infarction (at the age of 39).

An estimated cumulative dose of 5.2 g MTX had been given up to this point. A liver biopsy was performed, which was normal. In 1989, after an additional 1.92 g of MTX, the drug was stopped for unknown reasons in favor of PUVA. After 16 PUVA treatments, the psoriasis flared to involve approximately 95% of the body skin with plaques (Fig. 15.3). The patient transferred his care to the Cleveland Clinic and was admitted to hospital for a modified Goeckerman regimen consisting of the application of 5% crude coal tar with 2% salicylic acid followed by whirlpool and UVB. Triamcinolone 0.1% ointment was applied to his extremities initially and

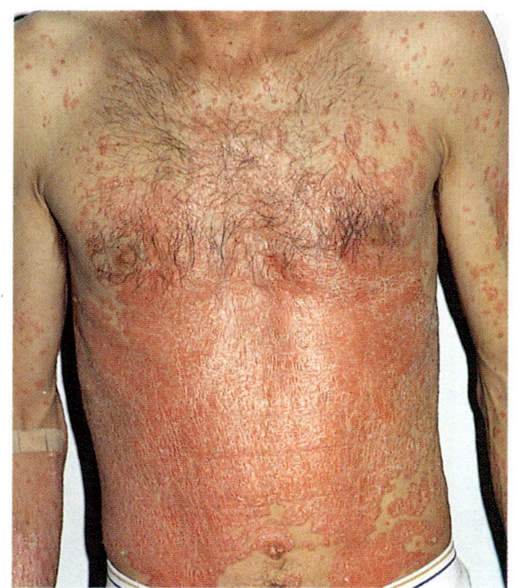

Fig 15.3 Case 1. Generalized plaque-type psoriasis.

later changed to 1% hydrocortisone and anthralin 0.25% (advanced to 1.0%) ointments. Etretinate was started at a dose of 50 mg daily (0.87 mg/kg per day). The extent of psoriasis decreased 50% at the time of discharge 16 days after admission.

Outpatient therapy consisted of topical anthralin 0.5%, 5% liquor carbonis detergens in petrolatum, and fluocinonide 0.05% and etretinate, later increased to 75 mg/day (1.3 mg/kg). After an initial rise in triglycerides and cholesterol of 20%, these laboratory abnormalities returned to baseline values, but his psoriasis still involved 50% of body surface area (BSA).

When he missed etretinate doses for a week and noted improvement in his skin, the dose was lowered to 50 mg/day. His psoriasis then flared to involve 65% BSA. Reinstitution of MTX was contemplated. The patient drank beer on weekends but agreed to abstain from further alcohol ingestion. Liver function tests had always been normal. A liver biopsy was performed showing mild periportal lymphocytic infiltration and no fibrosis (histologic grade I/IV).

MTX was restarted at 15 mg orally weekly. Marked improvement was noted after only three doses; after eight doses (total 120 mg) his trunk had completely cleared, and a few thin scaling plaques remained on the extremities. Another liver biopsy is planned after an additional 1.5 g cumulative dose of MTX.

Comments

This case illustrates the following points.

1 Methotrexate, while potentially more toxic than hydroxyurea or etretinate, is generally more effective than either drug for extensive chronic plaque-type psoriasis.

2 Hydroxyurea at 1.5 g daily is indicated for severe plaque-type psoriasis and may be nearly as effective as MTX, but long-term safety and monitoring criteria have not been as well established. The treating dermatologist stopped MTX after an additional 1.92 g instead of ordering a repeat liver biopsy.

3 PUVA was not sufficient to prevent the severe post-MTX flare. If the goal were to convert MTX to PUVA in a patient with extensive disease, it would be desirable to continue the MTX for the first 3–5 weeks while increasing the UVA dose; however, phototoxicity may be an added nuisance in managing the PUVA with MTX [13].

4 Etretinate may induce rises in blood lipids of 10–25% even in thin persons. In this patient with a history of atherosclerotic heart disease and low high density lipoprotein-cholesterol the theoretical risk of retinoids may have been reduced by concomitant administration of fish oil containing eicosapentaenoic acid (cholesterol-free Max-EPA).

5 In this patient, the optimal dose of etretinate lay between 50 and 75 mg/day, where the higher dose caused "retinoid dermatitis" mimicking psoriasis and the lower dose permitted a flare of psoriasis.

6 This patient began taking MTX in 1970 before treatment guidelines were published, but complete documentation allowed summation of the

total dose received. Later, following AAD revised guidelines, a liver biopsy showed minimal change after a total cumulative dose of over 7 g in a moderate drinker! This allowed for resumption of the most effective treatment for this particular patient 22 years after it was first used. Abstinence from alcohol and repeat liver biopsies after each additional 1.5–2 g MTX will afford a comfortable measure of safety.

7 Phototherapy combined with etretinate may have allowed better maintenance of psoriasis without the risk of MTX hepatotoxicity, but the patient's occupation (traveling salesman) and the distance between his home and our center made this a practical impossibility.

Case 2

Monitoring MTX therapy in a patient with alcoholic liver disease.

A 48-year-old white man was referred to the Cleveland Clinic for progressive psoriasis of 10 months' duration. Various topical corticosteroids, sulfasalazine, and oral antibiotics had been ineffective. Examination showed 80% BSA involvement with inflamed plaques with mild to moderate scaling (Fig. 15.4).

Treatment options were discussed with the patient. He lived too far from our facility for PUVA. He stated that he had "high cholesterol" and did not want to take etretinate. He was a moderate drinker but agreed to the following requirements for MTX treatment:

1 baseline blood tests;

2 abstinence from ethanol;

3 a liver biopsy 2–3 months after starting MTX if long-term therapy was planned.

The only abnormalities on routine laboratory testing were serum aspartate aminotransferase 50 U (normal range 7–40 U) and cholesterol 235. MTX was started at 7.5 mg p.o. weekly and gradually increased to 12.5 mg weekly with excellent clearing of psoriasis. A few resistant plaques remained on the pretibial areas. The serum aspartate aminotransferase normalized and the rest of the laboratory tests were unchanged. A liver biopsy was performed without complications 3 months after starting MTX. It showed mild to moderate portal and centrilobular fibrosis consistent with a histologic grade of IIIA/IV. MTX was continued along with monthly intralesional injections of triamcinolone acetonide 5 mg/ml into persistent plaques. A slight rise in serum alanine aminotransferase was noted at 36 U (normal range 0–30 U). According to AAD guidelines [22], I ordered a repeat liver biopsy in 6 months; it again showed a histologic grade of IIIA/IV.

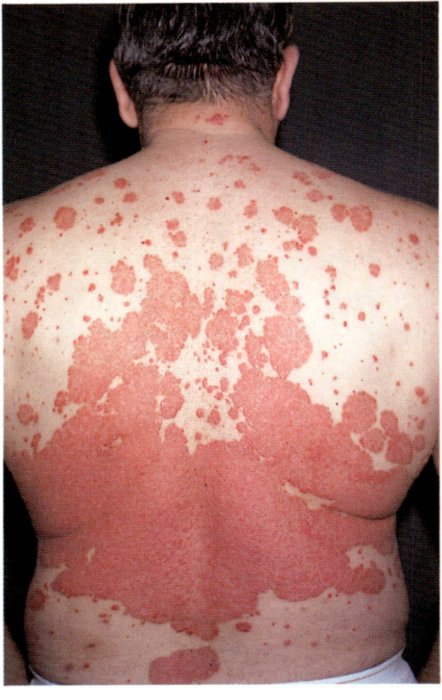

Fig 15.4 Case 2. Plaque psoriasis prior to methotrexate treatment.

Comment

Physicians are understandably reluctant to use MTX in patients with liver enzyme elevations who drink alcohol. If, as in this case, the clinical situation questions the use of methotrexate, then it is necessary to obtain a liver biopsy before or shortly after initiating therapy if the drug is to be beneficial for psoriasis.

Because this patient's cumulative MTX dose prior to the first biopsy was only 120 mg, we believe the grade IIIA mild fibrosis represented a pretreatment ethanol effect. The MTX was continued and we rebiopsied the liver after an additional 6 months of treatment (total cumulative dose of 445 mg). He has recently admitted to occasional use of hard liquor and will undergo another liver biopsy in 6 months. He understands that if the histologic grade progresses to IIIB/IV (moderate to severe fibrosis), we will discontinue MTX.

REFERENCES

1 Peckham PE, Weinstein GD, McCullough JL. The treatment of severe psoriasis. A national survey. *Arch Dermatol* 1987;123:1303–7.

2 Weinstein GD, Goldfaden G, Frost P. Methotrexate mechanism of action on DNA synthesis in psoriasis. *Arch Dermatol* 1971;104:236–43.

3 Olsen EA. The pharmacology of methotrexate. *J Am Acad Dermatol* 1991;25: 306–18.

4 Rees RB, Bennett JH, Maibach HI, Arnold HL. Methotrexate for psoriasis. *Arch Dermatol* 1967;95:2–11.

5 Callaway JL, McAfee WC, Finlayson RG. Management of psoriasis using methotrexate orally in a single weekly dose. *South Med J* 1966;59:424–61.

6 Roenigk HH, Bergfeld WF, Curtis GH. Methotrexate for psoriasis in weekly oral doses. *Arch Dermatol* 1969;99:86–93.

7 Van Scott EJ, Auerbach R, Weinstein GD. Parenteral methotrexate in psoriasis. *Arch Dermatol* 1964;89:550–6.

8 Auerbach R. Parenteral vs oral folic acid antagonists. *Arch Dermatol* 1964;90: 553–7.

9 Weinstein GD, Frost P. Methotrexate for psoriasis. A new therapeutic schedule. *Arch Dermatol* 1971;103:33–8.

10 Halprin KM, Fukui K, Ohkawara A. Blood levels of methotrexate and the treatment of psoriasis. *Arch Dermatol* 1971;103:243–9.

11 Collins P, Rogers S. The efficacy of methotrexate in psoriasis — a review of 40 cases. *Clin Exp Dermatol* 1992;17:257–60.

12 Paul BS, Momtaz-T K, Stern RS, *et al.* Combined methotrexate–ultraviolet B therapy in the treatment of psoriasis. *J Am Acad Dermatol* 1982;7:758–62.

13 Morison WL, Momtaz-T K, Parrish JA, Fitzpatrick TB. Combined methotrexate–PUVA therapy in the treatment of psoriasis. *J Am Acad Dermatol* 1982;6:46–51.

14 Van de Kerkhof PCM, Mali JWH. Methotrexate maintenance following Ingram therapy in "difficult" psoriasis. *Br J Dermatol* 1982;106:623–7.

15 Tuyp E, Mackie RM. Combination therapy for psoriasis with methotrexate and etretinate. *J Am Acad Dermatol* 1986;14:70–3.

16 Vanderveen EE, Ellis CN, Campbell JP, *et al.* Methotrexate and etretinate as concurrent therapies in severe psoriasis. *Arch Dermatol* 1982;118:660–2.

17 Larsen FG, Nielsen-Kudsk F, Jakobsen P, *et al.* Interaction of etretinate with methotrexate pharmacokinetics in psoriatic patients. *J Clin Pharmacol* 1990;30: 802–7.

18 Harrison RV, Peat M, James R, Orrell D. Methotrexate and retinoids in combination for psoriasis (Letter). *Lancet* 1987;i:512.

19 *MTX-Treatment Series.* Portland: National Psoriasis Foundation, Inc., 1989.

20 *Methotrexate in Psoriasis.* Pearl River: American Cyanamid Co., 1983.

21 *Methotrexate Package Insert.* Pearl River: American Cyanamid Co., 1989.
22 Roenigk HH, Auerbach R, Maibach HI, Weinstein GD. Methotrexate in psoriasis: revised guidelines. *J Am Acad Dermatol* 1988;19:145–56.
23 Stewart KA, Mackenzie AH, Clough JD, Wilke WS. Folate supplementation in methotrexate-treated rheumatoid arthritis patients. *Semin Arthritis Rheum* 1991; 20:332–8.
24 Duhra P. Treatment of gastrointestinal symptoms associated with methotrexate therapy for psoriasis. *J Am Acad Dermatol* 1993;28:466–9.
25 Comaish S, Juhlin L. Site of action of methotrexate. *Arch Dermatol* 1969;100: 99–105.
26 Lowe NJ, Stoughton RB, McCullough JL, Weinstein GD. Topical drug effects on normal and proliferating epidermal cell models. *Arch Dermatol* 1981;117:394–8.
27 Weinstein GD, McCullough JL, Olsen E. Topical methotrexate therapy for psoriasis. *Arch Dermatol* 1989;125:227–30.
28 Guzzo C, Benik K, Lazarus G, Johnson J, Weinstein G. Treatment of psoriasis with piritrexim, a lipid-soluble folate antagonist. *Arch Dermatol* 1991;127:511–4.
29 Morgan SL, Baggott JE, Vaughn WH, *et al.* The effect of folic acid supplementation on the toxicity of low-dose methotrexate in patients with rheumatoid arthritis. *Arthritis Rheum* 1990;33:9–18.
30 Kozlowski RD, Steinbrunner JV, Mackenzie AH, *et al.* Outcome of first-trimester exposure to low-dose methotrexate in eight patients with rheumatic disease. *Am J Med* 1990;88:589–92.
31 Bedrossian CWM, Miller WC, Luna MA. Methotrexate-induced diffuse interstitial pulmonary fibrosis. *South Med J* 1979;72:313–8.
32 Kremer JM, Lee RG, Tolman KG. Liver histology in rheumatoid arthritis patients receiving long-term methotrexate therapy. *Arthritis Rheum* 1989;32:121–7.
33 Zachariae H, Grunnet E, Sogaard H. Liver biopsy in methotrexate-treated psoriatics — a re-evaluation. *Acta Derm Venereol* 1975;55:291–6.
34 Warin AP, Landells JW, Levene GM, Baker H. A prospective study of the effects of weekly oral methotrexate on liver biopsy. *Br J Dermatol* 1975;93:321–7.
35 Zachariae H, Kragballe K, Sogaard H. Methotrexate induced liver cirrhosis. *Br J Dermatol* 1980;102:407–12.
36 Gilbert SC, *et al.* Methotrexate-induced cirrhosis requiring liver transplantation in three patients with psoriasis. *Arch Intern Med* 1990;150:889–91.
37 Janes CH, Lindor KD. Outcome of patients hospitalized for complications after outpatient liver biopsy. *Ann Intern Med* 1993;118:96–8.
38 Geronemus RG, Auerbach R, Tobias H. Liver biopsies vs liver scans in methotrexate-treated patients with psoriasis. *Arch Dermatol* 1982;118:649–51.
39 Miller JA, Dodd H, Rustin MHA, *et al.* Ultrasound as a screening procedure for methotrexate-induced hepatic damage in severe psoriasis. *Br J Dermatol* 1985;113: 699–705.
40 McHenry PM, Bingham EA, Callender ME, *et al.* Dynamic hepatic scintigraphy in the screening of psoriatic patients for methotrexate-induced hepatotoxicity. *Br J Dermatol* 1992;127:122–5.
41 Zachariae H, Aslam HM, Bjerring P, *et al.* Serum aminoterminal propeptide of type III procollagen in psoriasis and psoriatic arthritis: relation to liver fibrosis and arthritis. *J Am Acad Dermatol* 1991;25:50–3.

sixteen Cyclosporine

INTRODUCTION

Cyclosporine is a cyclic polypeptide consisting of 11 amino acids isolated from the soil fungus *Tolypocladium inflatum Gams* in 1972. Cyclosporine is a unique immunosuppressant because it interferes directly with T-cell function by inhibiting the cytokine cascade (interleukins-1 (IL-1) and -2 (IL-2) and IL-2 receptor (IL-2R)) without myelosuppressive effects [1]. The drug has been proved superior to azathioprine, cyclophosphamide, and corticosteroids in the prevention of graft rejection in patients receiving allogeneic kidney, liver, heart, and bone marrow transplants [2]. Many diseases with putative autoimmune etiologies besides psoriasis have been treated with cyclosporine in double-blind trials [3]. Efficacy has been shown for the mucocutaneous manifestations of dermatologic diseases such as atopic dermatitis, oral lichen planus, and Behçet's disease.

MECHANISM OF ACTION

Oral cyclosporine is absorbed rapidly from the small intestine, but it is incomplete (about 30%) and highly variable (4–89%). The bioavailability of the soft gelatin capsules is equivalent to the oral solution. Peak plasma concentrations are achieved in 2–4 hours.

The drug is metabolized extensively in the liver by the microsomal P450 oxidase system. The metabolites are primarily excreted into the bile and enter the enterohepatic circulation. About 6% of the dose is excreted in the urine, and only 0.1% of the dose is excreted as unchanged cyclosporine. There is great variability in the metabolism, with an average terminal half-life of 19 hours (range: 10–27 hours).

Cyclosporine is widely distributed in all body tissues. Owing to its lipophilic nature, it remains in the tissues long after dosing has been discontinued. In blood the distribution is concentration-dependent, that is, at high concentrations leukocytes and erythrocytes become saturated. In the plasma, approximately 90% of cyclosporine is bound to lipoproteins.

The individual variation in plasma concentration can be accounted for in part by differences in concentrations of high and low density lipoproteins. Bioavailability of the drug appears to increase during the first 2 weeks of oral administration apparently after the "first-pass effect," as tissues become saturated, and as the enterohepatic recirculation reaches equilibrium.

CLINICAL USE

Efficacy

The first reports of cyclosporine's remarkable efficacy in psoriasis were the serendipitous results of treating patients for psoriatic arthritis and allogeneic kidney transplantation. During the next decade, numerous reports of open and controlled studies of cyclosporine in the treatment of more than a thousand patients with psoriasis have helped to define the selection, dosing, toxicity, and monitoring of patients with the drug [4,5]. The report of a consensus conference was published in 1992 [6].

Because of the great individual variability in absorption, bioavailability, and responsiveness of psoriasis to cyclosporine, doses ranging from 1 to 14 mg/kg per day have reportedly been effective. As expected, the higher doses are associated with a more rapid onset of improvement, greater efficacy, and more significant toxicity.

The efficacy of high-dose cyclosporine was shown in a double-blind study; 14 mg/kg per day was significantly better than placebo at improving psoriasis ($P < 0.0001$) [7]. After 4 weeks of treatment, the onset of subjective and objective improvement occurred rapidly, as soon as 1 and 7 days later, respectively. The authors recognized that high-dose cyclosporine was not the optimal regimen for psoriasis however. The study was important because it confirmed efficacy as well as the significant toxicities to be monitored in future protocols employing lower doses for longer periods of time. They demonstrated statistically significant elevations in diastolic blood pressure, serum creatinine, blood urea nitrogen, bilirubin, cholesterol, triglycerides, potassium, and uric acid. Magnesium was reduced. Interestingly, there were no alterations in any of the liver enzymes tested.

Subsequent dose-finding studies performed in multiple European centers and the University of Michigan (USA) have given results that are in agreement. The conclusions for standard therapy are still left to the interpretation and judgment of the experienced clinician and will be discussed at the end of this section.

"Success" was defined as a reduction in psoriasis area and severity index (PASI) score of 75% or more or a score of 8 or less after 3 or more months of cyclosporine treatment of severe plaque-type psoriasis. Success rates were about 21, 54, and 88% for 1.25, 2.5 or 3, and 5 mg/kg per day. When the cyclosporine dose was escalated from a starting dose of 1.25 or 2.5 mg/kg per day, 28% of cases achieved a dose of 5 mg/kg per day because of insufficient therapeutic response at the lower doses [8]. In another multidose double-blind trial with placebo, success was defined as complete clearing or trace psoriasis (almost clear). After 8 weeks of fixed-dose therapy, success was achieved for 0, 36, 65, and 80% of patients receiving vehicle, 3, 5, and 7.5 mg/kg per day of cyclosporine [9].

Cyclosporine does not cure psoriasis and does not induce remissions that are more durable than, e.g., psoralen UVA (PUVA) or the Ingram regimen; therefore, continuous cyclosporine administration or conversion to alternative systemic therapy is necessary in order to maintain prolonged remission. Discontinuation of cyclosporine or a suboptimal dose allows skin lesions to recur at a rate and severity consistent with the natural history of an individual's disease. In a study of 24 of 30 patients who cleared completely with 5 mg/kg per day cyclosporine within 3 months, eight (33%) relapsed by 8 months [10]. (Relapse was defined as return of rash to 50% of the area involved prior to cyclosporine therapy.) The relapse rate for cyclosporine (67%) was comparable to that for anthralin-treated patients (75%). Moreover, continuing cyclosporine for an additional 4 weeks after clinical clearance, to "consolidate" remission, appeared to confer no advantage. A maintenance dose-finding study suggested that cyclosporine doses could be titrated down to a range of 1.1–7.2 mg/kg per day according to disease activity.

Clinical studies

Combination therapy

PUVA was added to cyclosporine therapy after relapse occurred upon reduction of the dose or if cyclosporine 5 mg/kg per day was considered ineffective as monotherapy. Combination therapy was effective in only one of four patients [11]. The well-documented increased risk of cutaneous squamous cell carcinoma is probably potentiated by cyclosporine. Therefore, combination treatment with cyclosporine and PUVA is not recommended.

Using a protocol similar to the above, etretinate was added to the therapy of five patients. No additive therapeutic effect of etretinate to cyclosporine therapy was observed [12]. The dose of etretinate was not stated; however, four of five patients developed typical mucocutaneous side effects. All five patients demonstrated reversible increases in serum creatinine (19–56%).

Isotretinoin has been used to treat severe acne in kidney and heart transplant patients taking cyclosporine [13,14]. The acne improved without evidence of graft rejection or cyclosporine toxicity. Cyclosporine trough levels remained within the recommended therapeutic range with the usual dosage adjustments required during monitoring. Therefore, while isotretinoin has limited usefulness in plaque-type psoriasis, there may be instances in women of childbearing potential, pustular psoriasis, or cyclosporine nephrotoxicity where combination therapy might be considered. The chief concern here is hyperlipidemia [15], a well-known side effect of both cyclosporine and retinoids.

Griffiths *et al.* [16] employed cyclosporine with and without the potent topical corticosteroid clobetasol propioniate. The combination cleared psoriasis faster (6 weeks vs 3.5 weeks) than cyclosporine alone, and there was no significant difference in relapse rates or side effects. Such an approach would be valuable if it allowed for a lower starting dose of cyclosporine.

The combination of methotrexate (MTX) and cyclosporine therapy has been considered dangerous [17] because the target organ of toxicity for one drug is the predominant organ of excretion of the other (liver/kidney). However, the combination has proved significantly more effective than either agent alone in reducing the incidence of acute graft-vs-host disease in patients receiving allogeneic bone marrow transplantation. Early toxicities include delayed engraftment, increased mucositis, and hepatotoxicity [18]. While survival with the combination is similar or improved, the relapse rate of leukemia is increased in some studies compared to monotherapy [19]. In an animal model of rheumatoid arthritis, rats immunized with native type II collagen manifested a significant decrease in the incidence and severity of arthritis when treated with the combination of MTX and cyclosporine compared to either agent alone. The liver and kidney demonstrated no histologic abnormalities after the study suggesting that combination therapy may be safe and effective for rheumatoid and psoriatic arthritis [20].

How to use cyclosporine

Consultation

Cyclosporine is a potent and toxic drug for patients with severe psoriasis. Physicians should consult a dermatologist with experience in the management of patients taking cyclosporine before initiating therapy. In patients with normal baseline renal function, monitoring is straightforward, and it is usually not necessary to enlist the aid of a nephrologist.

Selection

Patients with extensive or disabling plaque-type, erythrodermic, or pustular psoriasis who have failed, cannot tolerate, or cannot obtain approved systemic therapies including PUVA, MTX, and etretinate.

Contraindications

1 Abnormal renal function.
2 Uncontrolled hypertension.
3 Primary or secondary immunodeficiency.
4 Severe hepatic dysfunction.

Relative contraindications

In psoriasis, other immunosuppressive or carcinogenic medications, including PUVA and UVB, should not be given during cyclosporine therapy because of the increased risk of skin cancer. Whenever possible, drugs known to interfere with the metabolism of cyclosporine and drugs known to be nephrotoxic including aspirin, ibuprofen, and other nonsteroidal antiinflammatory drugs (NSAIDs) should be avoided. Patients with a previous or concomitant noncutaneous malignancy should obtain clearance from their own general practitioner or oncologist before receiving cyclosporine.

How to evaluate patient prior to initiation of cyclosporine
The patient should receive (preferably written) educational material about cyclosporine, and the risk/benefit ratio for the individual should be discussed with the physician or consultant. If the decision is made to proceed with cyclosporine treatment, the patient should undergo a complete physical examination to include routine screening tests for cancer where appropriate (rectal exam, stool guaiac, cervical cytologic smear, mammogram) and a thorough examination of the integument to include the oral cavity and genitalia for tumors as well as an estimation of BSA involved, type of psoriasis, and degree of disability. Blood pressure should be recorded on two or more occasions prior to therapy. Routine laboratory tests include 12-hour fasting serum electrolytes, liver enzymes, and lipids, complete blood count, and urinalysis. A baseline serum creatinine level should be recorded on two or more occasions. We do not believe it is necessary to measure the glomerular filtration rate (GFR) or calculate creatinine clearance because these tests are not practical to obtain in an office setting and will not be used to monitor nephrotoxicity during therapy except in controlled experimental protocols.

How to initiate cyclosporine therapy

It is clear now that the starting dose should not exceed 5 mg/kg per day, but controversy exists as to whether the dose should be even that high. Several studies have shown that administration of 3 mg/kg per day for 3 months reduces the PASI score in the majority of patients. Such a conservative approach spares 30–40% of patients of ever having to receive a higher dose of cyclosporine (and presumably a greater risk of nephrotoxicity). In patients in whom it is desirable to obtain a more rapid response to therapy, such as acute inflammatory forms of psoriasis, patients in hospital and patients with disabling arthropathy, it is appropriate to use 4 or 5 mg/kg per day (Fig. 16.1). Because the plasma half-life is less than 24 hours, it is logical to administer cyclosporine in divided doses 12 hours apart.

Maintenance dose of cyclosporine

If the patient started at 3 mg/kg per day and continued this dose for 3 months, taper or increase the dose by 0.5–1 mg/kg per day monthly depending upon the response. Do not exceed 5 mg/kg per day. If this dose produces an insufficient therapeutic response, then consider cyclosporine a failure and convert the patient to alternative therapy. If the patient's psoriasis is well maintained at 1 mg/kg per day consider stopping cyclosporine as less than half the patients will relapse in 6 months. If the

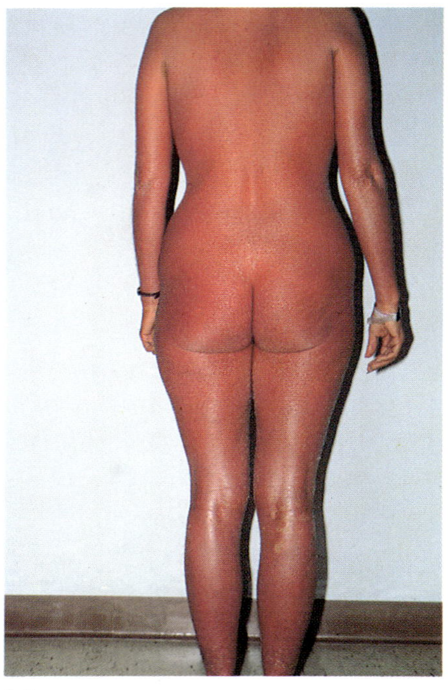
(a)

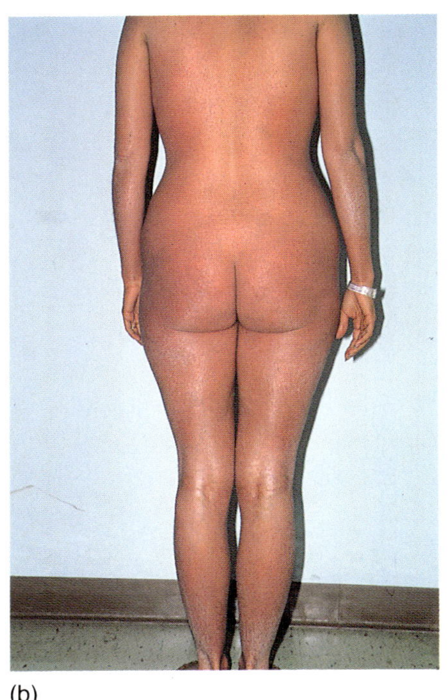
(b)

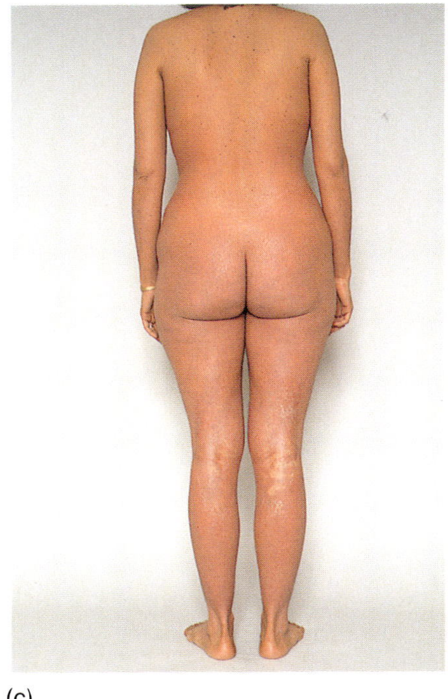
(c)

Fig 16.1 Psoriatic erythroderma (a) before treatment and (b) after 1 week and (c) 2 weeks of cyclosporine 5 mg/kg per day.

psoriasis flares during the taper, revert to the previous higher dose and consider chronic maintenance. Provided that the monitoring recommendations are followed, cyclosporine may be used safely and continuously for at least 2 years [21].

Renal monitoring

During the first 3 months of cyclosporine therapy, blood pressure and serum creatinine should be assessed every 2 weeks. After that, if these parameters are acceptable and stable, a monthly determination will suffice.

The maximal serum creatinine level is most closely associated with decreased GFR and serious morphologic changes. Cyclosporine-induced nephropathy developed in only 7% of patients with a maximal increase in serum creatinine of less than 30% above baseline values and in 59% of patients with an increase of 100% or more [22]. Therefore, if serum creatinine rises above 30% of baseline value (not the upper limit of the normal range), the dose of cyclosporine must be reduced. If the serum creatinine does not decrease below 130% of baseline value after 1 month, discontinue cyclosporine. If the reduced cyclosporine dose improves the creatinine to a "safe" level but fails to maintain the psoriasis, then the patient must be considered a cyclosporine failure. The drug should be discontinued rather than accepting the risk of irreversible nephropathy in the treatment of a nonlife-threatening disease.

It is believed that cyclosporine increases the synthesis of thromboxane A_2, a potent vasoconstrictor [23]. In the hope of decreasing thromboxane A_2 production, fish oil concentrate 12 g (containing eicosapentaenoic acid and docosahexaenoic acid in a ratio of 3 : 2) was given to eight patients receiving cyclosporine 5 mg/kg per day [24]. The fall in GFR in this group (9%) was significantly less than the patients treated with either 2.5 or 5 mg/kg per day cyclosporine alone (18%). The differences in increases of serum creatinine, however, were not statistically significant. Fish oil, still in search of a therapeutic niche, added to the diet of patients may attenuate cyclosporine-induced renal dysfunction.

What is the role of cyclosporine blood levels in psoriasis?

There is no role for cyclosporine blood levels in the routine monitoring of uncomplicated cases. In the treatment of psoriasis, there is no significant correlation between cyclosporine level and efficacy or renal dysfunction [25].

Cyclosporine dosing, efficacy, and toxicity are monitored as follows:

1 monitor the dose of cyclosporine taken by writing detailed limited prescriptions;

2 monitor efficacy by examining the skin and asking patients about subjective symptoms such as pruritus at periodic followup visits;

3 monitor toxicity by measuring blood pressure and serum creatinine.

Plasma cyclosporine levels by radioimmunoassay are now widely available in hospital and commercial laboratories. Consider obtaining cyclosporine trough levels (right before the next dose is due) in cases of unexpected inefficacy, suspected noncompliance, unexpected toxicity, and drug interactions. However, it is more important to increase the frequency of serum creatinine determinations if drugs known to increase cyclosporine concentration (e.g., ketoconazole, erythromycin) or nephrotoxic drugs (e.g., NSAIDs) are prescribed. In practice, we have found that cyclosporine trough levels of about 100 ng/ml are efficacious and levels over 200 ng/ml may be nephrotoxic.

TOXICITY

The mild common adverse effects of cyclosporine are generally well tolerated and accepted by patients: gingival hyperplasia or overgrowth of the interdental papillae (can also be associated with calcium channel blockers used to treat hypertension); hypertrichosis [26] affecting face, scalp, and extremities; tremor, paresthesia, headache; and nausea. These symptoms are dose-dependent and usually disappear upon cessation of therapy.

As with all immunosuppressive medications, there is a theoretical increased risk of infections and malignancy, particularly lymphoma, squamous cell carcinoma, and Kaposi's sarcoma [27]. The incidence of lymphoma in transplant patients is about 0.1–0.4%, but is lower in patients with autoimmune diseases (<0.1%). In a population of 950 patients with psoriasis treated with cyclosporine for an average of 6 months, one case each of B-cell lymphoma and T-cell lymphoma (mycosis fungoides) was reported.

Many patients with severe psoriasis are already at risk for squamous cell carcinoma because of previous exposure to arsenic, X-rays, solar radiation, therapeutic UVB, and/or PUVA. In the same group of 950 patients there were nine squamous cell carcinomas. The rate of incidence of skin tumors in psoriasis treated with cyclosporine has been calculated to be 0.5–0.8/1000 patients per month [21]. No cases of Kaposi's sarcoma in psoriasis have been observed. The frequency and severity of bacterial, viral, and opportunistic infections in psoriatics appear not to be increased by cyclosporine alone. Infections in psoriatics occurred at the same rate with placebo, cyclosporine, and etretinate and were uncomplicated.

The two most important side effects of cyclosporine, requiring baseline evaluation, constant monitoring, and intervention (medical treatment, dose reduction, or discontinuation of cyclosporine) are hypertension and nephrotoxicity [21,28]. Cyclosporine causes vasoconstriction of the afferent glomerular arteriole, which leads to decreased renal blood flow and a decrease in the GFR [28,29]. The increase in serum creatinine and urea is a direct reflection of decreased GFR. In the fixed multidose studies by Ellis *et al.* [7,9] the percent increase of creatinine for 0, 3, 5, 7.5, and 14 mg/kg per day was 0, 5, 10, 22, and 25%, respectively. For BUN, it was 0, 25, 44, 42, and 95%, respectively. The GFR was measured before and after 8 weeks of cyclosporine therapy in 34 patients by clearance of ^{125}I iodothalamate sodium clearance. It decreased by 2, 6, 15, and 19% with the 0, 3, 5, and 7.5 mg/kg per day doses, respectively. Only 19% was a significantly decreased result compared to the others. Using multiple linear regression analysis the authors determined that change in the serum urea nitrogen concentration was the best single predictor of change in the GFR. Gilbert *et al.* [30] emphasized that the rise in serum creatinine was a poor predictor of the decrease in GFR in five patients treated with a mean dosage of 4.7 mg/kg per day for 9 weeks. Serum creatinine rose 10%, but the GFR decreased 37%. However, these results may be aberrant because of the small sample and concomitant antihypertensive medications that were not calcium channel blockers. Lewis *et al.* [22] and Ellis *et al.* [9] have independently reported a median decline of 16% in GFR for patients receiving an average dose of 3.3 and 5.2 mg/kg per day. The GFR increased toward its baseline level concomitant with a moderate reduction in average dose over a period of 1–3 months.

Chronic cyclosporine-induced nephropathy is characterized histopathologically by moderate to severe focal (striped) interstitial fibrosis and tubular atrophy. Renal arteriolar abnormalities such as intimal hyalinosis may also be seen. Zachariae *et al.* [29] performed pretreatment and posttreatment renal biopsies in 12 psoriasis patients treated with cyclosporine 1.8–6 mg/kg per day for 6–18 months. Increases in serum creatinine and blood pressure required a dose reduction in several patients. The increases were reversible, and none required antihypertensive medications. Serum creatinine increased in eight of 12 and creatinine clearance decreased in nine of 12. Ten had a normal biopsy before treatment. After treatment, 11 of 12 had an abnormal kidney biopsy. Blinded morphometric evaluation showed a significant increase in the amount of interstitial fibrous tissue and a nonsignificant increase in arteriolar hyaline wall thickening. The percent decrease in creatinine clearance correlated significantly with the degree of fibrosis. This study demonstrated slight to moderate morphologic renal damage in patients receiving relatively low doses of cyclosporine. Similarly, Powles *et al.* [31] found morphologic evidence of cyclosporine nephrotoxicity in six of eight renal biopsies performed after 48–66 months of chronic maintenance cyclosporine therapy at a mean dose of 3.3 (range: 2–5) mg/kg per day. They noted that the best predictor of adverse biopsy results was failure of renal function to return to baseline after the month of therapy.

Renal biopsies were performed in 192 patients with autoimmune or inflammatory diseases during cyclosporine therapy to assess the safety of continuing treatment [32]. Eleven patients with psoriasis were included in this study and were treated with a mean dose of 3.9 mg/kg per day for a median of 17 months before the biopsy. Forty-one of the 192 patients showed evidence of cyclosporine-induced nephropathy, but none of the psoriatics was affected.

An advisory board of seven kidney pathologists recommended that the presence of cyclosporine-induced nephropathy as defined should result in discontinuation of treatment in nonlife-threatening conditions such as psoriasis. The relevance of the milder lesions reported by Zachariae *et al.* [29] to continued treatment is uncertain. The incidence of cyclosporine-induced nephropathy was significantly related to the maximal increase in serum creatinine or urea [32]. Serum uric acid, potassium, magnesium, and bilirubin concentrations were not related to nephropathy. The multivariate analysis showed that in adults the maximal increase in serum creatinine, the initial dose of cyclosporine, and increased age all contributed significantly to the risk of cyclosporine-induced nephropathy. The duration of treatment, the cumulative dose of cyclosporine, the duration of the increase in serum creatinine, or the occurrence of elevated blood pressure did not have an additional significant influence on the risk of nephropathy. The patients with cyclosporine nephropathy were compared to those who did not develop it: the maximal increase in serum creatinine was 101% vs 50%; initial dose of cyclosporine 9.3 mg/kg per day vs 8.0 mg/kg per day; age 31 years vs 23 years [32].

There is consensus among all investigators that while changes in renal function do not always reflect morphologic changes, if serum creatinine rises to more than 30% above an individual patient's baseline value, then the dose of cyclosporine should be reduced [6,22,28,29]. The likelihood of developing nephropathy can be minimized by limiting the dose of cyclosporine to a maximum of 5 mg/kg per day and adhering to the lowest possible maintenance dose.

Hypertension

Cyclosporine induces a dose-related rise in diastolic blood pressure almost equal to 1 mmHg for every 1 mg/kg per day of drug [21]. Hypertension develops in 10–15% of patients within weeks of initiating treatment at

2–5 mg/kg per day. Lewis *et al.* [22] reported hypertension (systolic blood pressure >160 mmHg or diastolic >95 mmHg) in 33% of patients after 0.5–62 (mean 11.5) months of treatment suggesting that the risk of developing hypertension increases with either duration of cyclosporine treatment or cumulative cyclosporine dose. It is usually reversible after cyclosporine is stopped.

How to treat hypertension

Hypertension commonly develops during cyclosporine therapy. If systolic pressure of 160 mmHg or diastolic pressures of 95 mmHg are documented on two or more occasions, there must be intervention. If the clinical situation permits reducing the dose or stopping cyclosporine, that should be done first. If medical treatment of hypertension is contemplated, consultation with an internist or nephrologist may be obtained, but the physician experienced with cyclosporine can usually treat hypertension.

The calcium channel blockers may be "renal protective," that is, they cause preferential vasodilation of renal afferent arterioles with increases in GFR and renal blood flow [33]. Verapamil had a renal-sparing effect when used in combination with cyclosporine in the rat [32]. Although some calcium antagonists increase cyclosporine levels (nicardipine, diltiazem), we have not had difficulty with verapamil and prescribe it as first-line therapy for cyclosporine-associated hypertension (Calan SR 120–240 mg/day). Nifedipine and isradipine have also been recommended. Inform patients that both cyclosporine and the calcium channel blockers have been reported to cause gingival hypertrophy.

It is best to avoid the diuretics. The popular combination of hydrochlorothiazide and triamterene, for example, increases the risk of hyperuricemia, gout [32], and hyperkalemia in patients taking cyclosporine.

Drug interactions

Several commonly prescribed drugs can alter the concentration of cyclosporine in blood or enhance certain cyclosporine toxicities synergistically or additionally by different mechanisms.

The plasma level of cyclosporine is influenced by drugs that affect hepatic microsomal P450 activity. Substances known to inhibit metabolism and increase cyclosporine levels are: danazol, ketoconazole, erythromycin, nicardipine, diltiazem, methyltestosterone, and oral contraceptives. Agents that induce cytochrome P450 enzymes increase hepatic metabolism and diminish cyclosporine levels include phenytoin, phenobarbital, carbamazepine, rifampin, and intravenous trimethoprim-sulfamethoxazole. Concomitant administration of potentially nephrotoxic drugs may accentuate cyclosporine effects by compromising renal blood flow or by a direct tubulointerstitial effect: aminoglycoside antibiotics, amphotericin B, NSAIDs, and diuretics. The addition of immunosuppressive drugs such as corticosteroids, azathioprine, and cyclophosphamide to cyclosporine increases the risk of severe infections and malignancies.

Topical cyclosporine

In an attempt to circumvent the systemic toxicity of cyclosporine, topical formulations of 5% in oil and ointment base have been applied to psoriasis with and without plastic film occlusion for 6 hours per day [34]. No clinical differences were observed between cyclosporine-treated and control lesions. Cyclosporine concentration in the topically-treated lesions was equivalent to that of psoriatic lesions after 7 days of systemic therapy [35]. The investigators demonstrated a reduction in the number of neutrophils in the epidermis and papillary dermis but not mononuclear cells and no effect on epidermal growth kinetics. Hypotheses to explain the failure of topical cyclosporine to improve psoriasis include: (i) cyclosporine does not reach the biologic target in skin in adequate concentrations (endothelial cells? fibroblasts?); (ii) cyclosporine does not reach circulating lymphocytes before they are recruited to enter the skin; and (iii) intradermal metabolism does not produce the hepatic metabolites that may be more immunosuppressive than the parent compound. Most of these hypotheses were disproved by Burns *et al.* [36] who showed that thrice-weekly intralesional injections of cyclosporine 17 mg/ml improved psoriatic plaques without affecting distant plaques or producing significant blood trough levels. The concentration in tissue was higher than the mean trough tissue levels in keratomes of psoriasis plaques from patients receiving high-dose cyclosporine (14 mg/kg per day) for 1 week. Metabolism of cyclosporine probably does not occur in the skin, so the parent compound is in fact active in psoriasis. The successful local use of cyclosporine may relate to a different mechanism of action than with systemic therapy or to a requirement for a higher drug level in skin in order to inhibit activation of T cells when they do arrive in the psoriatic epidermis. The high tissue levels required for successful local cyclosporine psoriasis therapy (5.6 ± 2.4 ng/mg wet tissue weight) cannot be achieved with topical preparations because of cyclosporine's poor penetration through skin. Pain on injection was the most common side effect. Topical therapy with cyclosporine is ineffective, and intralesional injections, while efficacious, are impractical.

TACROLIMUS (FK506)

The macrolide antibiotic FK506 is a new immunosuppressive drug that is chemically unrelated to cyclosporine but also inhibits helper T-lymphocyte activation and the synthesis and expression of cytokines. The University of Pittsburgh (USA) [37] has reported that FK506 is highly effective in the prevention and treatment of whole organ transplant rejection.

Seven patients with psoriasis, four receiving organ transplants, were reported recently who cleared completely by 4 weeks with full antirejection doses of FK506 [38]. The remissions have been substained for 5.5–14 months. Improvement of psoriatic arthritis occurred simultaneously in the three patients who had it. Efforts to reduce the dose of FK506 resulted in relapse of psoriasis.

Serial biopsies from active psoriatic plaques revealed rapid disappearance of dermal inflammatory cells and neutrophils in the stratum corneum. Hyperkeratosis and acanthosis were slower to return to normal.

Immunophenotypic analysis during remission showed reductions in epidermal and dermal CD4+, CD8+, CD25+ (IL-2R+ activated T cells), and CDW60+ (disease-associated T cells); striking rise in CD1+ epidermal Langerhans cells; and persistence of CD54 (intercellular adhesion molecule-1; ICAM-1) on residual lymphocytes and vascular endothelium [39]. These results are similar to those reported for cyclosporine.

While the efficacy of FK506 in psoriasis is exciting, the serious adverse effects of this agent seem to be identical to those of cyclosporine: hypertension and nephrotoxicity. Three patients developed arterial hypertension controlled with a single drug. In the four patients who underwent organ transplantation serum creatinine levels increased 100–200% (mean 152%) above baseline. These patients may have had some degree of preexisting renal compromise. The three patients with psoriasis only experienced serum creatinine increases of 27–111% (mean 68%) above baseline [38]. If the "> 30% rule" for cyclosporine-induced nephropathy applies to FK506, then the therapeutic window for FK506 in patients with psoriasis as the primary diagnosis may be very narrow indeed because of the risk of permanent impairment of renal function in order to keep the skin clear. Mild neurotoxicity was noted in three patients. Infections, hypertrichosis, and gingival hyperplasia were not observed.

Topical application of FK506 at 0.04–0.4% to domestic pig skin (which resembles human skin more closely than rodent skin) caused pronounced inhibition of contact hypersensitivity reactions to dinitrofluorobenzene [40]. The response was similar to the activity of 0.13% clobetasol. Cyclosporine was inactive at 10%. The authors suggested that topical FK506 may be effective for skin diseases such as psoriasis that respond to topical corticosteroids and systemic cyclosporine, but a more logical conclusion is that the lower molecular weight FK506 (804 Da) is able to penetrate skin better than cyclosporine (1202 Da). Studies on the topical application and intralesional injection of FK506 in psoriasis should be performed.

CASE STUDIES

Case 1

Low-dose cyclosporine is successful for severe plaque-type psoriasis after failure of Goeckerman regimen, MTX, and re-PUVA.

A 33-year-old white man was admitted to the Cleveland Clinic in 1987 for a Goeckerman regimen for severe psoriasis vulgaris with 80% BSA involved. He had had psoriasis for 13 years without arthritis. He was treated briefly with MTX in 1985 but developed severe headaches. He was next treated with re-PUVA consisting of isotretinoin with an initial positive

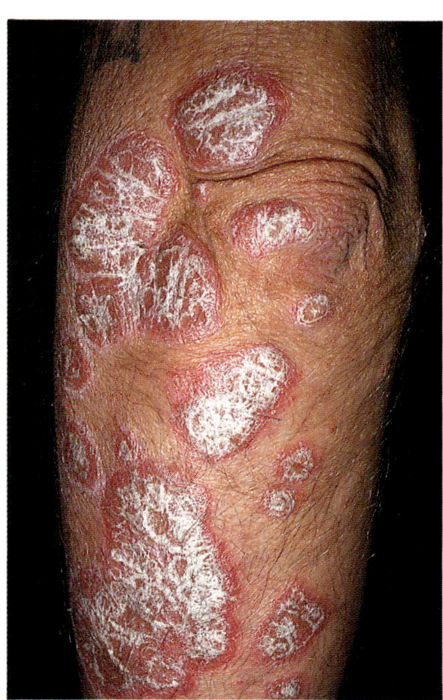

Fig 16.2 Case 1. Severe plaque-type psoriasis upon admission to day-treatment center.

effect that gradually deterioriated. In 1987 etretinate was substituted for isotretinoin at 100 mg/day (0.9 mg/kg per day), but the mucocutaneous side effects became intolerable. The dose was decreased to 25 mg/day. This low dose of etretinate was continued during the Goeckerman treatment. Corticosteroids were not used. He was discharged after 2 weeks in improved condition and maintained on UVB b.i.w. Etretinate was subsequently stopped because of soreness of his ankles and knees that was proved to be drug related by stopping and rechallenging with etretinate.

He was admitted to the psoriasis day-care center in October 1991 with 90% BSA involvement (Fig. 16.2) including the face. An empiric course of penicillin VK 1 g/day for 10 days was given. His anti-DNAse B was subsequently found to be elevated at 1 : 170. The Goeckerman regimen (3% crude coal tar and UVB starting at 30 mJ/cm^2, increasing by 10 mJ/cm^2 daily, and giving 100% extra dose to extremities) resulted in a modest response. His skin was still 55% involved. By January 1991 his skin had flared back to 80% involvement including highly inflamed plaques covered with large bran-like scales.

He was evaluated for cyclosporine therapy. He was normotensive and weighed 114 kg. His creatinine was 1.3 mg%, and his potassium was 5.0 mmol/l. He was started on cyclosporine 300 mg b.i.d. (5.3 mg/kg per day) and monitored at 3–4-weekly intervals. At each of the next three visits his skin showed further improvement, and the dose was decreased by 100 mg/day. After 13 weeks of cyclosporine treatment his skin was almost clear. Creatinine and potassium rose to 1.4 and 5.7, respectively. There was no change in blood pressure. After 1 month of taking 300 mg/day (2.6 mg/kg per day), a few new guttate lesions with fine scaling appeared on the trunk and extremities. The dose was held at this level. Creatinine and potassium returned to normal: 1.2 and 4.7, respectively. His cyclosporine trough level at this dose was 171 ng/ml after 2 months.

Comments

1 Headache is a common side effect of MTX that rarely leads to discontinuation of therapy.

2 Musculoskeletal symptoms such as bone ache and arthralgias are common side effects of etretinate that rarely lead to discontinuation of therapy.

3 The measurement of serum creatinine at regular intervals is the cornerstone of efficient monitoring for cyclosporine nephropathy. It is rarely necessary to measure creatinine clearance or GFR by inulin clearance or isotopic methods.

4 Cyclosporine induces alterations in tubular function, which result in hyperkalemia. Hypomagnesemia and increased serum uric acid may also occur, but these effects are seldom clinically relevant and do not require any intervention unless symptomatic gout occurs [41].

5 We prefer starting cyclosporine at about 5 mg/kg per day and decreasing until the lowest nontoxic dose that is still effective for psoriasis is reached and maintained. As with MTX, a small amount of residual psoriasis is desirable to ensure that a potent medicine is not overdosed.

6 It is generally not necessary to measure cyclosporine blood levels because efficacy can be monitored by skin examination and toxicity by serum creatinine and blood pressure determinations. Nevertheless, we have found that a trough level of about 150 ng/ml is optimal for both parameters.

Case 2

Severe pustular psoriasis, alcoholism, and combination cyclosporine/isotretinoin therapy.

A 51-year-old white man had severe psoriasis without arthritis for 5 years. He was admitted for treatment at another university dermatology program and received a Goeckerman regimen, PUVA, and etretinate. He admitted to heavy smoking and ethanol ingestion. He stated that he was only able to receive light therapy while hospitalized because he lived too far from the facility to continue outpatient maintenance treatments. Moreover, etretinate had been discontinued because of a rise in liver enzymes, and coal tar caused intolerable folliculitis.

Examination showed extensive involvement with indurated plaques involving about 65% BSA with scattered pustules (Fig. 16.3). Blood pressure was 140/72 mmHg; creatinine 0.8 mg%; liver enzymes were normal; calcium 8.8 mg%, uric acid 5.0, cholesterol 202, triglycerides 186, and high density lipoprotein-cholesterol 20, and white blood cell count 10 100/mm^3. He was treated with fluocinonide 0.05% under occlusion for the palms, UVB, and cyclosporine 6 mg/kg per day in two divided doses. His blood pressure rose to 176/110. A diuretic was started, and the diastolic pressure decreased to 96. Verapamil (a calcium channel blocker) was added, and the dose of cyclosporine was reduced. His blood pressure improved. After 7 months his hands were cleared. The patient stated that he was overall "the best ever" (Fig. 16.4).

Three months later, while taking 5 mg/kg per day of cyclosporine, his psoriasis flared on the palms and soles, and he complained of headaches. His blood pressure was 210/120, and his serum creatinine had risen to 1.7 (100% above baseline). Cyclosporine was discontinued because a clinically ineffective dose caused hypertension and renal insufficiency. The cyclosporine trough level was 83 ng/ml. He subsequently developed a

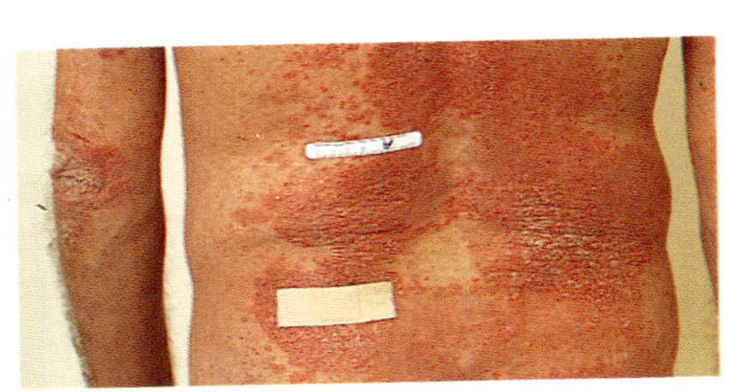
(a)

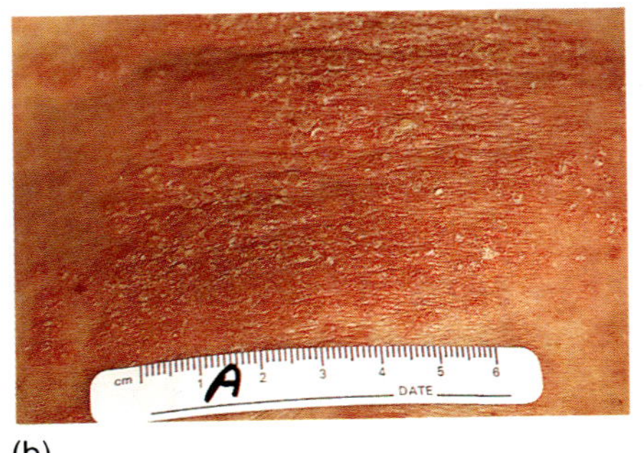

(b)

Fig 16.3 Case 2. (a) Generalized inflammatory plaque disease with (b) pustule formation.

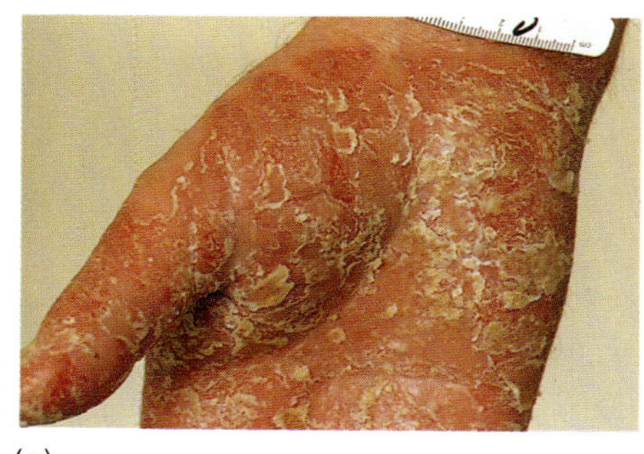
(a)

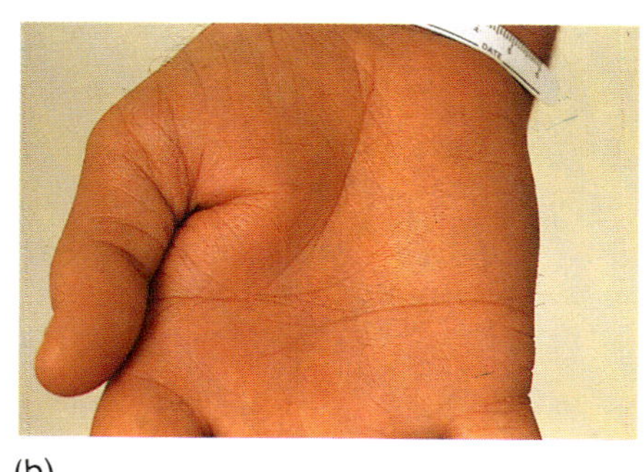
(b)

Fig 16.4 Case 2. Severe pustular psoriasis of the palm (a) before and (b) after cyclosporine treatment.

severe pustular flare and was admitted to hospital because involvement of the hands and feet had completely disabled him. Lakes of pus were present on the palms, soles, and thighs. Large red scaly plaques were present on the trunk and extremities. His skin was 80% involved, and he had a low grade fever. The white blood cell count was 12 800; uric acid 9.0, and creatinine 1.5. Cultures of pus grew Staphyloccus aureus. *Blood cultures were negative. He was treated with oral cephalexin 500 mg q.i.d.. PUVA with extra doses to the palms and soles was given in hospital, but the patient again declined outpatient light therapy. His blood pressure was well-controlled in hospital presumably because of a low salt diet and no alcohol.*

Hydroxyurea was started in May 1990 and increased to 1 g daily. It was stopped in July 1990 when no therapeutic response was observed. Sulfasalazine 500 mg t.i.d. was tried next. It was discontinued 2 weeks later when a papular eruption with diffuse erythema developed. It could be distinguished from psoriasis as a drug eruption. He continued to develop severe pustular flares and was hospitalized on five separate occasions during the next 15 months. He acknowledged that alcohol abuse aggravated his skin and blood pressure problems, and he agreed to speak with the chemical dependence consultant. He was diagnosed with "alcohol dependence, chronic phase," but he refused to be transferred to the detoxification unit.

He was treated with a series of empiric combinations (Table 16.1). Anti-DNAse B, an indicator of prior streptococcal infection, was elevated at 1 : 240.

Table 16.1 Empiric combination treatments

Plan A	Plan B	Plan C
PUVA + UVB Triamcinolone 0.1% Cefazolin i.v. 1 g q8h Fluconazole p.o. 100 mg/day	PUVA + UVB Fluocinolone 0.025% Ciprofloxacin p.o. 750 mg b.i.d. Calcitriol (vitamin D3) 1 μg q.h.s.	PUVA + UVB Oxacillin i.v. 1 g q6h Cyclosporine p.o. 200 mg b.i.d. Isotretinoin p.o. 40 mg/day

While receiving calcitriol (Plan B), 24-hour urinary calcium excretion increased from 37 to 312 mg and serum calcium increased to 10.9 before any improvement in his psoriasis was seen. Calcitriol was therefore stopped. After the "Plan C" admission he abstained from alcohol for a few months and remained markedly improved while continuing on cyclosporine 200 mg/day (2.5 mg/kg per day) and isotretinoin 40 mg/day. He remained normotensive with a cyclosporine trough level of 136 ng/ml. Unfortunately, when he began to drink about four-fifths of a liter of whiskey daily, he decreased the dose of cyclosporine to 100 mg/day on his own and flared within 3 weeks. He took high doses of over-the-counter ibuprofen for skin pain. His uric acid and his creatinine rose to 13.0 and 3.2, respectively. Intravenous infusion of normal saline partially improved these levels. The cyclosporine trough level while taking 100 mg/day was 70 ng/ml. Verapamil was reintroduced for hypertension, this time without a diuretic.

When last examined 4 months after discharge, he was still drinking. His psoriasis, while severe by any standard, was improved and manageable for him with 50% BSA with thin red plaques and light branny scale. The palms were not pustular and were functional. The soles were covered with thick scales but no pustules. His treatment consisted of cyclosporine 2.5 mg/kg per day, isotretinoin 40 mg/day, verapamil 240 mg/day, and 0.1% triamcinolone ointment. Uric acid was 8.7, creatinine 1.8, calcium 9.6, cholesterol 294, and triglycerides 534. The cyclosporine trough level was 143 ng/ml.

Comments

This case is remarkable because it demonstrates how difficult it is to treat severe psoriasis in an alcoholic patient without the benefit of outpatient UV light maintenance. In addition, this patient seemed to develop an adverse reaction to almost every systemic antipsoriatic medication given. The complications were not always completely reversible.

Case 2 illustrates many points relating to the various treatment modalities.

1 Coal tar: folliculitis is a common local reaction that usually does not preclude its continued use.

2 Corticosteroids: this patient's reliance on potent topical corticosteroids between hospital admissions may have contributed to pustular flares.

3 Etretinate: causes elevations in transaminase levels in about 20% of cases. Severe idiosyncratic acute hepatitis resulting in chronic active hepatitis or death may occur in 1.5% of cases.

4 Hydroxyurea: was ineffective, but the optimal dose of 1.5 g/day was not used. No side effects were encountered.

5 Sulfasalazine: cutaneous eruptions are relatively common (17% in one series) [42] and occur within 1–6 weeks of initiating therapy.

6 Calcitriol: caused a marked increase in serum calcium and urinary calcium excretion within 1 week of receiving 1 μg in a single dose at night. A "low calcium diet," that is, omitting foods with a known high

calcium content such as milks, cheeses, and yogurts was not specifically recommended.

7 The patient was not a candidate for MTX because of alcoholism.

8 Cyclosporine: this patient was treated with cyclosporine before guidelines for use of the drug were published [6]. Patients now receive 2.5 mg/kg per day and this dose is increased as needed, or they are given 5.0 mg/kg per day which is tapered as tolerated. Apparently this patient's metabolism of cyclosporine was affected by preexisting liver damage, ethanol intake, and/or concomitant medications.

9 As hypertension and renal dysfunction are the most predictable side effects of cyclosporine, we now decrease the dose of cyclosporine if the creatinine rises 30% or more above baseline. Surprisingly, 5 mg/kg per day had no effect on psoriasis in this patient but caused severe hypertension and doubled the serum creatinine.

10 Calcium channel blockers are indicated for hypertension caused by cyclosporine. Verapamil 240 mg/day seemed to increase the trough level of cyclosporine while controlling blood pressure, allowing us to give a lower daily dose of cyclosporine.

11 The diuretic combination hydrochlorthiazide–triamterene which was used initially alone then in combination with verapamil probably contributed to the patient's dehydration and elevated uric acid levels without improving the cyclosporine-induced hypertension. Despite a uric acid level of 13.0 mg %, gouty arthritis did not develop, and no treatment other than stopping the diuretic and rehydration was necessary.

12 The combination of cyclosporine 2.5 mg/kg per day and isotretinoin 0.5 mg/kg per day with verapamil presently affords this patient the greatest relief. Serum creatinine and blood pressure are stable. Hypertriglyceridemia which can be caused by both cyclosporine [15] and isotretinoin is undoubtedly aggravated by his alcoholism. As we grapple with this problem, we recognize that abstinence, low fat diet, weight loss, dietary fish oil supplementation, and lipid lowering drugs may all be helpful.

13 The patient's unrestricted use of over-the-counter NSAIDs may have been additive to cyclosporine-induced nephrotoxicity. Prostaglandin synthetase inhibitors such as aspirin and ibuprofen are relatively contraindicated during cyclosporine therapy and should be limited or not used at all.

REFERENCES

1 Keown PA, Stiller CR. Cyclosporine: a double-edged sword. *Hosp Pract* 1987; 22:207–20.

2 Kolansky G. Cyclosporine: pharmacokinetics, administration, and efficacy in organ transplantation and other applications. *Hosp Formul* 1989;24:583–97.

3 Page EH, Wexler DM, Guenther LC. Cyclosporin A. *J Am Acad Dermatol* 1986; 14:785–91.

4 Timonen P, Friend D, Abeywickrama K, *et al.* Efficacy of low-dose cyclosporine A in psoriasis: results of dose-finding studies. *Br J Dermatol* 1990;122(Suppl. 36): 33–9.

5 Meinardi M, Derie MA, Bos JD. Oral cyclosporine A in treatment of psoriasis:

overview of studies performed in the Netherlands. *Br J Dermatol* 1990;122(Suppl. 36):27–91.
6 Mihatsch MJ, Wolff K. Consensus conference on cyclosporin A for psoriasis February 1992. *Br J Dermatol* 1992;126:621–3.
7 Ellis CN, Gorsulowsky DC, Hamilton TA, *et al.* Cyclosporine improves psoriasis in a double-blind study. *JAMA* 1986;256:3110–6.
8 Christophers E, Mrowietz U, Henneicke H-H, *et al.* Cyclosporin A in psoriasis: interim results of a multicentre dose-finding study in severe chronic plaque-type psoriasis. In Wolff K, ed. *Cyclosporin A and the Skin.* London: Royal Society of Medicine Services, 1992:21–6.
9 Ellis CN, Fradin MS, Messana JM, *et al.* Cyclosporine for plaque-type psoriasis. Results of a multidose, double-blind trial. *N Engl J Med* 1991;324:277–84.
10 Level NJ, Munro CS, Higgins EM, *et al.* The absence of rapid relapse of psoriasis treated with cyclosporin A: a comparison with dithranol. *Br J Dermatol* 1992;127(Suppl. 40):18(Abstract).
11 Korstanje MJ, Hulsmans RFHT. Combination therapy: cyclosporin A: PUVA in psoriasis. *Acta Derm Venereol* 1990;70:89–90.
12 Korstanje MJ, Van de Staak WFBM. Combination-therapy cyclosporin-A – etretinate for psoriasis. *Clin Exp Dermatol* 1990;15:172–3.
13 Bunker CB, Rustin MHA, Dowd PM. Isotretinoin treatment of severe acne in post-transplant patients taking cyclosporine (Letter). *J Am Acad Dermatol* 1990;22: 693–4.
14 Abel EA. Isotretinoin treatment of severe cystic acne in a heart transplant patient receiving cyclosporine: consideration of drug interactions (letter). *J Am Acad Dermatol* 1991;24:511.
15 Grossman RM, Delaney RJ, Brinton EA, *et al.* Hypertriglyceridemia in patients with psoriasis treated with cyclosporine. *J Am Acad Dermatol* 1991;25:648–51.
16 Griffiths CEM, Powles AV, Baker BS, *et al.* Combination cyclosporine A and topical corticosteroid in the treatment of psoriasis. *Transplant Proc* 1988;30(Suppl. 4):50–2.
17 Korstanje MJ, van Breda Vriesman CJP, van de Staak WJBM. Cyclosporine and methotrexate. A dangerous combination. *J Am Acad Dermatol* 1990;23:320–321.
18 Yau JC, Dimopoulos MA, Huan SD, *et al.* An effective acute graft-vs-host disease prophylaxis with minidose methotrexate, cyclosporine, and single-dose methylprednisolone. *Am J Hematol* 1991;38:288–92.
19 Aschan J, Ringden O, Sundberg B, *et al.* Methotrexate combined with cyclosporin A decreases graft-vs-host disease, but increases leukemic relapse compared to monotherapy. *Bone Marrow Transplantation* 1991;7:113–9.
20 Brahn E, Peacock DJ, Banquerigo ML. Suppression of collagen-induced arthritis by combination cyclosporin A and methotrexate therapy. *Arthritis Rheum* 1991;34: 1282–8.
21 Feutren G, Laburte C, Krupp P. Safety and tolerability of cyclosporin A in psoriasis. In Wolff K, ed. *Cyclosporin A and the Skin.* London: Royal Society of Medicine Services, 1992:3–12.
22 Lewis HM, Powles AV, Garioch JJ, *et al.* Six years experience of cyclosporin A in the treatment of chronic plaque psoriasis. *Br J Dermatol* 1992;127(Suppl. 40): 18(Abstract).
23 Korstanje MJ. How to improve the risk–benefit ratio of cyclosporin therapy for psoriasis. *Clin Exp Dermatol* 1992;17:16–19.
24 Stoof TJ, Korstanje MJ, Bilo HJG, *et al.* Does fish oil protect renal function in cyclosporin-treated psoriasis patients? *J Int Med* 1989;226:437–41.
25 Feutren G, Friend D, Timonen P, Laburte C. Cyclosporin monitoring in psoriasis (Letter). *Lancet* 1990;335:866–7.
26 Wysocki GP, Daley TD. Hypertrichosis in patients receiving cyclosporine therapy.

Clin Exp Dermatol 1987;12:191–6.
27 Benaini PL, Marchesi L, Cainelli T, Crosti C. Kaposi's sarcoma in kidney transplant recipients treated with cyclosporin. *Br J Dermatol* 1988;118:709–14.
28 Margolis DJ, Guzzo CY, Johnson J, Lazarus GS. Alterations in renal function in psoriasis patients treated with cyclosporine, 5 mg/kg/day. *J Am Acad Dermatol* 1992;26:195–7.
29 Zachariae H, Hansen HE, Kragballe K, Olsen S. Morphologic renal changes during cyclosporine treatment of psoriasis. *J Am Acad Dermatol* 1992;26:415–9.
30 Gilbert SC, Emmett M, Menter A, *et al.* Cyclosporine therapy for psoriasis: serum creatinine measurements are an unreliable predictor of decreased renal function. *J Am Acad Dermatol* 1989;21:470–4.
31 Powles AV, Cook T, Hulme B, *et al.* Renal function and biopsy findings after 5 years' treatment with low-dose cyclosporine for psoriasis. *Br J Dermatol* 1993; 128:154–65.
32 Feutren G, Mihatsch MJ. Risk factors of cyclosporine-induced nephropathy in patients with autoimmune diseases. *N Engl J Med* 1992;326:1654–60.
33 Kaplan NM. Calcium entry blockers in the treatment of hypertension. *JAMA* 1989;262:817–23.
34 Gilhar A, Pillar T, Etzionni A. Cyclosporin in dermatologic disorders. *Int J Dermatol* 1989;28:425–5.
35 Schulze H-J, Mahrle G, Steigleder GK. Topical cyclosporine A in psoriasis (Letter). *Br J Dermatol* 1990;122:113–4.
36 Burns MK, Ellis CN, Eisen D, *et al.* Intralesional cyclosporine for psoriasis. *Arch Dermatol* 1992;128:786–90.
37 Abu-Elmagd K, Van Thiel D, Jegasothy BV, *et al.* FK506: a new therapeutic agent for severe recalcitrant psoriasis. *Transplant Proc* 1991;23:3322–4.
38 Jegasothy BV, Ackerman CD, Todo S, *et al.* Tacrolimus (FK506) — a new therapeutic agent for severe recalcitrant psoriasis. *Arch Dermatol* 1992;128:781–5.
39 Thomson AW, Nalesnik M, Abu-Elmagd K, Starzl TE. Influence of FK506 on T lymphocytes, Langerhans' cells and the expression of cytokine receptors and adhesion molecules in psoriatic skin lesions: a preliminary study. *Transplant Proc* 1991;23:3330–1.
40 Meingassner JG, Stutz A. Immunosuppressive macrolides of the type FK506: a novel class of topical agents for treatment of skin diseases? *J Invest Dermatol* 1992;98:851–5.
41 Lin H-Y, Rocher LL, McQuillan MA, *et al.* Cyclosporine-induced hyperuricemia and gout. *N Engl J Med* 1989;321:287–92.
42 Gupta AK, Ellis CN, Siegel MT, *et al.* Sulfasalazine improves psoriasis. *Arch Dermatol* 1990;126:487–93.

seventeen Vitamin D and Analogs

INTRODUCTION

Vitamin D_3 is not a vitamin in the classic sense, that is, it is not a nutritional requirement. It can be photosynthesized in the epidermis from 7-dehydrocholesterol when exposed to the UVB spectrum (290–320 nm) of natural sunlight. It must then be bound to plasma vitamin-D-binding protein and transported via the circulation to the liver and kidney for successive hydroxylations before it becomes active 1,25-dihydroxy vitamin D_3. Its two main physiologic functions are stimulation of intestinal calcium absorption and the mobilization of calcium from bone [1].

Specific nuclear receptors for 1,25-dihydroxy vitamin D_3, hereafter referred to as calcitriol, were demonstrated in normal human epidermis and cultured keratinocytes (KCs) indicating that the skin is a target organ. Receptors have also been found in melanocytes, Langerhans cells, fibroblasts, endothelial cells, activated T lymphocytes, macrophages, and granulocytes.

MECHANISM OF ACTION

A monoclonal antibody to the vitamin D receptor (VDR) labeled VDR antigens were expressed in KCs of all viable layers of the epidermis in normal and nonlesional skin. In psoriasis, there was a significant increase in VDR expression in the basal and suprabasal layers as well as a marked increase in the density of VDR-positive intraepidermal and perivascular T cells and macrophages. Increased VDR expression of psoriatic KCs could be a reflection of high proliferative activity and the altered differentiation pattern in psoriasis. Lesional skin may respond more readily to therapeutic doses of vitamin D because of increased numbers of receptors, assuming that they are functional. Epidermal KCs and activated macrophages can convert 25-hydroxy vitamin D_3 into the bioactive metabolite *in vitro*. Upregulation of the VDR may reflect higher local levels of the hormone. It is not known whether cytokines modulate VDR expression in KCs or leukocytes, but calcitriol does inhibit interleukin-2 and interferon-γ production by T lymphocytes [3].

The expression of VDR by neutrophils in the inflammatory infiltrate of psoriasis makes the following *in vitro* findings intriguing. Calcitriol significantly decreased phagocytosis and the generation of reactive oxygen species by both normal and psoriatic polymorphonuclear leukocytes (PMNLs), but chemotaxis of only the psoriatic PMNLs was significantly inhibited [4]. The metabolically inactive vitamin D_2 had no effect in these assays. Thus, calcitriol may exert both antiproliferative as well as local antiinflammatory actions that ultimately result in improvement of the psoriatic lesion.

In normal human KC cultures calcitriol inhibits cell proliferation and induces terminal differentiation [5]. Growth inhibition caused by calcitriol was accompanied by marked inhibition of DNA synthesis and a decrease in the number of high-affinity receptors for epidermal growth factor (EGF)/transforming growth factor-α (TGF-α). The cells were viable; calcitriol was not cytotoxic at the concentrations used.

Cultured KCs from involved and uninvolved psoriatic skin were not resistant to the antiproliferative effect of calcitriol [6]. Inhibition of all growth was virtually complete at 10^{-6} mol/l. Similarly, DNA synthesis was inhibited in KC cultures in a dose–response fashion from 10^{-8} to 10^{-6} mol/l. The growth of psoriatic fibroblasts in culture can also be inhibited by calcitriol, but some cultures may be resistant to it [7].

It has been proposed that another mechanism of action of calcitriol in psoriasis is that by increasing free intracellular calcium in KCs, normal differentiation may be induced [8]. Bittiner and coworkers [9] showed that calcitriol at very low concentrations (10^{-11}–10^{-9} mol/l) in normal human KC cultures caused rapid transient increases in intracellular free calcium independent of protein synthesis.

CLINICAL USE OF VITAMIN D

There are many examples of the serendipitous use of a medication or procedure used for another indication which helps psoriasis. Such an anecdotal finding usually generates an open trial of the treatment in a small number of patients with psoriasis to assess toxicity as well as efficacy. The true test of efficacy is the double-blind placebo-controlled trial or the bilateral paired comparison (for topical agents) where the patient serves as his or her own control. The development of vitamin D analogs in the treatment of psoriasis illustrates this orderly progression well: serendipity, *in vitro* work, open trials to assess toxicity and efficacy, double-blind trials, topical formulations, and development of analogs with higher safety profile and equal or greater efficacy.

Oral vitamin D

A patient receiving 1α-hydroxy vitamin D for osteoporosis demonstrated dramatic clearing of her psoriasis. This was followed by several open studies using oral calcitriol which showed promise, some with dramatic results and significant toxicity [7,10]. To my knowledge, a placebo-controlled study has not been performed with calcitriol; however, a trial consisting of two treatment arms is currently in progress, i.e., suberythemogenic UVB with calcitriol or placebo.

Calcitriol can cause hypercalciuria, hypercalcemia, kidney stones, nephrocalcinosis, and soft tissue calcification. Pincus and Holick [11] reported that 76% of 55 patients improved markedly without significant toxicity for up to 3 years when a maximum daily dose of between 1.5 and 2.5 μg was given. They further recommended administering the drug as a single dose at bedtime because there is less dietary calcium remaining in the intestine at this time. Patients were asked to limit their dietary calcium intake to under 800 mg/day. Table 17.1 lists various foods with a relatively high calcium content. Calcium, vitamin D supplements, and antiacids containing calcium must not be taken.

Calcitriol is a drug in which the therapeutic level and toxic level are very close and overlap in some patients.

How to use calcitriol

1 Calcitriol should probably be relegated to fourth-line adjuvant status and combined with UVB or psoralen UVA (PUVA) in severe or recalcitrant cases.

2 Do not treat patients with a personal or immediate family history of kidney stones.

Table 17.1 Dietary calcium sources*

Very high (> 250 mg)	High (150–249 mg)	Intermediate (75–149 mg)	Low (< 75 mg)
Milk, (includes whole, low fat, and skim)	Most solid cheeses (e.g., American Blue, Cheddar, Colby, Mozzarella, Muenster)	Cottage cheese (2% low fat)	Cottage cheese, creamed
Milkshakes	Salmon with bones	Ice cream	Brazil nuts
Yogurt (plain or fruit)	Collards	Icemilk	Filberts
Ricotta cheese	Waffle	Beans, dried	Meatloaf
Swiss cheese	Macaroni and cheese	Oysters	Broccoli stalk
Sardines with bones	Cream soups	Shrimp	Tortilla, corn
Cheese pizza	Beef taco	Kale	Beans, baked with tomato sauce
		Turnip greens	
		Cornbread	
		Pancakes	
		Chili con carne	
		Custard	
		Chocolate pudding	
		Spaghetti, meatballs, tomato sauce, and cheese	

* Per serving.

3 Measure baseline serum calcium, phosphorus, albumin, and 24-hour urinary calcium excretion; the maximum allowed throughout the treatment period is 250 mg for women and 300 mg for men.

4 Initiate treatment at 0.5 μg at bedtime. Increase by 0.25 μg every 2 weeks based on calcium levels and skin condition to a maximum of 1.5 μg/day.

5 Limit calcium intake to 800 mg daily.

6 Monitor 24-hour urinary calcium, and serum calcium and phosphorus every 2 weeks before increasing the dose of calcitriol. Monitor monthly after dose and calcium levels have stabilized.

Topical calcitriol and analogs

Holick *et al.* [12] compounded calcitriol in petrolatum 15 μg/g and asked patients to apply 0.1 g over less than 100 cm^2 area once daily. About 90% of patients showed marked improvement or clearing in 4–6 weeks. In some patients, areas as large as 2000 cm^2 were treated, applying the equiv-

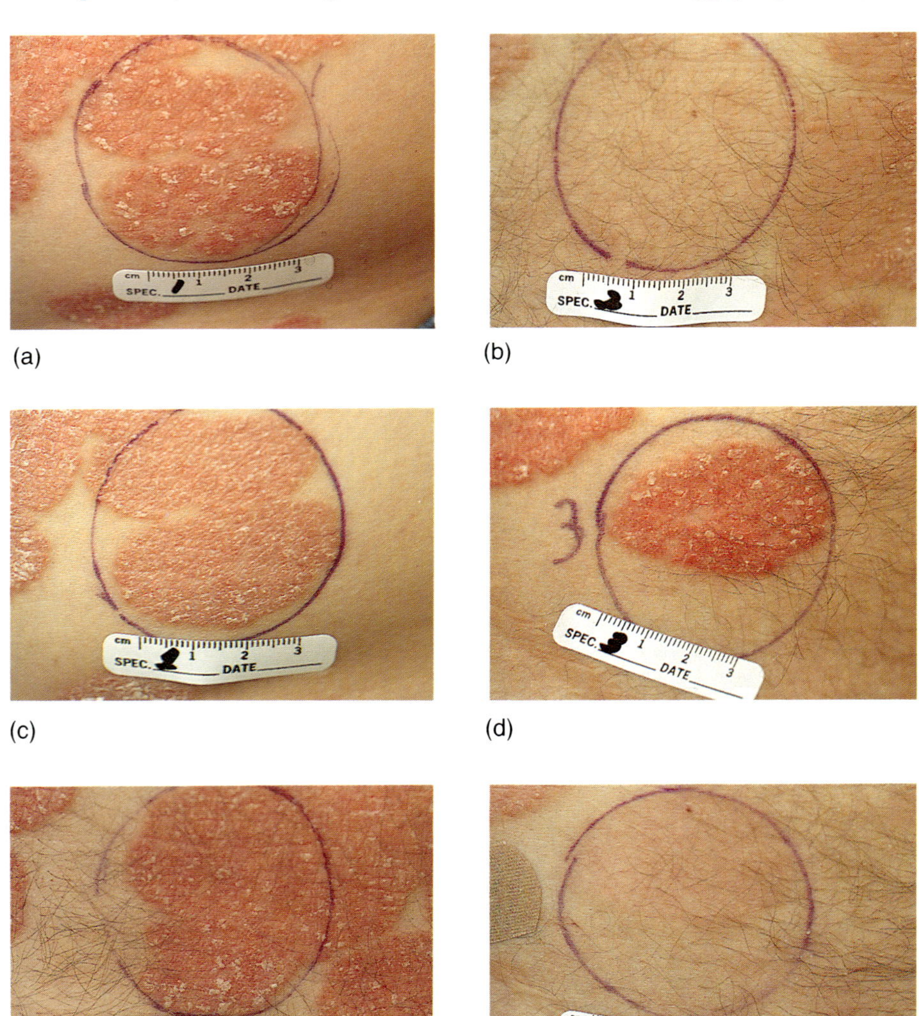

Fig 17.1 Calcitriol or placebo cream was applied once daily for 4 weeks. Pre- and posttreatment results are shown for (a) and (b) placebo, (c) and (d) 0.0025% calcitriol, and (e) and (f) 0.0005% calcitriol.

alent of 45–60 μg calcitriol per day. No toxicity has been observed for up to 3 years of use [11].

Topical treatment with calcitriol has yielded variable results depending on concentration, vehicle, and frequency of application. Calcitriol 0.5 μg in a medium-chain triglyceride vehicle showed no clinical efficacy compared to vehicle alone [13]. Calcitriol cream (Topitriol) was significantly more effective than vehicle at 0.005 and 0.0025% (Fig. 17.1), but only 35% of lesions were clear or almost clear compared to 12% for vehicle [14].

Calcitriol 0.1 μg/g in petrolatum applied t.i.d. led to 11 of 16 (69%) patients improved compared to the vehicle control side, but only two of the patients were markedly improved or cleared [15]. Interestingly, the calcitriol ointment had no clinical effect on ichthyosis vulgaris or X-linked ichthyosis, disorders of keratinization in which epidermal proliferation is normal or diminished. The author suggested that the most plausible mechanism of action of calcitriol was suppression of epidermal hyperproliferation.

An analog of calcitriol, also known as MC903, calcipotriol, and calcipotriene, has been developed which acts via the same VDR but is 100 times less calciotropic than calcitriol. It is equally as effective in induction of differentiation and inhibition of proliferation of human KC *in vitro*. Its efficacy and acceptability have been confirmed in double-blind placebo-controlled trials [16]. The optimal concentration was found to be 50 μg/g of ointment, and this product is now commercially available in Canada, UK, and other European countries as Dovonex or Daivonex.

A double-blind right to left comparison of calcipotriol 50 μg/g and betamethasone valerate 0.1% ointments showed that calcipotriene was slightly superior for mild to moderate psoriasis vulgaris [17]. At 6 weeks the mean psoriasis area and severity index score reduction was 68.8% with calcipotriol and 61.4% with betamethasone ($P < 0.001$). Both preparations were well tolerated; the most common adverse event, lesional or perilesional irritation, was slightly but not significantly more common with calcipotriol. At the end of treatment, patients considered 82% of calcipotriol sides greatly improved or cleared compared to 69% of betamethasone sides. Similar results were observed in open studies comparing calcipotriol with short-contact anthralin therapy [18].

In short-term studies of the effects on calcium metabolism of topical calcipotriol (3 g or 150 μg daily), no increase in serum calcium, 24-hour urinary calcium, or change in other special markers of calcium/bone metabolism was detected [19]. After stopping calcipotriol for 7 days, nine patients received 1.5 μg/day oral calcitriol for 7 days. Their relapse of psoriasis was not prevented and they developed a significant increase in serum calcium, calcitriol, and 24-hour urinary calcium, and a significant decrease in parathyroid hormone compared with pretreatment values. Despite a possible 1% systemic absorption of calcipotriol, no effects on calcium metabolism were observed.

In an immunohistologic study of lesional biopsies during calcipotriol treatment the earliest change noted was a decrease in PMNLs after 1 week

[20]. The number of actively cycling epidermal cells (Ki-67-positive nuclei) showed a statistically significant decrease after 2 weeks. There was a trend toward diminished cytokeratin K16, a marker for aberrant differentiation, in the suprabasal layers between week 4 and 12. The number of T cells was decreased by 4 weeks. In this study, the antineutrophil and antiproliferative effects of calcipotriol occurred first, were significant, and persisted. Berth-Jones and colleagues [21] found that there was a marked normalization of cytokeratin expression (K5, K10, K16) during treatment with either calcipotriene or betamethasone valerate.

Topical calcipotriol will undoubtedly find its place as first- or second-line therapy along with topical corticosteroids for mild to moderate cases of psoriasis vulgaris covering up to 20% of the body surface area. Most of the improvement occurs during the first 4–6 weeks of treatment and is maintained with continuous application. While mild irritant dermatitis of the face and anogenital area have been reported frequently, these unwanted effects generally do not lead to withdrawal of calcipotriol [22], thus giving the clinician a safe and effective alternative for the face and body folds where fluorinated topical corticosteroids are contraindicated. Allergic contact dermatitis to calcipotriol has been reported with possible cross-sensitivity to other vitamin D analogs [23].

It is conceivable that tachyphylaxis may occur with calcipotriol if VDRs become saturated. It is not known whether the KC VDRs are downregulated during treatment, but neither tachyphylaxis nor dermal atrophy have occurred after 6 months [24]. Rest periods off calcipotriene can be combined with other antipsoriatic therapies such as topical corticosteroids, anthralin, UV light, or retinoids. To avoid potential hypercalcemia, the weekly dosage should not exceed 100 g of ointment (5000 μg calcipotriol) [10].

REFERENCES

1 Holick MF. The cutaneous photosynthesis of previtamin D_3: a unique photoendocrine system. *J Invest Dermatol* 1981;76:51–8.
2 Milde P, Hauser U, Simon T, *et al.* Expression of 1,25-dihydroxyvitamin D_3 receptors in normal and psoriatic skin. *J Invest Dermatol* 1991;97:230–9.
3 Rigby WF, Hamilton BJ, Waugh MG. 1,25-Dihydroxyvitamin D_3 modulates the effects of interleukin 2 independent of IL-2 receptor binding. *Cell Immunol* 1990; 125:396–414.
4 Bigardi AS, Legori A, Mozzanica N, Altomare GF. Effects of vitamin D_3 on the neutrophil functions in psoriasis. *Fifth International Psoriasis Symposium Proceedings, San Francisco*, July 1991:111.
5 Smith EL, Walworth NC, Holick MF. Effect of 1 alpha, 25-dihydroxyvitamin D_3 on the morphologic and biochemical differentiation of cultured human epidermal keratinocytes grown in serum-free conditions. *J Invest Dermatol* 1986;86:709–14.
6 Hashimoto K, Matsumoto K, Higashiyama M, *et al.* Growth-inhibitory effects of 1,25-dihydroxyvitamin D_3 on normal and psoriatic keratinocytes. *Br J Dermatol* 1990;123:93–8.
7 Smith EL, Pincus SH, Donovan L, *et al.* A novel approach for the evaluation and treatment of psoriasis. *J Am Acad Dermatol* 1988;19:516–28.

8 Sharpe GR, Gillespie JI, Greenwell JR. Changes in intracellular free calcium of human keratinocytes during differentiation and stimulation with EGF. *Br J Dermatol* 1990;122:269–70.

9 Bittiner B, Bleehen SS, MacNeil S. 1 alpha,25 $(OH)_2$ vitamin D_3 increases intracellular calcium in human keratinocytes. *Br J Dermatol* 1991;124:230–5.

10 Berth-Jones J, Hutchinson PE. Vitamin D analogues and psoriasis. *Br J Dermatol* 1992;127:71–8.

11 Pincus S, Holick M. 1,25-Dihydroxyvitamin D_3: rationale for its use in the treatment of psoriasis. In Roenigk HH Jr, Maibach, HI, eds. *Psoriasis*, 2nd edn. New York: Marcel Dekker, Inc., 1991:791–807.

12 Holick MF, Pochi P, Bhawan J. Topically applied and orally administered 1,25-dihydroxyvitamin D_3 is a novel, safe, and effective therapy for the treatment of psoriasis; a three year experience and histologic analysis. *J Invest Dermatol* 1989; 92:446.

13 Van de Kerkhof PCM, van Bokhoven M, Zultak M, Czarnetzki BM. A double-blind study of topical 1 alpha, 25-dihydroxyvitamin D_3 in psoriasis. *Br J Dermatol* 1989;120:661–4.

14 Ashenfelter A, Coutinko J, Gwo J, *et al.* Calcitriol cream in the treatment of psoriasis: efficacy and safety considerations. *Fifth International Psoriasis Symposium Proceedings, San Francisco*, July 1991:108.

15 Okano M. 1 alpha,25-$(OH)_2D_3$ use on psoriasis and ichthyosis. *Int J Dermatol* 1991;30:62–4.

16 Dubertret L, Wallach D, Sontegrand P, *et al.* Efficacy and safety of calcipotriol (MC 903) ointment in psoriasis. *J Am Acad Dermatol* 1992;27:983–8.

17 Kragballe K, Gjertsen BT, deHoop D, *et al.* Double-blind, right/left comparison of calcipotriol and betamethasone valerate in treatment of psoriasis vulgaris. *Lancet* 1991;337:193–6.

18 Kragballe K. Treatment of psoriasis with calcipotriol and other vitamin D analogues. *J Am Acad Dermatol* 1992;27:1001–8.

19 Gumowski-Sunek D, Rizzoli R, Saurat J-H. Effects of topical calcitriol on calcium metabolism in psoriatic patients: comparison with oral calcitriol. *Dermatologica* 1991;183:275–9.

20 DeJong EMGJ, Van de Kerkhof PCM. Simultaneous assessment of inflammation and epidermal proliferation in psoriatic plaques during long-term treatment with the vitamin D_3 and analogue MC903: modulations and interrelations. *Br J Dermatol* 1991;124:221–9.

21 Berth-Jones J, Fletcher A, Hutchinson PE. Epidermal cytokeratin and immunocyte responses during treatment of psoriasis with calcipotriol and betamethasone valerate. *Br J Dermatol* 1992;126:356–61.

22 Cunliffe WJ, Berth-Jones J, Claudy A, *et al.* Comparative study of calcipotriol (MC903) ointment and betamethasone 17-valerate ointment in patients with psoriasis vulgaris. *J Am Acad Dermatol* 1992;26:736–43.

23 Bruynzeel DP, Hol CW, Nieboer C. Allergic contact dermatitis to calcipotriol (Letter). *Br J Dermatol* 1992;127:66.

24 Kragballe K, Fogh K, Sogaard H. Long-term efficacy and tolerability of topical calcipotriol in psoriasis. Results of an open study. *Acta Derm Venereol* 1991;71: 475–8.

eighteen Miscellaneous Treatments

FISH OIL

The rationale for using fish oil dietary supplements as a therapeutic modality for psoriasis is sound. Phospholipase A_2 activity is increased in the entire body skin of psoriatics. Arachidonic acid (AA), leukotriene B_4 (LTB_4), and 12-hydroxyheptadecatrienoic acid (12-HETE) are markedly elevated in lesional skin. Marine fish oil contains ω-3 polyunsaturated fatty acids, which could theoretically substitute for AA as substrate for the lipoxygenase and cyclooxygenase enzymes. The less chemotactically active LTB_5 may be formed as well as the relatively noninflammatory but more vasodilatory prostaglandins of the 3-series (PGE_3, TXA_3, PGI_3) [1].

Unfortunately, in open-label and double-blind placebo-controlled trials, fish oil has shown only minimal to modest improvement of plaque-type psoriasis when used as monotherapy in doses ranging from 1.8 to 13.5 g daily [2–4]. Fish oil may be slightly more effective when combined with suberythemogenic UVB. When combined with topical betamethasone dipropionate cream 0.05%, the same level of improvement occurred for both groups treated with fish oil (4 g/day) or olive oil. When betamethasone cream was discontinued but the oils were continued, there was no difference in the relapse rate [5]. In some studies the ratio of $LTB_5 : LTB_4$ in polymorphonuclear leukocytes (PMNLs) increased. LTB_4 produced by PMNLs decreased by 50%, and the ratio of eicosapentaenoic acid (EPA) : AA increased in psoriatic plaques, but there was no correlation with clinical improvement. Purified EPA without docosahexanoic acid (which is also in fish oil) at 3.6 g/day gave similar results; the production of 5-hydroxyeicosapentaenoic acid by stimulated PMNLs was also significantly increased without dramatic improvement of psoriasis [6]. These results suggest that the precise regulatory control of proliferation and inflammation by AA and its metabolites is more complex than originally postulated or that leukotrienes and eicosanoids play minor or secondary roles in these processes.

Topical fish oil under occlusion (6 hours per day) was superior to paraffin oil at improving the thickness of plaques [7]. Both oils improved scaling and erythema to an equal extent, but neither helped pruritus. The beneficial effects plateaued after 7 days of treatment and were maintained with further treatment. Despite the unpleasant odor, patients judged the fish oil treatment to be acceptable.

Because of the relatively high oral doses of fish oil required to attain a mild effect, or the need for daily occlusion of the malodorous substance, it is doubtful that fish oil will ever be accepted by patients or their doctors as monotherapy. A preliminary study suggested that four to six meals with fish per week may have the same effect on lipids as 7.5 g fish oil daily [8].

Fish oil may be most beneficial as adjunctive therapy to retinoids [9] or cyclosporine [10], because of its sparing of side effects rather than its own therapeutic effects. Lower doses of fish oil supplementation (1.8–2.6 g EPA daily) decrease the hypertriglyceridemic effects of etretinate and acitretin. Hypertriglyceridemia also occurs during cyclosporine therapy, and fish oil may be useful here as well. More importantly, fish oil added to the diet of psoriatics may attenuate the hypertension and nephrotoxicity caused by cyclosporine, possibly by decreasing production of the vasoconstrictive mediators PGE_2 and PGI_2. Aside from the smell and the aftertaste, fish oil is very safe. Because EPA can prolong bleeding time, it should be prescribed with caution to any patient who has a bleeding tendency or who is taking anticoagulants.

HYDROXYUREA

When Leavell and Yarbro [11] reported the first therapeutic trial of hydroxyurea in patients with severe recalcitrant psoriasis in 1970, an alternative to methotrexate (MTX) was being sought. In a double-blind crossover study, hydroxyurea at 500 mg b.i.d. "improved" nine of 10 patients clinically and histologically after 4 weeks of treatment. Further treatment cleared six of nine patients.

Two decades later, the antimetabolite hydroxyurea has certainly not supplanted MTX, but it has a role in a minority of patients. The drug is mainly used today by hematologists in the treatment of chronic myelogenous leukemia (CML) and polycythemia rubra vera.

Hydroxyurea is a simple compound with the empirical formula: $CH_4N_2O_2$. It is well absorbed from the gastrointestinal tract and serum concentration peaks in about 2 hours. Excretion is primarily renal. The parent compound is probably the active drug. Hydroxyurea inhibits cell proliferation by blocking DNA synthesis but does not impair RNA or protein synthesis.

Using hydroxyurea for severe widespread chronic plaque psoriasis refractory to conventional topical therapy, 60% (51 of 85) of patients achieved "complete to near complete clearing" [12]. The starting dose was usually 1.5 g daily, and the maintenance dose ranged from 0.5 to 1.5 g daily. Adverse reactions occurred in 37 of 85 (43%) patients, the majority being hematologic — anemia, leukopenia, thrombocytopenia, and pancytopenia. Macrocytosis was observed in all patients. Treatment was discontinued because of adverse effects in 16 patients (18%). Other side effects that occurred in a small number of patients included diffuse hyperpigmentation of involved and uninvolved skin, photosensitivity of psoriasis, alopecia, elevation of liver enzymes, and nausea. Recall erythema localized to previously X-irradiated areas has been reported. Other cutaneous reactions have included fixed drug reactions, poikiloderma, and leg ulcerations; the latter two have occurred only in patients with CML. Guidelines for the use of hydroxyurea were proposed in a recent review [13].

All of the following treatments for psoriasis vulgaris should be tried where appropriate before considering hydroxyurea: conventional topical therapy, UVB phototherapy, psoralen UVA (PUVA), MTX, and etretinate. Only cyclosporine which is equally or more toxic, much more expensive, and not Food and Drug Administration-approved for psoriasis should take a second berth to hydroxyurea. Hydroxyurea is not effective for pustular or erythrodermic psoriasis or psoriatic arthritis. It is contraindicated in pregnancy and lactation. Significant hepatic or renal disease are relative contraindications.

How to use hydroxyurea

1 Complete blood count (CBC), chemistry profile, and urinalysis should be performed at baseline.
2 Repeat CBC weekly for the first month and then every 2–4 weeks thereafter.
3 Repeat liver profile and urinalysis monthly.
4 Start therapy at 1 g daily. About half of the hematologic side effects relating to myelosuppression and megaloblastic erythropoiesis can be avoided at this dose.
5 Reduce the dosage if hemoglobin drops more than 2 g/dl, the white blood cell count decreases to less than $3500/mm^3$, or the platelet count decreases to less than $100\,000/mm^3$.
6 Improvement is usually evident at 6–8 weeks of therapy. If no improvement occurs by this time, and the hematologic parameters remain acceptable, increase the dose to 1.5 g daily and follow counts weekly.

Hydroxyurea has been effective as short-term continuous treatment for up to 28 weeks, and as intermittent treatment for up to 18 months. In general, an attempt should be made to decrease or stop the drug after maximal improvement has been achieved. While it is not known what total dose of hydroxyurea is toxic, cumulative doses should be charted periodically.

Since hydroxyurea is only mildly to moderately effective in most cases of extensive plaque-type psoriasis, it is a good choice for intermittent treatment when rotating systemic drugs every 1–2 years [14] that have different target organs of toxicity such as etretinate (skeleton, lipids); MTX (liver); and cyclosporine (kidneys).

SULFASALAZINE

Sulfasalazine (salicylazosulfapyridine, Azulfidine) is used as a steroid-sparing agent for inflammatory bowel disease. It has also been shown to be effective as second-line disease-modifying therapy for rheumatoid arthritis or ankylosing spondylitis. It may have antiinflammatory activity in these diseases and psoriasis by inhibiting 5-lipoxygenase.

After oral administration one-third of the sulfasalazine is absorbed in the small intestine and two-thirds passes to the colon where it is split by bacteria into its components, sulfapyridine (SP) and 5-amino salicylic acid (5-ASA). Most of the SP and about one-third of the 5-ASA is absorbed. Serum concentrations of SP and metabolites tend to be greater in patients with a slow acetylator phenotype. These patients are more likely to have adverse reactions to sulfasalazine.

Sulfasalazine has been evaluated as monotherapy in the treatment of psoriasis in open-label [15] and double-blind [16] trials by the same group of investigators. In the former study 24 of 32 patients completed 8 weeks of therapy receiving 3–4 g sulfasalazine daily. Of these, 50% had a marked to excellent response (50–100% improvement) and 50% had a minimal to modest response (0–50% improvement). In the followup double-blind analysis, 17 of 23 patients randomized to receive sulfasalazine completed 6 weeks of treatment compared to 26 of 27 placebo-treated patients. Significant improvement in global severity, scale, erythema, thickness, and total body surface area involved was evident at 4 weeks and further improvement was noted at 8 weeks. The placebo-treated patients were unchanged or worse. Overall, of the 17 evaluable patients in the sulfasalazine group, seven had a marked response (60–89%), seven moderate (30–59%) and three minimal (0–29%).

AA and eicosanoids were measured in lesional plaques prior to therapy and following 1 and 8 weeks of sulfasalazine treatment. There were no significant changes in the levels of AA, LTB_4, 12-HETE, and 15-HETE after 1 week. At 8 weeks there was a trend towards AA reduction and a significant decrease in LTB_4 only. Keratinocyte intercellular adhesion molecule-1 (ICAM-1) expression was unchanged at 1 week and significantly reduced at 8 weeks [16]. Unfortunately, the changes in LTB_4 and ICAM-1 were detected after significant clinical improvement had occurred and do not help to elucidate the mechanism of action of sulfasalazine in psoriasis.

In an open-label trial of sulfasalazine 1 g t.i.d. in Thailand, 22 of 27 patients completed 12 weeks of therapy. Of these, one-half showed complete clearing and one-half showed moderate to marked improvement [17].

Side effects of sulfasalazine occur frequently. While usually not severe, the most common side effects, anorexia, nausea, vomiting, fatigue, headaches, and cutaneous eruptions, frequently lead to discontinuation of sulfasalazine before any therapeutic benefit can be expected. Enteric-coated tablets (Azulfidine EN-tabs) are indicated for patients who cannot take regular sulfasalazine tablets because of gastrointestinal side effects, i.e., nausea and vomiting after the first few doses. In the studies cited, the incidence of a cutaneous eruption was 18%. The drug-induced rash is the typical generalized erythematous maculopapular pruritic variety and is reversible. The authors warn that photosensitivity can occur with sulfasalazine and UV light should be used with caution. They observed a transient macular eruption in a photosensitive distribution in two patients. A psoriasiform dermatitis developed in a patient after the initiation of sulfasalazine therapy for classical rheumatoid arthritis [18]. Transient neutropenia and elevated liver enzymes have been reported. Mild hemolytic anemia with decreased hemoglobin or cyanosis may occur. Other adverse reactions occur rarely but are more likely with a daily dosage of 4 g or more, or in slow acetylators who have a total serum SP level above 50 μg/ml.

Although not specifically studied, some patients treated with sulfasalazine experienced improvement of their psoriatic arthritis [15,16]. Several groups of investigators have evaluated sulfasalazine in the treatment of ankylosing spondylitis and psoriatic arthritis. The results have been variable, but data suggest that sulfasalazine is less effective for spinal disease than for peripheral joint involvement [19]. Newman and colleagues [20] treated 10 patients with polyarticular psoriatic arthritis with sulfasalazine 2 g daily for 16 weeks. Joint count score, morning stiffness, and global assessments of disease activity were significantly improved. A lower dose of sulfasalazine may be effective for arthropathy than is needed for cutaneous psoriasis. Elevated percentages of circulating B cells and immunoglobulin levels decreased during sulfasalazine therapy suggesting that its mechanism of action may relate to B-cell activation.

Despite the relatively high dropout rate during 8 weeks of therapy (25%), Gupta and coworkers [15,16] emphasize that an equal proportion of patients may experience efficacy of sulfasalazine comparable to PUVA, MTX, or etretinate. A trial of sulfasalazine is therefore justified for patients with moderate to severe psoriasis who are no longer controlled by topical or UVB phototherapy. In the long-term, if effective, sulfasalazine at 3–4 g/day is less costly and less toxic than PUVA, MTX, etretinate, or cyclosporine.

How to use sulfasalazine

1 Obtain baseline CBC, urinalysis, liver function, and renal function tests; repeat at 2 weeks, 1 month, then every 3 months thereafter.

2 Instruct patient to take 500 mg t.i.d. for 3 days; if tolerated, increase to 1 g t.i.d.

3 If gastrointestinal symptoms occur, reduce the dose by 500 mg decrements until a tolerable dose is attained.

4 If the patient cannot tolerate at least 1.5 g/day, switch to enteric-coated tablets.

5 If a symptomatic drug rash or urticaria develop, discontinue sulfasalazine.

6 Treat for at least 4–6 weeks before making final judgments about efficacy.

7 Do not increase the dose to 4 g/day because toxicity is much more likley to supervene and improved efficacy has not been confirmed.

HISTAMINE-2(H2)BLOCKERS

Limited experience has suggested that histamine type 2 receptor antagonists such as cimetidine and ranitidine are either ineffective [21] or worsen psoriasis in the short term but may improve it with chronic administration [22]. In an open prospective trial with ranitidine 300 mg p.o. b.i.d. for 16 weeks, there were 12/20 responders [23], defined as a 40% reduction of PASI compared to baseline. The mean PASI reduction of the responders was 67%. Randomized double-blind placebo-controlled trials should be undertaken to confirm the efficacy of this generally well-tolerated class of drugs in the long-term treatment of psoriasis.

CASE STUDY

Severe recalcitrant generalized psoriasis in a noncompliant patient.

A 30-year-old morbidly obese woman with psoriasis vulgaris for 10 years developed an erythrodermic and pustular flare of psoriasis in October 1992 and was admitted to the hospital for systemic treatment combined with the Goeckerman regimen. She had a history of recurrent streptococcal throat infections during the past few years. Examination revealed 90% body skin involvement with bright erythema, mild scaling, and tiny pustules on the periphery of plaques on the legs and abdomen. There was prominent facial erythema and edema. The scalp was crusted. Erosions were present in the submammary region and groins. She also had deep-seated, tender pustules on the palms. She weighed 116 kg; her height was 152 cm.

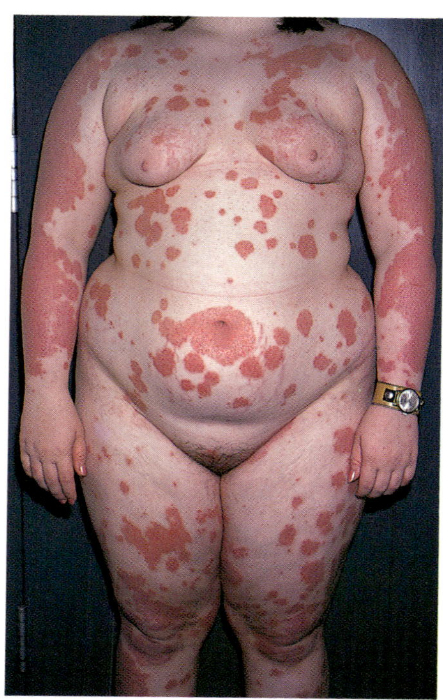
(a)

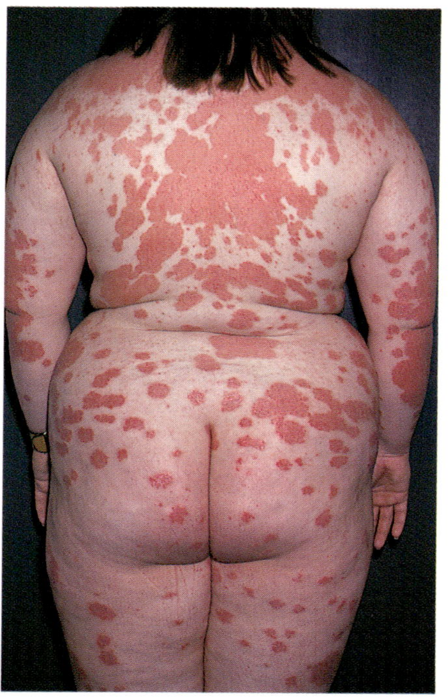
(b)

Fig 18.1 Severe inflammatory plaque disease upon admission to hospital: (a) anterior and (b) posterior views.

In 1987, she was admitted to the hospital for Goeckerman treatment (Fig. 18.1). She showed a good response but had a flare in her disease shortly after discharge. While taking birth control pills, she became pregnant and subsequently had a miscarriage. In 1988, she was treated in the hospital by the Goeckerman regimen with the addition of anthralin cream 0.25%. During this admission, she inadvertently applied anthralin to the eyes causing severe chemical conjunctivitis. Shortly after discharge from the hospital, her psoriasis flared again. In December 1988, her psoriasis was so severe that she was again admitted to the hospital and given a weekly oral dose of MTX 25 mg along with the Goeckerman regimen.

MTX was stopped after 4 months of treatment because she refused to have a liver biopsy. PUVA therapy was initiated with an early response in her plaques, but it had to be discontinued because she lived 90 miles from the nearest PUVA facility and found it impractical to combine her employment with this treatment. A home UVB unit was then prescribed because the Goeckerman had been temporarily successful each time it was given. Unfortunately, she did not return for appointments as frequently as requested, did not keep a log of exposure times, and her psoriasis continued to flare.

Cyclosporine therapy 5 mg/kg per day was initiated in 1991 with a good response, but her skin did not clear completely even at this dose. She developed mild hypertension and was treated with a calcium channel blocker. She did not return for frequent measurements of blood pressure and renal function tests as requested. Because of our inability to safely monitor cyclosporine, therapy was discontinued. Her blood pressure subsequently normalized. Serum creatinine did not rise above her baseline level of 0.8 mg%.

Sulfasalazine treatment was next initiated at 500 mg t.i.d. Within 3 days of taking this medication, she discontinued it because of nausea and stomach upset. An erythrodermic flare ensued, and she was admitted to hospital in early 1992. After a long discussion about remaining treatment options, the patient consented to liver biopsy. The liver biopsy was performed and showed no pathologic change. The hospitalization was complicated by a deep vein thrombosis for which she was heparinized.

Upon discharge, she was placed on MTX at 20 mg weekly in addition to home UVB. She was given only enough pills to last until the next clinic appointment. She began to see another dermatologist closer to her home who administered intramuscular MTX unaware that she was also taking our prescription for oral MTX.

During the last admission in 1992, the anti-DNAse B was elevated. We prescribed whirlpool treatments, isotretinoin 40 mg/day (after ruling out pregnancy), intravenous cefazolin 1 g q8h, 25 mg MTX by intravenous bolus, 0.1% triamcinolone acetonide, and UVB increased to 2 min daily. Pustulation ceased within days. Liquor carbonis detergens 10% ointment was added on the 10th day in hospital. Erythema and induration decreased by 75% after 14 days and she was discharged.

Comments

This patient would benefit most from a retinoid–PUVA combination or cyclosporine, but she cannot be treated with any of these.

1 Etretinate cannot be used because she is a woman of childbearing potential.

2 Isotretinoin cannot be prescribed to her as an outpatient because she will possibly not keep followup appointments for laboratory testing. We fear that she might get pregnant while taking isotretinoin, especially because she is no longer a candidate for oral contraceptive pills (history of thromboembolic phenomenon). She is currently contemplating elective sterilization.

3 She is not a candidate for PUVA because the distance from her home to a facility is prohibitive.

4 She is not a candidate for cylosporine because she has demonstrated noncompliance with regard to followup visits for blood pressure and renal function checks.

The case illustrates several additional points:

5 Home UVB was unsuccessful; we are uncertain if the patient ever actually employed it.

6 Sulfasalazine was not tolerated at the starting dose of 1.5 g/day and discontinued after 3 days. Despite the positive reports in the literature [15–17] we have not been able to successfully treat a single patient with sulfasalazine because of nausea, rash, or inefficacy.

7 Anthralin can no longer be prescribed because the patient inadvertently rubbed it into her eyes causing severe conjunctivitis on two occasions.

8 Isotretinoin can be used to rapidly stop pustulation, but additional therapy is usually necessary to maintain a remission.

9 The patient deliberately took MTX from two physicians simultaneously, unknown to each other and perhaps on different days of the week, thus increasing the cumulative dose and making it difficult to calculate; she therefore exposed herself to serious cutaneous, hematologic, and hepatic toxicity. A liver biopsy should be performed annually in this patient.

10 The patient is morbidly obese, a risk factor for MTX-induced hepatotoxicity, liver biopsy morbidity, and possibly for increasing the severity of psoriasis. In a questionnaire study of 536 patients in southern Germany, Braun-Falco and colleagues [24] found that when asked about the influence of weight gain on psoriasis, 8% stated that there was an improvement and 55% noted deterioration. He noted that during the "lean years" of World War II, manifestations of psoriasis patients improved. Braun-Falco writes, "A decreased delivery of energy-rich substances appears to work favorably on the skin manifestations of psoriasis. The psoriatic patient should live on the edge of hunger." We will enlist the help of a dietician to design an isocaloric weight loss diet for this patient. Unfortunately, she admits that she is not highly motivated to follow it.

REFERENCES

1 Wilkinson DI. Do dietary supplements of fish oils improve psoriasis? *Cutis* 1990; 46:334–6.

2 Kettler AH, Baughn RE, Orengo IF. The effect of dietary fish oil supplementation on psoriasis. *J Am Acad Dermatol* 1988;18:1267–73.

3 Kragballe K. Dietary supplementation with a combination of *n*-3 and *n*-6 fatty acids (Super gamma-oil marine) improves psoriasis. *Acta Derm Venereol* 1989;69:265–8.

4 Kragballe K, Fogh K. A lowfat diet supplemented with dietary fish oil (Max-EPA) results in improvement of psoriasis and in formation of leukotriene B_5. *Acta Derm Venereol* 1989;69:23–8.

5 Gupta AK, Ellis CN, Goldfarb MT, *et al.* The role of fish oil in psoriasis. A randomized, double-blind, placebo-controlled study to evaluate the effect of fish oil and topical corticosteroid therapy in psoriasis. *Int J Dermatol* 1990;29:591–5.

6 Kojima T, Terano T, Tanabe E, *et al.* Long-term administration of highly purified eicosapentaenoic acid provides improvement of psoriasis. *Dermatologica* 1991;182: 225–30.

7 Escobar SO, Achenbach R, Iannantuono R, Torem V. Topical fish oil in psoriasis — a controlled and blind study. *Clin Exp Dermatol* 1992;17:159–62.

8 Fahrer H, Hoeflin F, Lauterburg BH, *et al.* Diet and fatty acids: can fish substitute for fish oil. *Clin Exp Rheumatol* 1991;9:403–6.

9 Ashley JM, Lowe NJ, Borok ME, Alfin-Slater RB. Fish oil supplementation results in decreased hypertriglyceridemia in patients with psoriasis undergoing etretinate or acitretin therapy. *J Am Acad Dermatol* 1988;19:76–82.

10 Stoof TJ, Korstanje MJ, Bilo HJ, *et al.* Does fish oil protect renal function in cyclosporin-treated psoriasis patients? *J Intern Med* 1989;226:437–41.

11 Leavell UW, Yarbro JW. Hydroxyurea: a new treatment for psoriasis. *Arch Dermatol* 1970;102:144–50.

12 Layton AM, Sheehan-Dare RA, Goodfield MJD, Cotterill JA. Hydroxyurea in the management of therapy resistant psoriasis. *Br J Dermatol* 1989;121:647–53.

13 Boyd AS, Neldner KH. Hydroxyurea therapy. *J Am Acad Dermatol* 1991;25:518–24.

14 Weinstein GD, White GM. An approach to the treatment of moderate to severe psoriasis with rotational therapy. *J Am Acad Dermatol* 1993;28:454–9.

15 Gupta AK, Ellis CN, Siegel MT, Voorhees JJ. Sulfasalazine: a potential psoriasis therapy? *J Am Acad Dermatol* 1989;20:797–800.

16 Gupta AK, Ellis CN, Siegel MT, *et al.* Sulfasalazine improves psoriasis. A double-blind analysis. *Arch Dermatol* 1990;126:487–93.

17 Suvarnapradip P, Jirundorn P, Jerasutus S, Suvanprakorn P. The beneficial effects of sulfasalazine in psoriatic patients. *Fifth International Psoriasis Symposium, San Francisco*, July 1991:179.

18 Bliddal H, Stangerup M. Psoriasis-like skin eruption in a patient with rheumatoid arthritis after sulphasalazine therapy. *Clin Rheumatol* 1991;10:178–80.

19 Kozin F. Medical and surgical treatment of seronegative spondyloarthropathies. *Curr Opin Rheumatol* 1991;3:592–6.

20 Newman ED, Perruquet JL, Harrington TM. Sulfasalazine therapy in psoriatic arthritis: clinical and immunologic response. *J Rheumatol* 1991;18:1379–82.

21 Long PR, Milleu OF. Cimetidine and psoriasis (Letter). *Arch Dermatol* 1981;117:523.

22 Nielsen HJ, Nielsen H, Georgson J. Ranitidine for improvement of treatment-resistant psoriasis. *Arch Dermatol* 1991;127:270.

23 Witkamp L, Velthuis PJ, Verhaegh ME, *et al.* An open prospective clinical trial with systemic ranitidine in the treatment of psoriasis. *J Am Acad Dermatol* 1993;28: 778–81.

24 Braun-Falco O, Burg G, Farber EM. Psoriasis: eine Fragebogenstudie bei 536 Patienten. *Munch Med Wochenschr* 1972;114:1–15.

Appendix

Table 1 UVB phototherapy units available for home use

Jordan light	Richmond Light Co. 6023 Newington Drive Richmond, VA 23224
Panasol	National Biological Corporation 1532 Enterprise Parkway Twinsburg, OH 44087
Spectra 724	Daavlin P.O. Box 626, 619 E. Trevitt St. Bryan, OH 43506
Panelite	Ultralite Enterprises, Inc. 390 Farmer Ct. Lawrenceville, GA 30245
Hot quartz Alpine lamp	Sperti KBD, Inc. 20 Kenton Lands Rd. Erlanger, KY 41018

Table 2 Sources of UVA protective optical equipment

Source	Address	Comment
Blak-Ray (goggles and spectacles)	UVP, Inc 5100 Walnut Grove Avenue San Gabriel, CA 91778 Tel: (818) 285–3123	Not documented or marketed for PUVA protection
Clear UVA Blocking Lens UV 400 (orcolite)	Dioptics Medical Products	Order through local optician; patient brochures available

Continued on p. 340

Table 2 *Continued*

Source	Address	Comment
UVL Filtering glasses	Dermalight Systems 13135 Ventura Blvd #306 Studio City, CA 91604 Tel: (818) 995–4274	
Essilor Orma UVX Coating	Essilor Ltd Cooper Road Thornbury, Bristol BS12 2UW Great Britain	
Disposable UV Goggles (DPE-1)	Cooper-Hewitt Corp 20 Kenton Lands Road Erlanger, KY 41018	
Goggle 200 A Goggle 100 B	DermaControl 9416 Gulfstream Road Frankfort, IL 60423	
UV Blocking Goggles UV Glasses	National Biological Corp 1532 Enterprise Parkway Twinsburg, OH 44087	
Noirettes (wrap-around glasses)	Recreational Innovations Co PO Box 159 South Lyon, MI 48170 Tel: (313) 769–5565 (800) 521–9746	11 colors for lenses are available in styles ranging from "fit-overs with side shields" to "wrap-arounds"
Orcolite UV 400 Coating	Norville Optical Co, Ltd Mogdala Road Gloucester GLI 4DG Great Britain	
Perfalit Lambda 400 Coating	Rudenstok (Scotland) Limited Clydeway Industrial Centre 8 Elliot Place Glasgow G3 8EP Great Britain	
Polaroid Polarizing Lenses	Poloroid UK Limited Vale of Leven Industrial Estate Dumbarton G82 3PW Great Britain	
Red Heads Goggles $20/dozen	Daavlin PO Box 626 Bryan, OH 43506	
Solar Shields	Same	
Sunnies Goggles	Same	

Continued

Table 2 *Continued*

Source	Address	Comment
Silver-Shield goggles	Dioptics Medical Products Suite C 15550 Rockfield Blvd Irvine, CA 92718 Tel: (714) 859–7111	
Sola UV Gard Lenses	Pilkington Ophthalmic Opticians Lens Wholesalers and Manufacturers Unit 1, Holdford Way Birmingham, Great Britain	
Spectroline UV-Absorbing Eyewear	Spectronics Corp 956 Brush Hollow Road PO Box 483 Westbury, New York 11590 Tel: (516) 333–4840	
Super Sunnies	Lucas Products Corp Toledo, OH 43612 Tel: (419) 476–5992	Goggles to be worn during therapy only

Table 3 Phototherapy equipment manufacturers: UV light sources

Manufacturer	Unit	Relative cost
Athrodax Great Western Court Ashburton Ross-on-Wye Herefordshire HR9 7DW Great Britain Tel: (0989) 66669 Fax: (0989) 768140	Fluorescent UVA/UVB and synchronous phototherapy cabinet UV8001K Fluorescent UVA, UVB Systems	
Cooper-Hewitt Corp 20 Kenton Lands Road Erlanger, KY 41018	Mercury UVA–UVB lamp PH-36	Inexpensive
Daavlin PO Box 626 Bryan, OH 43506 Tel: 1–800–322–8546 Ohio: (419) 636–6304	Spectra 726–2X 12 lamp UVB Spectra 728–2X 16 lamp UVA Spectra Minil UVA Hand Foot Unit with Electromechanical Timer Spectra 305/350 UVA/UVB Cabinet	
DermaControl Inc (Division of Ultramedics) 9416 Gulfstream Road Frankfort, IL 60423 Tel: (815) 469–8027	UVA Model 56 Phototherapy Cabinet UVB Model 56 Phototherapy Cabinet Combination UVA/UVB Phototherapy Cabinet Model 42–14	

Continued on p. 342

Table 3 *Continued*

Manufacturer	Unit	Relative cost
Dermalight Systems 13135 Ventura Blvd, #306 Studio City, CA 91604 Tel: (818) 995–4274	Dermalight 6000 UVB&UVA or UVA alone Radiation cabinet, filters, UVAmat-1, UV Met Dermalight column System with two filters, UV meter, UVAMat computer control Dermalight 2001 has interchange filters allowing UVA or UVB radiation — used for face, hand, or foot treatment Psora-comb hand-held UVA/UVB light source Halide lamps	Very expensive
Dixwell Zone Industrielle DuPontet 69360 Saint Symponien d'ozon (lyon-Sud), France Tel: 78020449 Fax: 78029260	Fluorescent UVA, UVB and hand units EMLY UVA–UVB/UVA+UVB Cabinet Tecimex UVA/UVB hand or foot unit	
Metec 1614 Barclay Blvd Buffalo Grove, IL 60089 Tel: 8–800–323–7697	Fluorescent Systems, UVA, UVB	
National Biological Corp 1532 Enterprise Parkway Twinsburg, OH 44087 Tel: 1–800–338–5045 Ohio: (216) 425–3535	Fluorescent Systems, UVB/UVA HOUVA II UVA/UVB Cabinet Hand/foot II UVA/UVB Unit	
Richmond Light Co 2301 Falkirk Drive Richmond, VA 23236 Tel: (804) 276–0559	UVB Jordan Light/Model 648-B (4′ unit) Model 672-B (6′ unit) (Uses 6 FS-40 or FS-72 UVB lamps)	
Spectronics 956 Brush Hallow Westbury, NY 11590 Tel: (516) 333–4840	Fluorescent UVB, UVA Systems for a variety of laboratory uses	

Continued

Table 3 *Continued*

Manufacturer	Unit	Relative cost
UltraDerm Systems Professional Arts Bldg 5090 State Street Saginaw, MI 48603 Tel: (517) 792–6100	UVB light box Model 102 UVB (Uses Westinghouse lamps FS20, FS40, or FS72)	
Ultralite Enterprises, Inc 277 Industrial Park Drive Lawrenceville, GA 30245 Tel: (404) 936–0594	UVA	

Table 4 Radiometry units

Manufacturer	Unit	Relative cost
Anthradax Surgical Ltd Great Western Court Ashburton Ross-on-Wye, Herefordshire HR9 7DW Great Britain Tel: (0989) 66669 Fax: (0989) 768140	Waldmann Lichttechnik UV Meter for UVA and UVB	
Daavlin PO Box 626 Bryan, OH 43506 Tel: 1–800–322–8546	IL-1300 UVA Radiometer IL-1300 UVB Radiometer IL-1300 Radiometer with UVA and UVB Sensors	
DermaControl Inc. 9416 Gulfstream Road Frankfort, IL 60423	IL-844A UVA Dosimeter IL-844B UVB Dosimeter IL-1350 UVA–UVB Radiometer	
Dermalight Systems 13135 Ventura Blvd Suite 306 Studio City, CA 91604 Tel: 1–800–882–8321	UV meter with A or B sensor	Inexpensive
EG and G Gamma Scientific 3777 Ruffin Road San Diego, CA 92123–1876 Tel: (619) 279–8034	UVA Measuring Device	

Continued on p. 344

Table 4 *Continued*

Manufacturer	Unit	Relative cost
The Eppley Laboratory, Inc. (EPLAB) 12 Sheffield Avenue PO Box 419 Newport, RI 02840 Tel: (401) 847–1020 Fax: (401) 847–1031	Ultraviolet Radiometer Model TUVR (used for measuring sun and sky ultraviolet radiation)	Expensive
National Biological Corp 1532 Enterprise Parkway Twinsburg, OH 44087 Tel: (216) 425–3535	UVB Measuring Device* XCLMB UVA Measuring Device* XCLMA-303	 Inexpensive
Spectronics Corporation 956 Brush Hollow Road PO Box 483 Westerbury, NY 11590 Tel: (516) 333–4840 Fax: (516) 383–4859	DM-365H Long-wave UVA Radiometer	Inexpensive

* Radiometers we have found most useful.

Index

Page numbers in *italic* refer to figures and/or tables